The Sclera and Systemic Disorders

Volume 2 in the Series

Major Problems in Ophthalmology

PATRICK D. TREVOR-ROPER, FRCS

Consulting Editor

OTHER MONOGRAPHS IN THE SERIES

PUBLISHED

Galloway: **Ophthalmic Electrodiagnosis**

The Sclera

and

Systemic Disorders

PETER G. WATSON, MA, MB, BChir., FRCS, DO

*Consultant Ophthalmic Surgeon, Addenbrooke's Hospital, Cambridge;
Scleritis Clinic, Department of Ophthalmology, Institute of Ophthalmology,
Moorfields Eye Hospital, London; Associate Lecturer, Faculty of Clinical
Medicine, University of Cambridge.*

BRIAN L. HAZLEMAN, MB, BS, MRCP

*Consultant Rheumatologist, Addenbrooke's Hospital and Strangeways
Research Laboratories, Cambridge; Associate Lecturer, Faculty of
Medicine, University of Cambridge.*

1976

W. B. Saunders Company Ltd   London · Philadelphia · Toronto

W. B. Saunders Company Ltd: 1 St. Anne's Road
Eastbourne, East Sussex BN21 3UN

West Washington Square
Philadelphia, Pa. 19105

833 Oxford Street
Toronto, Ontario M8Z 5T9

To our families

The Sclera and Systemic Disorders   ISBN 0-7216-9134-X

Library of Congress Catalog Card Number 76-26776

Photoset, printed and bound in Great Britain by R. J. Acford Ltd,
Industrial Estate, Chichester, Sussex.

Print No: 987654321

Contents

Foreword

Our "Major Problems in Ophthalmology" are inevitably most copious in those areas of our specialty where disorders of the eye have their roots in alien fields of medicine. The niceties of these are often hard for ophthalmologists to comprehend, and our limited knowledge of them may well have been overtaken by more recent physiopathological concepts.

In our first monograph of this series, Nicholas Galloway dealt ably with the march-land of "Ophthalmic Electrodiagnosis". It is fitting that this second offering should cover an issue which is equally on the borders of ophthalmology, although one of major ophthalmic importance.

Disorders of the sclera are widespread and damaging, yet they are generally ill-understood, and for that reason receive rather summary treatment in text-books and scant attention in research institutes. This admirable treatise by Peter Watson and Brian Hazleman should redress the balance; and, taking off from the mists of medieval nomenclature and the vagaries of evolutionary 'improvisation' they lead us painlessly through the complexities of connective-tissue pathology, to a wider comprehension of scleral disorders. We are fortunate in having such lively and understanding guides.

London, 1976

Patrick Trevor-Roper

Preface

Scleral disease is rare, but not so rare that it is not seen at some time or another by every ophthalmologist or physician involved in the management of the connective tissue diseases. Some forms of scleral and episcleral disease are innocent and harmless, whereas others are severe and destructive. Scleral disease is often, moreover, the presenting feature of many serious and potentially fatal systemic diseases; indeed 27 per cent of patients who develop necrotising scleritis are dead within five years. It is therefore vital that the correct diagnosis is made and that the most effective treatment is given as early as possible in the course of the disease. Again, because of the comparative rarity of scleral disease the diagnosis is often missed and in one series was unsuspected in 40 per cent of eyes enucleated with a primary histological diagnosis of scleritis.

We have therefore felt it to be important that there should be a source to which both physicians and ophthalmologists could refer when they encounter a patient with scleral disease. To this end, we have brought together in this book all the diagnostic features which enable one to differentiate between the various conditions which affect the sclera and, particularly for the ophthalmologist, the salient features of those systemic diseases which are commonly associated with scleral inflammation. A study of Chapters 3 and 4 should enable anyone to recognise the majority of conditions affecting the sclera. Those who are confronted by a patient with scleritis, or who are studying for a higher degree in ophthalmology or medicine, should find Chapters 7 to 10 of value, not only as a guide to the diagnosis and the treatment, but also as an indication of the other associated conditions.

Finally we have also included a discussion of the aetiology, pathogenesis and the rationale of treatment based on our experience of over 300 cases of severe scleral disease in the Scleritis Clinic at Moorfields Eye Hospital, London. This clinic was set up in 1963 to study the clinical features and the natural history of conditions which affect the sclera and to develop effective methods of management.

The bibliography, though lengthy, is not intended to be exhaustive. We have therefore concentrated on those references which review certain aspects of the work or which are classic papers, or else which state a point of view which is either controversial or compensates for our lack of personal experience.

Cambridge, 1976   Peter G. Watson
                                                       Brian L. Hazleman

Acknowledgements

It gives us the greatest pleasure to be able to acknowledge the help we have had from so many sources in the preparation of this book, particularly those colleagues who have referred patients to us, to Professor Barrie R. Jones for his interest and use of facilities of the Professorial Unit at Moorfields Eye Hospital, London, where most of the work was undertaken, to Professor Norman Ashton at the Department of Pathology, Institute of Ophthalmology, London, to Professor L. Zimmerman at the Armed Forces Institute of Pathology, Washington, and to Dr D. G. Cogan at the Massachusetts Eye and Ear Hospital, for allowing us to examine their collections of histological material. Without them we could not have accumulated the experience necessary to complete this work.

Particular thanks are also due to Mrs Barbara Evans for typing the difficult manuscript and Miss Joan Lewry for all her hard labour in checking the references, and to Peter Page Thomas, Alan Lyne, R. Watson and Mrs M. Pettifer for reading parts of or all of the manuscript. We would also like to acknowledge the help we have received from the medical illustration departments of both Moorfields Eye Hospital and Addenbrooke's Hospital, particularly T. Tarrant and J. Trotman who have been bombarded over the years and have always responded with great cheerfulness and effectiveness, as the quality of the illustrations shows. None of those who have helped in the Scleritis Clinic over the past 13 years have been asked to do so, and all have contributed greatly to its work. Many of their ideas have been incorporated in this volume. To single out any for special mention is perhaps unfair but we would particularly like to thank David Lobascher, Sohan Hayreh, Alan Lyne and Sandy Holt-Wilson for the tremendous amount of work which was done during the period of time they spent with us.

Apart from those illustrations which have been acknowledged in the text or in captions, we would like to thank the following editors and publishers for their permission to publish the following illustrations and tables:

Blackwell Scientific Publications (Figure 3.36 from *Clinical Aspects of Immunology*, 1976 (Ed.) Gell, Coombs and Lachmann); *British Journal of*

Acknowledgements

Ophthalmology (Figures 3.7, 3.8, 3.9, 4.4, 4.15, 4.38, 4.44 and 4.50 from Watson, Hayreh and Awdry, 1968, and Figure 7.4, Table 4.4 and Table 4.5 from Watson and Hayreh, 1976); Churchill Livingstone (Figures 3.20, 3.29, 3.32, 3.33, 4.3, 4.25, 4.33, 4.37, 7.3, 7.12, 7.14, 7.18, 7.20, 7.21, 7.22, 7.23, 7.24, 7.31, 7.41, 7.44, 8.18 and 8.19 from Watson in *Recent Advances in Ophthalmology*, 1976 (Ed.) Trevor-Roper); *Hospital Update* (Plates I to VI from Lachmann and Hazleman, 1975); *Klinische Monatsblatter für Augenheilkunde* (Figure 2.8 from Kokott, 1934); *Transactions of the Ophthalmological Societies of the United Kingdom* (Figure 7.30 from Watson, 1974); Williams and Wilkins (Figure 4.41 from Watson in *Contemporary Ophthalmology*, 1972 (Ed.) Bellows).

CHAPTER ONE

Historical Introduction

'*Every physician, almost, hath his favourite disease, to which he ascribes all the victories obtained over human nature. The gout, the rheumatism, the stone, the gravel and the consumption have all their several patrons in the faculty.*' *Tom Jones* (Henry Fielding, 1707–1754).

Sclera. Why sclera? Fortunately for us, in 1865 Thomas Windsor was goaded by a colleague who objected to the use of the word sclera or scleral, into writing a paper on its etymology, because 'purity of the language is so much to be desired that we do not think it will be a waste of time to endeavour to justify our use of these terms'.

The word sclera was certainly used by the Greeks and Romans. Aulus Cornelius Celsus who lived at the start of the Christian era used the same word κερατοειδες (Gr. *keratoeides* = horn-like) for both cornea and sclera. Galen (AD 130), in *De Usu Partium* uses the term σκληρα μηνιγξ (Gr. *sklera meninx* = hard membrane) to describe how this thick membrane goes round the choroid in the same way that the dura mater covers the brain. It seems that the word sclera was changed to sclerotica in the Middle Ages, possibly by Mundinius in 1325. In 1535 Carpus said, 'Posterior to the cornea is a membrane, not transparent but opaque and hard. So it is called sklerotica which covers the whole eye behind.' This change of word was not entirely approved of even then because Joubert in 1585 said in his dictionary, 'Sclerotique .... by the Greeks called skleros which signifies hard, from this barbarians have invented the word sclerotica'. The word sclerotica persisted in general use, however, until its use was discouraged, first in German by Kraus (1844) in his medical dictionary in which he says: 'Sclerotica— μηνιγξ σκληρα (Gr. *meninx sklera* = the hard membrane)—die feste Augenhaut, von scleros: würde besser Sclera heissen!' The final nail in 'sclerotica's' coffin came from Thomas Windsor who changed the word in English by pointing out that 'sclera and sclerotica are both adjectives agreeing with tunica, understood. The tunica sclera would signify hard membrane, a denomination sufficiently expressive; the tunica sclerotica might mean hardening membrane, a term devoid of sense'.

1

Although some older anatomists continued to use terms like the 'dura oculi tunica' of Vesalius or dura tunica, sclera has become the word universally accepted as referring to the collagenous coat of the eye.

Galen, the master anatomist and surgeon to the gladiators, knew of the fascial coats of the eye, calling them 'tunica adnata'. He also introduced the term 'rheumatism' to designate pain which he believed to be caused by one of the four cardinal 'humours' which constituted the human organism being in faulty combination with the others and being eliminated or discharged from the blood into one of the many cavities of the body, including the joints. It was in this way—a humour dripping into a joint cavity—that the word gout arose (L. *gutta* = a drop).

The generic term rheumatism was, until the time of Sydenham (1676), practically interchangeable with catarrh, since it was believed that local collections of fluid within the body were due to discharge of a thin humour from the blood which also gave rise to pain, the onset of which was usually associated with changes in the weather. The word 'rheum', the watery secretion of any tissue, was in the Middle Ages originally applied to the normal secretions, such as the tears, but later came to descibe any pathological state accompanied by excessive secretions, such as catarrhal colds. Rheumatism assumed an identity of its own through the work of the Parisian physician Baillou (1643). He defined catarrh as a disease of mucous membranes associated with inflammatory secretion and clearly separated from this 'rheumatism', as marked by migratory pains.

Galen only lived long enough to lay the basis of scientific medicine, which unfortunately could not be developed sufficiently to cope with the plagues which followed the move to city life. The people's faith in doctors declined and passed to the Church who viewed the care of the sick as a moral obligation incumbent on its members regardless of whether they were trained or not.

As both Christians and Arabs forbade dissection of the human corpse, no further anatomical advances were made until the 14th century when the Graeco-Roman era of speculation concerning the nature of disease, based on 'humours' of the organism, yielded slowly to reasoned observation in the early schools of anatomy by Leonardo da Vinci and Vesalius. This explains why Hippocrates was familiar with the clinical signs of joint disease, but said little of the structural changes in the affected connective tissues—a reflection of the fact that anatomical dissection had not become accepted practice.

With the Renaissance came a new interest in study of the human form in painting and sculpture. The study of anatomy thus became essential and produced a wealth of material not only from Leonardo da Vinci and Vesalius but also from Giovanni Ferrara, Gabriele Falloppio, Fabricius and later Harvey. Because the configuration of the lids and the lustre of the eye is so important in facial expression, the changes which occur with age and suffering were intensively studied and accurately reproduced by the artists of the Renaissance, but the actual anatomy of the minutiae such as the sclera and episclera was left till later. In fact it was not until the French Revolution that Jacques René Tenon (1724–1816) described his capsule (Tenon, 1806), later called 'tunica vaginalis oculi' by Andrée Bonnet (1842).

That great figure of the Renaissance Galileo-Galilei was probably the first patient to have the combination of eye disease with rheumatic disease properly documented. From letters still extant it would seem that in October 1606 Galileo developed a severe febrile illness after he had become severly chilled making his astronomical observations. Following the initial acute phase of the illness, Galileo developed chronic progressive rheumatoid disease associated with recurrent iritis, iridocyclitis, possibly scleritis and corneal degeneration from which he eventually became almost blind (Germani, 1964).

Coinciding with accurate anatomical descriptions came accurate descriptions of disease, but these overlapped with galenic or mediaeval concepts of aetiology with their plethora of humours and vapours, making it difficult to discover what was meant by some of the descriptions of inflammatory disease. It was not until clinicopathological correlation became established practice under Morgagni (1761) that systemic pathological study of the connective tissue and rheumatic and ocular disease became widespread.

Hunter (1759) appears to have recognised the changes of osteoarthritis, Pott (1779) to have identified the features of tuberculous arthritis, and Morgagni and Monro Secundus the anatomical changes of gout. Sydenham (1676) had already described the clinical features of chorea, when Cullen (1778) identified rheumatic fever. The first description of systemic sclerosis is attributed to Curzio (1754).

The first clinical description of scleral disease was probably that of Sir William Read, Royal Ophthalmologist to Queen Anne (1702–1714): 'For it is most certain that this horny membrane .... by how much deeper the blister is hidden in the membrane .... in danger to make an ulceration by breaking through the membrane, whereupon may ensue an utter loss and decay of all the humours'. Although Scarpa (1801) decribed anterior and posterior staphylomata, these were anatomical descriptions of the results of disease rather than a description of the disease itself. Scleral inflammation was described as part of 'rheumatic diseases of the eye' by Wardrop (1818) but the term 'rheumatic' is imprecise and it is difficult to know whether or not he was describing the scleral changes in what we call now 'rheumatoid arthritis'. He said that scleritis comes 'from the patient's having kept wet clothes on his head when overheated. In another patient the disease came on after travelling during the night in a carriage with one side of his head close to an open window'. He added that scleritis not infrequently occurs 'in patients who have previously had rheumatism in other parts of the body. Rheumatism may frequently be observed to attack a joint or part that has been injured.' He also recognised, it seems, that scleritis could arise from other causes: 'but there are other kinds of inflammation which derive their character, not from the peculiarity of the texture inflamed, but from being produced from some specific virus. ("Virus" is used here in the sense given in the *Shorter Oxford Dictionary*: a morbid principle or poisonous substance produced in the body as a result of some disease, especially one capable of being introduced into other persons or animals.) Hence the gonorrheal, the syphilitic, the scrofulous, the gouty and the rheumatic inflammations of the eye; all of which are accompanied with symptoms different from those of simple inflammation of one of the textures which compose that organ.' He also noted 'how difficult it is to distinguish in many instances between venereal, gouty and rheumatic affections of the joints'.

It is surprising how little mention there is of affections of the locomotor system, other than gout, in the medical articles of the past. Why should it be that physicians did not consider these disorders worthy of more than perfunctory mention? It may have been due to a feeling of therapeutic helplessness on their part, as all emphasis was concentrated upon the discovery of a specific medicine for each disease and the concept of patient management or physical treatment was seldom considered.

The seventeenth-century revival by Sydenham of the Hippocratic ideals of close clinical observation of the patient and his symptoms in preference to a purely academic reliance by the physicians upon the recorded opinions of their forerunners was beginning to result in the recognition of specific disease syndromes. Following the lead of the famous botanist Linnaeus, who was busy classifying the plant world, medical men such as William Cullen were soon producing similar over-elaborate classifications of disease: gout and allied rheumatic disorders accounted for nearly 20 categories. Sydenham (1624–1689) distinguished between 'chronic' rheumatism and gout, although the latter term continued to embrace a large and undefined collection of syndromes throughout most of the eighteenth-century. Sydenham's classical description of the acute and chronic ravages of gout, which he described after 30 years of painful personal experience, has never been bettered. In his *Treatise on Gout* (1683) he showed how to differentiate between gout and rheumatic fever. He also noted and rationalised the connection of the gout with the formation of gravel and calculus. For treatment he advised dietetic restriction, particularly of meat, and regular exercise.

True gout has influenced the course of history. It caused the Roman General Agrippa to commit suicide; it soured the disposition of the great reformer, Martin Luther. It is also said to have been instrumental in the loss of the American colonies in that Pitt, who could have dealt with the crisis, was prevented from going to the House of Commons because of an acute attack of gout.

A major step forward came in 1848 when Sir Alfred Garrod (1819–1907) showed that the gouty tophus consisted of sodium biurate and with his classical demonstration using his thread test he proved that the blood of the gouty patient contained an excess of uric acid. W. H. Wollaston (1797) had previously shown that the tophaceous material from his own gouty ear contained sodium biurate. Garrod demonstrated that uric acid in the serum crystallised along a cotton thread left in it overnight. He reported this in his book *Gout and Rheumatic Gout* (1859). Also in this book he differentiated between the various arthritic conditions saying, 'The term "rheumatic gout" is widely used by the medical profession of a disease having a special pathology in no way related to true gout and not necessarily rheumatism ... although unwilling to add to the number of names ... perhaps "rheumatoid arthritis" would answer the object, by which term I would wish to imply an inflammatory condition of the joints not unlike rheumatism in some of its characters, but differing materially from it'. Later, his son, Sir Archibald Garrod (1857–1936) differentiated the pathological characteristics of rheumatoid arthritis from those of osteoarthritis in his book *A Treatise on Rheumatism and Rheumatoid Arthritis* (1890).

'Rheumatoid arthritis' was first clearly described as an entity by Landré-

Beauvais in 1800; he was physician to the Saltpetrière Hospital in Paris and published his observations in his doctoral thesis. He noticed that it mostly affected women, and described its most striking clinical features under the name of 'goutte asthénique primitive des jointures'. Further precision was given to the concept of chronic arthritis by the work of Heberden (1802). In 1867, in a doctoral thesis, Jean Charcot gave a further description of what we now know as rheumatoid arthritis. This was illustrated by Charcot himself to show the various types of joint contractures which may be produced. He still appeared to subscribe to the hypothesis that the underlying aetiology was gouty. As Stockman (1920) pointed out, from the earliest times until recently, medical writers made little or no distinction between the different types of 'chronic rheumatic arthritis' so that today it is practically impossible to disentangle their descriptions.

There is certainly no convincing description of rheumatoid arthritis in mediaeval writing (Short, 1974) except perhaps the description of arthritis in Constantine IX (980–1055) who suffered from a progressive inflammatory polyarthritis with involvement of the soft tissues and increasing deformities (Caughey, 1974).

Although Garrod (1859) introduced the term rheumatoid arthritis there was no clear clinical recognition until 1906 when the Bath physician, G. A. Bannatyne, in the fourth edition of his monograph, stated that the disease affected joints in a manner different from osteoarthrosis. He reproduced the first x-ray photograph ever to appear in a medical book. Indeed Virchow (1858) and Charcot (1867) positively delayed progress by insisting upon the identity of degenerate and rheumatoid joint disease under the misleading title of 'arthritis deformans'. It was not until 1857 that Robert Adams of Dublin convincingly separated the osteoarthritic type of arthropathy from the others.

Several authors have commented on the absence of rheumatoid deformities in painting or sculpture before 1800 (Snorrason, 1952; Boyle and Buchanan, 1971). Recently Dequeker (1975) examined the hands in Flemish primitive paintings, and although there were changes suggestive of rheumatoid-like lesions, there was in no case absolutely convincing evidence of symmetrical rheumatoid arthritis.

The anatomical features of rheumatoid arthritis did not appear to engage the interest of surgeons preoccupied with tuberculous and other forms of infective joint disease (Brodie, 1813). It seems very likely that the superficial similarities of the diseases, the frequency and age incidence of tuberculous arthritis and the low mean expectation of life in the years when Hunter, Brodie, Baillie and other great pioneers of morbid anatomy were at work, effectively disguised the problem of rheumatoid arthritis, a disorder much more conspicuous in ageing populations such as our own, among whom infectious arthritis is now rare.

Although evidence exists that ankylosing spondylitis affected the human race from prehistoric times and was recognised by Hippocrates and even certain members of the English Royal Family in Plantagenet times, there is no written description of the disease before the end of the seventeenth century, when Connor (1691) described a skeleton with signs of ankylosing spondylitis. Widespread clinical recognition of the disorder did not materialise until the late 1800s when the Russian Bechterew (1893), Strumpell (1897) and Charcot's successor Marie (1898) reported several cases. Benjamin Brodie (1813) included descriptions of the joint changes in ankylosing spondylitis together with what is apparently the first description of the triad of urethritis, arthritis and conjunctivitis, now called Reiter's syndrome (Reiter, 1916). Cazenave (1850) drew attention to the skin changes of discoid lupus erythematosus and Kaposi (1872) subsequently described the disseminated form of this disease and emphasised the widespread involvement of viscera. The first clear recognition of polyarteritis nodosa came at almost the same time (Kussmaul and Maier, 1866).

In the latter half of the nineteenth century, progress in understanding the pathology of these diseases was slow. Perhaps because of the introduction of the compound microscope by Charles Chevalier (1804–1854), and the identification of microorganisms as the cause of disease by Pasteur from 1857, interest was diverted to those diseases which had a bacteriological basis and lack of any direct evidence that the rheumatic diseases were infective discouraged further investigation.

Virchow (1858) expounded the doctrine of 'omnus cellula e cellula', that is, the seat of disease should always be sought in the cell, and this has been the basis of investigation into this group of diseases and their eye complications ever since.

The search for microorganisms as a cause of eye disease started as soon as methods for their detection became readily available; tuberculosis was soon added as a cause of scleral disease to those chronic granulomatous conditions already recognised. Koch (1843–1910) had shown how difficult it was to recognise certain organisms, even when cultured under ideal conditions (Koch, 1882). It was not, therefore, regarded as strange that no organisms could be cultured from the chronic granulomas found in the sclera.

Similarly, streptococci were identified by Ogston in 1881 and Poynton and Paine (1913) conducted an extensive series of investigations to see whether rheumatic fever was the result of an infection. By the time their monograph was published, an immune origin for the disease was suspected. Klinge (1933) established an association between an immune arthritis in rabbits injected with horse serum and the presence in the affected tissues of fibrinoid material. This classic work laid the foundations for the theory which postulates the existence of the systemic collagen or connective tissue diseases (Klemperer, Pollack and Baehr, 1942).

Klemperer described widespread foci of fibrinoid change in connective tissues in systemic lupus erythematosus and systemic sclerosis and suggested that both diseases be regarded as diffuse disorders of connective tissue. As rheumatic fever, rheumatoid arthritis, dermatomyositis and polyarteritis nodosa have similar basic changes, they were also grouped together.

As a result of the foundations laid by Ehrlich (1854–1915), Pfeiffer (1858–1945), Hamowitz and many others, and by drawing analogies from the appearances in other tissues such as those in the joints, it became obvious that most of the reactions seen as a result of disease in the sclera could also be the result of immune processes of a similar type.

Klemperer used the term 'collagen disease', but in 1954 he emphasised that he meant to refer in his original description to the complete intercellular connective tissue, both fibres and ground substance, but had used the word collagen in a nonspecific sense for the sake of brevity. He also pointed out the danger that the term 'diffuse collagen disease' may become applied to any illness with puzzling clinical and anatomical features, rather than those conditions affecting connective tissue.

This group of diseases was then considered to be due to a derangement of the immune response. The demonstration of antibodies in the serum of patients which reacted with antigens present in their own tissues led to the idea that these antibodies were capable of damaging host tissues. This concept has been based largely on the work of Sir Macfarlane Burnett (1959). It is considered that a 'forbidden' clone of cells arising from a single immunocyte on account of a combination of somatic mutation and genetically determined characteristics, proliferates and produces antibody. This was claimed to be the basic abnormality leading to the initiation of autoimmune disease.

Having produced a reasonable explanation for the pathological changes seen in both eye and joint, the search has since continued for trigger factors which could initiate and perpetuate changes and the factors which determine the particular features of each disease. The search, which has implicated trauma, bacteria, mycoplasma, viruses, genetic factors, or combinations of these, still continues. The primary antigen may not be an infectious agent or a specific antigen produced in response to it, but may be other components of connective tissue altered immunologically by the inflammatory response to a virus or other agent. Indeed the interaction of viruses with cells can lead to the release of hydrolytic enzymes from sublethally infected cells; these enzymes could be the first auto-antigens towards which immune responses are directed.

Before the cause of any disease can be established, it must fulfil either the criteria laid down by Koch in 1882 or, if the condition is thought to be autoimmune, it must fulfil the criteria defined by Milgrom and Witebsky (1962). These criteria have not been satisfied for any of the connective tissue diseases or for many of the nonspecific causes of scleral disease. Our interest in scleral disease will continue until they have.

REFERENCES

Adams, R. (1857) *Illustrations of the Effects of Rheumatic Gout or Chronic Rheumatic Arthritis on all the Articulations.* London: Churchill.

Baillou, G. de (1643) *Liber de Rheumatismo.* Paris: Quesnet.

Bannatyne, G. A. (1906) *Rheumatoid Arthritis: its Pathology, Morbid Anatomy and Treatment.* 4th edition. Bristol: Wright.

Bechterew, V. von (1893) Steifigkeit der Wirbelsäule und ihre Verkrümmung als besondere Erkrankungesform. *Neurologisches Zentralblatt,* **12,** 426–434.

Bonnet, A. (1842) *Traité des Sections Tendineuses et Musculaires dans la Strabisme.* Lyons.

Boyle, J. A. & Buchanan, W. W. (1971) *Clinical Rheumatology.* pp. 71–72. Philadelphia: Davis.

Brodie, B. C. (1813) Pathological researches respecting the diseases of joints. *Medico-chirurgical Transactions,* **4,** 207–277.

Brodie, B. C. (1818) *Pathological and Surgical Observations on the Diseases of Joints.* London: Longman.

Burnett, F. M. (1959) *The Clonal Selection Theory of Acquired Immunity.* Cambridge: Cambridge University Press.

Carpus, A. (1535) *Anatomica Carpi*, quoted by Windsor, T. (1865) Notes on the terms sclera and sclerotica. *Ophthalmic Review*, 1, 149–151.

Caughey, D. E. (1974) The arthritis of Constantine IX. *Annals of the Rheumatic Diseases*, 33, 77–80.

Cazenave, P. L. (1850) Des principales formes du lupus et de son traitement. *Gazette des Hôpitaux de Paris*, 3, 393.

Celsus, Aulus Cornelius (30 AD) *De Medicina*, quoted by Windsor, T. (1865) Notes on the terms sclera and sclerotica. *Ophthalmic Review*, 1, 149–157.

Charcot, J. M. (1867) *Leçons sur les Maladies des Vieillards et les Maladies Chroniques*. Paris: Delahaye.

Connor, B. (1691) *Sur la Continuité de Plusiers Os, à l'Occasion d'un Tronc et les Os des Iles, qui Naturellements sont Distincts et Separés, ne font qu'un Seul Os Continué et Inséperable*. Thesis, Rheims.

Cullen, W. (1778) *First Lines on the Practice of Physic for the Use of Students in the University of Edinburgh*. Edinburgh: Creech.

Curzio, C. (1754) An account of an extraordinary disease of the skin and its cure. *Philosophical Transactions of the Royal Society*, 48, 579–587.

Dequeker, J. (1975) Arthritis in the Flemish primitive paintings. *Proceedings of the Heberden Society*, November issue.

Galen of Pergammon (130 AD) *De Usu Partium*, translated Adams, F., London (1844–1847). Notes on the terms sclera and sclerotica, quoted by Windsor, T. (1865) in *Ophthalmic Review*, 1, 149–151.

Garrod, A. (1859) *The Nature and Treatment of Gout and Rheumatic Gout*. London: Walton and Maberly.

Garrod, A. B. (1890) *A Treatise on Rheumatism and Rheumatoid Arthritis*. London: Griffin.

Germani, G. M. (1964) Rheumatoid disease and the blindness of Galileo-Galilei. *Ospedale Maggiore*, 59, 193–196.

Heberden, W. (1802) *Commentaries on the History and Cure of Disease*. London: Payne.

Hunter, J. (1759) Manuscript 54. In the possession of the Royal College of Surgeons of London.

Joubert, J. (1585) *Interpretatio Dictionum Anatomicum*, quoted by Windsor, T. (1865) Notes on the terms sclera and sclerotica. *Ophthalmic Review*, 1, 149–151.

Kaposi, M. (1872) Neue Beiträge zur Kenntnis der Lupus Erythematosus. *Archiv für Dermatologie und Syphilis*, 4, 36–78.

Klemperer, P. (1950) The concept of collagen diseases. *American Journal of Pathology*, 26, 505–519.

Klemperer, P. (1954) *Connective Tissue in Health and Disease* (Ed.) Asboe-Hansen, G. p. 251. Copenhagen: Munksgard.

Klemperer, P. (1955) The significance of the intermediate substances of the connective tissue in human disease. *Harvey Lectures Series*, 49, 100–123.

Klemperer, P., Pollack, A. D. & Baehr, G. (1942) Diffuse collagen disease: acute disseminated lupus erythematosus and diffuse scleroderma. *Journal of the American Medical Association*, 119, 331–332.

Klinge, F. (1933) *Der Rheumatismus; pathologisch-anatomische und experimentell-pathologische Tatsachen und ihre Auswertung für das ärtzliche-Rheumaproblem*. pp. 163–176. Munich: Bergmann.

Koch, E. (1882) Die aetiologie der Tuberkulose. *Berliner klinische Wochenschrift*, 19, 221–230.

Kraus, J. (1844) *Kritisch-etymologisches medizinisches Lexicon*, 3rd edition, Göttenberg.

Kussmaul, A. & Maier, R. (1866) Über eine bischer nicht beschreibene eigenthümliche Arterienerkrankung die mit Morbus Brightii und rapid fort-schreitender allgemeiner Muskellämung einhergeht. *Deutsche Archiv für klinische Medizin*, 1, 484–578.

Landré-Beauvais, A-J. (1800) *Doit-on Admettre une Nouvelle Espèce Goutte sous la Denomination de Goutte Asthênique Primitive*. Paris: Brosson.

Marie, P. (1898) Sur la spondylose rhizomelique. *Revue de Medecine*, 18, 285–315.

Milgrom, F. & Witebsky, E. (1962) Auto-antibodies and autoimmune diseases. *Journal of the American Medical Association*, **181**, 706–716.

Monro, A. 'Secundus', quoted by Copeman, W. B. (1964) *A Short History of the Gout and the Rheumatic Diseases*. Berkeley, Los Angeles: University of California Press.

Morgagni, G. B. (1761) *De Sedibus et Causis Morborum per Anatomen Indagatis*. Venice: Remondiniana typog.

Mundinius (1325) quoted by Windsor, T. (1865) Notes on the terms sclera and sclerotica. *Ophthalmic Review*, **1**, 149–157.

Ogston, A. (1881) Report upon microorganisms in surgical diseases. *British Medical Journal*, **i**, 369–375.

Pott, W. (1779) *Remarks upon that Kind of Palsy of the Lower Limbs which is Frequently Found to Accompany a Curvature of the Spine*. London: Johnson.

Poynton, F. J. & Paine, A. (1913) *Research on Rheumatism*. London: Churchill.

Read, W. (1702–1714) *A Short but Exact Account of all Diseases Incident to the Eyes*. London: Baker.

Reiter, H. (1916) Ueber eine bischer unerkannte Spirochäten Infektin. *Deutsche medizinische Wochenschrifte*, **42**, 1535–1536.

Scarpa, A. (1801) *Saggio di Osservazioni e d'Esperienze sulla Principale Malattie degli Occhi*. Pavia.

Short, C. L. (1974) The antiquity of rheumatoid arthritis. *Arthritis and Rheumatism*, **17**, 193–205.

Snorrason, E. (1952) Landré-Beavais and his 'Goutte Asthenique Primitive'. *Acta Medica Scandinavica*, **142**, Supplement 266, 115–118.

Stockman, R. (1920) *Rheumatism and Arthritis*. Edinburgh: Green.

Strumpell, A. (1897) Bermerkungen über die chronische ankylosirende Entzundung der Wirbelsäule und der Huftgelenke. *Deutsche Zeitschrift fur Nervenheilkunde*, **11**, 338–343.

Sydenham, T. (1676) *Medical Observations Concerning the History and Cure of Acute Disease*. Translated by Latham, R. G. (1848). London: The Sydenham Society.

Sydenham, T. (1683) *Tractatus de Podogra et Hydrope*. London: Kettilby.

Tenon, J. R. (1806) *Memoires et Observations sur l'Anatomie, la Pathologie et la Chirurgie*. p. 193. Paris.

Vesalius (1519) quoted by Windsor, T. (1865) Notes on the terms sclera and sclerotica. *Ophthalmic Review*, **1**, 149–751.

Virchow, R. (1858) *Die Cellular-pathologie in ihre Begründing auf physiologische und pathologisches Gewebelehre*. Paris: Hirschwald.

Wardrop, J. (1818) Account of the rheumatic inflammation of the eye with observations on the treatment of the disease. *Medico-chirurgical Transactions*, **10**, 1–15.

Windsor, T. (1865) Notes on the terms sclera and sclerotica. *Ophthalmic Review*, **1**, 149–151.

Wollaston, W. H. (1797) On gouty and urinary concretions. *Philosophical Transactions of the Royal Society*, **87**, 386–400.

CHAPTER TWO

Anatomical and Physiological Considerations

'Anatomy is to physiology as geography is to history; it describes the theatre of events.' On the Natural Part of Medicine (Jean Fernel, 1497–1558).

The human sclera, although metabolically relatively inert, is nevertheless a remarkable structure as it permits the eyeball to be rotated through nearly 180° by quite powerful muscles without significant distortion. If the sclera were deformed when the eyes moved, the image on the retina to which the sclera is indirectly attached would become very blurred, not only because of wrinkling of the retina itself but also through irregular distortion of the lens iris diaphragm. The shape is in part maintained by the presence of the intraocular contents and the intraocular pressure. However, the sclera must be rigid enough to provide relatively constant conditions for the intraocular pressure so that, when the eyeball is moved, the intraocular pressure does not fluctuate and affect vision. In addition, the opacity of the sclera ensures that the internal light scattering does not affect the retinal image and, of course, the sclera must protect the intraocular contents from injury.

Theoretically these objects could be achieved by a rigid globe, by pot eyeballs. The problem has been solved in different ways throughout the animal kingdom. Frogs, turtles and most fish have a rigid globe of cartilage and birds, which have an irregular, non-globular eyeball, have a further reinforcement of bony ossicles around the posterior pole (Figures 2.1, 2.2 and 2.3). The rigid globe is relatively immobile; the bird overcomes this by moving its head, and the shark by putting the eye on a pedicle from the orbit, forming a ball and socket joint. Although the rigid globe allows extremely high visual resolution it has been abandoned in all placentals in favour of the largely fibrous globe. This fibrous tissue can be remarkably thick, as occurs in dolphins, porpoises and whales (Figure 2.4), the sclera of the hump-back whale being 30 mm thick at the posterior pole and only 3 mm thick at the limbus. Duke Elder (1958) considers this thick sclera is necessary to maintain the non-spherical

10

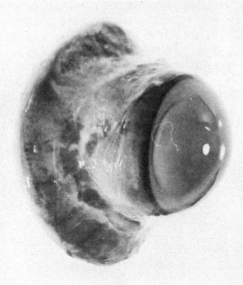

Figure 2.1. The eye of the eagle owl (*Bubo bubo*). The sclera, rather than passing backwards in a gentle curve as in the human eye, is almost at right angles to the limbus before it expands into a flask shape posteriorly.
Courtesy of Dr Keith Barnett, Newmarket.

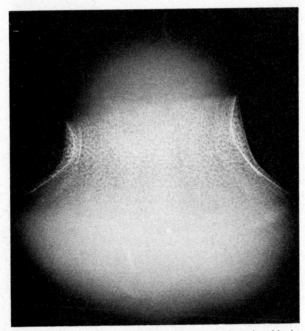

Figure 2.2. Sagittal plane x-ray photograph of the same eye to show that this shape is maintained by bony ossicles.
Courtesy of Dr Keith Barnett, Newmarket.

shape of the huge cestacean globe rendered mechanically weak by its size. In most mammals the globe is circular and the sclera thin and even throughout. It is possible that a less rigid fibrous structure allows a more even distribution of the blood supply to the choroid and thence the retina during the large excursions of voluntary ocular movement. Certainly, when the eye becomes

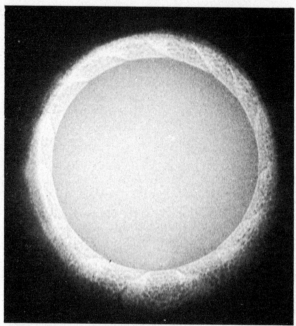

Figure 2.3. Coronal plane x-ray photograph showing how these ossicles overlap each other around the eye.
Courtesy of Dr Keith Barnett, Newmarket.

soft for any reason, be it due to injury or inflammation, then the vision falls disproportionately more than might be expected from the distortion of the intraocular contents alone, probably part of the fall in vision being due to the inefficient nutrition of the retina and the optic nerve. Conversely, when patients with dysthyroid ophthalmopathy look upwards, their intraocular pressure rises because of the pressure of the rigid recti muscles on the globe, and, in some cases, the vision will also fall dramatically on movement of the eyeball. Scleral folding on its own does not dramatically affect vision unless the macula is involved, as can be seen sometimes after retinal detachment surgery when the intraocular pressure and the vision are normal. The sclera fulfils its function partly by the arrangement of the fibres of the stroma and partly by the inherent physical properties of the structures of which it is composed.

It has long been recognised that conditions which affect the joints affect the sclera also. Superficially there is little resemblance between the structure of the joint and that of the sclera except that both consist of collagenous tissue derived from mesoderm and are acted upon by muscles. However, close inspection reveals many likenesses and it is not too far-fetched to suggest that the eye is a highly specialised form of joint used for seeing, the most obvious difference being the lack of articular cartilage, because the eye has no weight to bear, and the consequent total lack of true synovial membrane

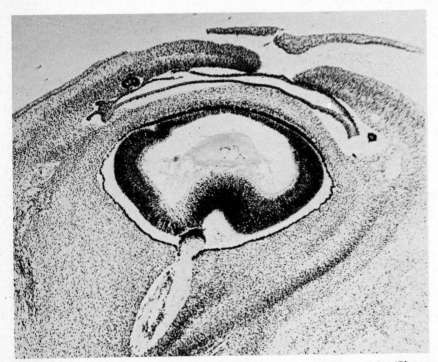

Figure 2.4.　Cross-section of the eye of the fetus of a common or harbour porpoise (*Phocaena phocaena*). The anterior sclera is thin, increasing greatly in thickness posteriorly. This configuration of the sclera may enable the eye to be held in shape as the animal dives to great depths.
Courtesy of Dr Anthony Greenwood, London.

in the eye socket. This absence of synovial membrane around the eye necessarily means that the effect of a disease affecting both structures will be different in the two cases. Effects due to trauma on a joint will not be seen in relation to the eye. Granulomatous changes which affect both structures will be seen firstly adjacent to vessels of the episclera and choroid on the one hand, and adjacent to the synovium on the other. Only later will the avascular tissues of the sclera and articular cartilage be involved. As the synovial changes are central to changes in the joint and much of what has been learned from the study of this tissue can be applied directly to that seen in the sclera and episclera, it will be described in detail, even though it has no direct counterpart around the eye. Just as it is mandatory for a general physician to understand the structure of the eye in order to comprehend its diseases, it is equally important for the ophthalmologist to understand the structure of connective tissues in order to understand connective tissue disease.

THE SCLERA AND ITS COVERINGS

The sclera consists almost entirely of collagen and comprises five-sixths of the outer tunic of the eye. It is covered by the fascia bulbi (Tenon's capsule) and by the episclera and is interrupted by the cornea in front and by the optic nerve behind. The sclera is traversed by the anterior ciliary vessels in front of the recti muscles and by the long and short posterior ciliary vessels and nerves behind these muscles. All these structures, with the exception of the nerves, can be identified with a slit-lamp microscope provided they are anterior to the equator of the eyeball.

The transparent cornea merges with the opaque sclera over an area of about 2 mm² at the limbus. As the cornea has a higher radius of curvature than the sclera a sulcus is formed at the limbus which is not readily visible as it is filled in by the overlying episclera and conjunctiva. Between the limbus and the tendinous insertions of the muscles, three fascial tissue layers can be distinguished, each containing a vascular network: the conjunctiva, Tenon's capsule and the episclera (Figure 2.5).

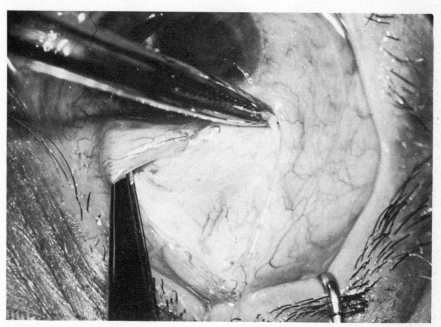

Figure 2.5. An incision has been made first vertically through the conjunctiva and then horizontally through Tenon's capsule revealing the episclera and the deep episcleral plexus of vessels. The conjunctival and superficial episcleral vessels can be seen over the tips of the scissors.

Bulbar Conjunctiva

The bulbar conjunctiva is a thin transparent mucous membrane, the epithelium of which is continuous with the corneal epithelium and lies on the conjunctival stroma which is a loosely arranged mobile connective tissue with some elastic fibres in its deeper layers. In front of the recti muscles the conjunctiva lies loosely on the underlying Tenon's capsule and can be readily moved over it, together with the vessels which lie within layers of the conjunctival stroma (Figure 2.5). About 3 mm from the limbus, the subconjunctival tissue and Tenon's capsule merge with each other and the fibres of each intermingle so that it is difficult to move the conjunctiva over the underlying tissue in this region. At the limbus itself, both conjunctiva and Tenon's capsule are inseparable from the underlying episclera and sclera.

Microscopically the surface epithelium contains goblet cells peripherally, but very few close to the limbus. At the limbus the epithelium is stratified and the basal cells form a single layer of cubical cells with large darkly staining nuclei. The pigment granules contained in these cells are especially marked in the pigmented races and readily visible on the slit-lamp microscope. The surface epithelial cells are similar to those found in the cornea except that they do not have such tight intercellular junctions.

The subconjunctival tissue contains vessels, a large number of fibroblasts, polymorphs, lymphocytes, plasma cells and melanocytes which increase in number close to the limbus. At the limbus four or five finger-like protrusions of the substantia bulge towards the surface forming limbar papillae.

Structurally and functionally the conjunctiva appears to be quite different from the tissues on which it lies, because the conjunctiva is only very rarely involved in underlying scleral disease when even the blood vessels which it contains stay uninflamed. Apparently normal conjunctiva can cover what appears to be complete dehiscences of scleral and episcleral tissue in necrotising scleral disease.

Fascia Bulbi: Tenon's Capsule

Tenon's capsule is a dense well-defined membrane which extends from the limbus backwards to ensheath the extraocular recti muscles and becomes continuous with their perimysium. It also passes backwards to ensheath the globe posteriorly and becomes inserted in the dural sheath of the optic nerve (Figure 2.6).

At the limbus Tenon's capsule is inseparable from the subconjunctival tissue and underlying episclera but becomes thicker about 3 mm from the limbus where it is freely mobile over the underlying episclera to which it is connected by fine trabeculae. The potential space between these two layers is readily found on surgical dissection (Figure 2.5). The thickness of Tenon's capsule in front of and over tendon insertions is responsible for the glistening bright eyes of children and young adults. It thins with age and in certain conditions, such as scleromalacia perforans, it disappears altogether.

Behind the muscle insertions the fascia bulbi becomes progressively thinner except below at the equator where it becomes very thick to form the 'ligament of Lockwood' on which the eye rests. As it passes backwards over the muscles it also thickens to form the so-called 'check ligaments', the longest and strongest of which are from the lateral rectus to the orbital tubercle, between the levator palpebrae and the superior rectus—so that the lid is retracted as well as raised when looking up—and between the inferior rectus to the lower lid, thus retracting the lower lid on looking down. Through its insertions into the conjunctival sac the fascia bulbi acts like the musculus articularis genu which pulls the synovial membrane out of the way in contraction of the quadriceps so that it is not torn by the patella (Wolff, 1968).

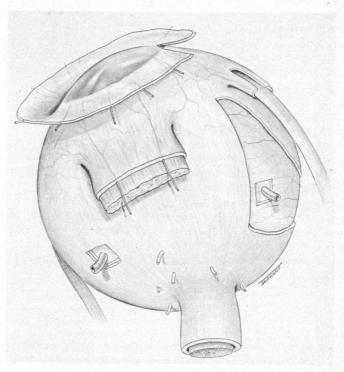

Figure 2.6.   A diagram of Tenon's capsule which extends from the limbus to ensheath the muscles and passes backwards to become continuous with the dural sheaths of the optic nerve. It is separate from the conjunctiva and from the episclera which is deep to it. Below the eye and anteriorly it thickens to form the check ligaments. It is penetrated by the long and short ciliary vessels and nerves, the lymphatics and the venae vorticosae.

Posteriorly Tenon's capsule is so thin that it is extremely difficult to distinguish where it ends in relationship to the optic nerve. It probably merges with the dural sheath of the nerve and with the fibrous bands which separate the orbital fat. Anteriorly Tenon's capsule consists of radially arranged compact collagen bundles parallel to the scleral surface, the cellular content of which is very low, comprising only a few fibroblasts. In this tissue lie the ramifications of the anterior ciliary vessels, the veins being the more superficial and the arteries coming close to the surface only near the limbal arcade. Towards the equator posteriorly, a fine tenuous network of vessels runs in this tissue from the posterior ciliary arteries.

Episclera

The episclera is a thin, dense, vascularised layer of connective tissue, the fibres of which are continuous with the underlying stroma of the sclera itself. In contrast with Tenon's capsule, the bundles of collagen are circumferentially arranged with tight attachments to the walls of the blood vessels, rendering the whole structure immobile when viewed with a slit-lamp microscope. The attachments to Tenon's capsule are dense near the limbus and weaken progressively towards the equator where the episclera is bound to the capsule only by very thin bands of collagen. Overlying the posterior sclera, both the episcleral tissue and the overlying Tenon's capsule are thin, which results in relative avascularity of the superficial layers of the posterior sclera. A small amount of elastic tissue can be found in the episclera together with melanocytes and a few macrophages. A few myelinated and unmyelinated nerve fibres ramify within the episclera. Their function is unknown; they do not seem to have any specialised nerve endings and they terminate mostly around the vessels.

Scleral Stroma

The episclera blends imperceptibly with the underlying scleral stroma whose fibres become progressively denser and more interlaced. This interlacing of the collagen fibres gives it its inherent strength, elasticity and resilience, making it resistant to injury. The fibrils themselves are like those found in a tendon or in non-articular surfaces of joints, interdigitating on various planes as well as in the same plane with elastic fibres at the end of each bundle. The extraocular muscle tendon fibres intermingle with the scleral fibres up to the limbus. Superficially the fibres are further apart, becoming closer and more compact in their deeper layers. The arrangement of the deep layers also differs in that they are arranged in a net-like fashion whereas the superficial fibres are laid down circumferentially at the equator and in circles or whorls near the macula.

Unlike the collagen fibrils in the cornea, the fibres vary in size in each bundle (10 to 16 μm in thickness and 100 to 140 μm in width according to Salzmann, 1912). They are strengthened by elastic fibres, particularly at the equator where the sclera is thinnest (0.3 mm) and at the limbus and optic disc (Figure 2.7). All the fibres are contoured away from the muscle insertions presumably to resist the stresses imposed by the muscles so that the eye will remain as a globe. These 'stress' lines have been carefully mapped by Kokott (1934) (Figure 2.8). The interdigitations are particularly dense and the sclera thickest (1 mm) around the posterior pole, presumably to hold that area rigid; they thin out again near the optic disc but some fibres pass across the disc at the lamina cribrosa. Changes in the collagenous structure here and near the posterior pole could account for the changes found in progressive myopia and for some cases of low tension glaucoma where the disc head collapses. Strangulation of the nerve fibres and blood vessels occurs with oedema of the disc as they run in fibrous channels within the scleral tissue. These fibrous channels penetrate the sclera at three main sites: around the optic nerve for the passage of the long and short posterior ciliary vessels and nerves, 4 mm behind the equator for the venae vorticosae, and between the limbus and the muscle insertions for the transmission of the anterior ciliary vessels, nerves and perivascular lymphatics (Figure 2.6).

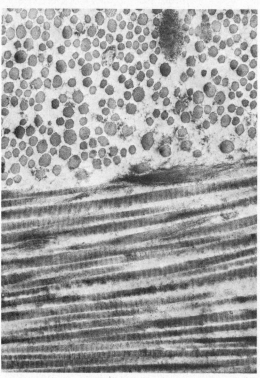

Figure 2.7.   Electron micrograph of human sclera showing variable diameter of collagen fibrils cut transversely (above) and longitudinally (below). A regular periodicity of 6 nm, typical of collagen fibrils, is apparent along their long axis. G.A./OsO$_4$ fixed, V.A./L.C. × 25 000.
Courtesy of Dr Ramesh Tripathi, London.

The innermost layer of the sclera is known as the lamina fusca. The scleral lamellae thin out in this region and blend with the suprachoroidal lamellae which have opened out to form the spaces occupied by the ciliary vessels and nerves and their branches. Fine strands of scleral collagen connect sclera to choroid and can be seen when the choroid and sclera are separated from each other as in choroidal effusions and detachments. The lamina fusca is dark and derives its name from the large number of melanocytes which have migrated into the deeper layers of the sclera, particularly in heavily pigmented individuals. These cells sometimes pass through the emissary foramen producing dark spots on the surface which can lead to mistakes in diagnosis and the suspicion of intraocular melanomas. The sclera can be diffusely pigmented, particularly in those races whose skin is darkly pigmented. Patchy pigmentation also occurs; it may be unilateral and may be associated with naevus formation (see Figure 3.1). Anteriorly, the superficial scleral fibres blend with the episcleral fibres at the limbus; the deeper fibres are continuous with those of the cornea and the deepest fibres condense in a ring which forms the scleral spur to which the trabecular tissue is inserted anteriorly and the longitudinal part

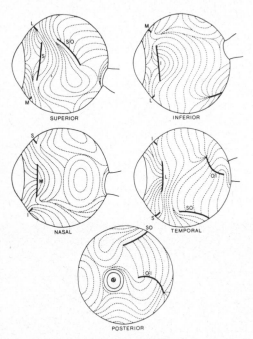

SUPERIOR   INFERIOR

NASAL   TEMPORAL

POSTERIOR

Figure 2.8. The arrangement of the scleral fibrils in different areas of the eye. Anterior to the equator the fibres are meridional, particularly in relation to the muscle insertions. They are densest at the posterior pole and circular around the optic nerve and scleral spur.

of the ciliary muscle posteriorly. The collagen fibres of the scleral spur, which are continuous with the fibres of the corneoscleral trabecular meshwork, increase in size from 40 nm in the trabecular sheets to 80 nm close to the sclera, so that the scleral spur feels hard and rigid when attacked surgically. The ciliary muscle is very strongly attached to its deep surface, but it is doubtful whether tendinous expansions pass through to the trabecular meshwork (Rohan, 1961; Hogan, Alvarado and Weddell, 1971).

BLOOD SUPPLY OF THE SCLERA AND EPISCLERA

The sclera has a low metabolic requirement because of the slow turnover of collagen of which it is composed. Scleral stroma contains no blood vessels in the normal healthy state although the long posterior ciliary arteries and nerves and the vortex veins are carried through it in fibrous canals. The stroma derives its nutrition from the episcleral and choroidal vascular networks; similarly the

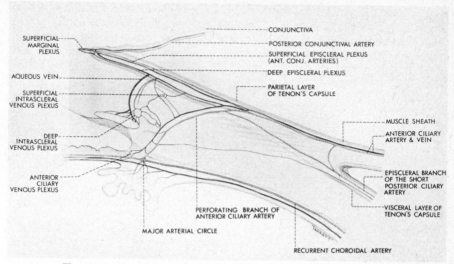

Figure 2.9.   Vascular supply of episcleral and anterior segment of the eye.

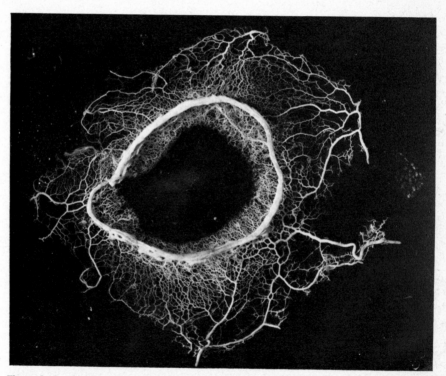

Figure 2.10.   Neoprene cast of the vessels of the anterior segment of the eye and Schlemm's canal. The major straight feeding arteries are the anterior ciliary arteries which overlie the recti muscles.

Courtesy of Professor Norman Ashton, London.

inflammatory cells found in inflammations of the sclera derive from both these sources. The episclera and Tenon's capsule are supplied by the anterior ciliary arteries anteriorly to the rectus insertions and the posterior ciliary arteries behind these insertions (Figure 2.9). The arterial supply to the episcleral tissue from the anterior ciliary artery is very rich, the veins lying superficial in the episcleral tissue and Tenon's capsule, whilst most of the arteries as they leave the depth of the muscle break up to form a meshwork deep in the episcleral tissue itself (two arteries to each muscle, except the lateral rectus which has one) (Figure 2.10). This arrangement gives rise to a very characteristic pattern when episcleral tissue is examined with the slit lamp (Figure 2.11). The arteries are deep-seated and are practically invisible in the normal eye but can be seen to break into a rete of fine vessels as it forms the limbal arcade when the eye is slightly congested. The veins, which may also receive aqueous from Schlemm's canal, run radially backwards from the limbus towards the muscle insertions where they amalgamate to form the anterior ciliary veins (Figure 2.12). There is an anastomosis with the posterior ciliary vessels between the muscles but these vessels are so fine that the connection is only rarely of significance. The posterior episclera is supplied by very fine vessels derived from the posterior ciliary circulation which form a thin network over the back of the globe. Two veins accompany each artery. Because the vessels are so small and the anastomosis with the anterior ciliary circulation so tenuous, there is a relatively poor blood supply to the sclera in the region of the equator, most of its requirements in this area being drawn from the choroidal and ciliary circulation.

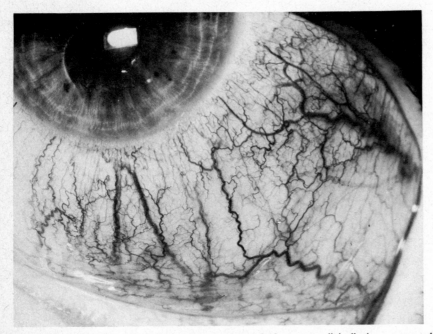

Figure 2.11. The same radial large vessels as Figure 2.10, as seen clinically in a congested eye with simple episcleritis.

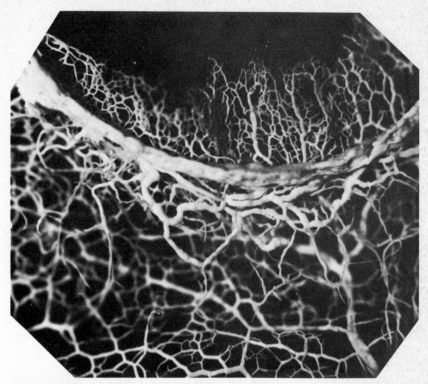

Figure 2.12.   The collector channels and vascular networks in the region of Schlemm's canal. The collector channels feed into deep scleral plexus and thence to the episcleral vessels. Neoprene cast. Courtesy of Professor Norman Ashton, London.

The blood supply is modified in the region of the limbus, the angle of the anterior chamber and Schlemm's canal to provide a rich vascular supply. Each ciliary artery dives into the sclera 4 to 6 mm from the limbus to join the circulus iridis major. The deep episcleral arteries leave the main trunk before they enter the sclera, anastomosing with each other to produce the limbal arterial arcade. Smaller branches of this arcade form the pericorneal plexus, the deep vessels of which can only be seen in the inflamed eye. The choroidal blood supply is not apparently modified in any way to take into account the requirements of the sclera; however, the sheer size and ready permeability of these vessels renders this unnecessary.

NERVE SUPPLY OF THE SCLERA

The nerve supply is surprisingly rich for a structure whose main function would appear to be supportive. As a result of this very rich nerve supply, inflammations of the sclera are extraordinarily painful due in part to direct stimulation of the nerve endings by the inflammatory process and in part to distension of the whole viscus and their subsequent stretching. The nerve supply of the posterior sclera is derived from the short ciliary nerves where they enter the sclera close to the optic nerve. More anteriorly it is derived from branches of the long ciliary nerves which accompany the long posterior ciliary arteries. At the equator the long ciliary nerves divide, some return posteriorly in the sclera itself to re-enter the choroid in the region of the lamina fusca. Of those which pass forward, most enter the ciliary body and some form the 'nerve loops of Axenfeld'. The latter is a nerve which has entered the ciliary body and then passes outwards through the whole thickness of the sclera and back into the ciliary body through the same canal. These nerves are found in 12 per cent of eyes and can form painful tumours when they come to lie in the episclera. The less obvious ones can often be detected on the slit lamp by their squashed mushroom appearance and the faint cuff of pigment which surrounds the nerve (see Figure 9.17). They are usually associated with blood vessels. Their function is unknown but they have caused anxiety on many occasions because they are pigmented and sometimes slightly painful. They should not, however, be removed.

The rest of the nerves pass upwards and outwards, penetrating the sclera about 3 mm from the limbus, and the branches end in the cornea, trabecular meshwork, Schlemm's canal, and episclera; they are very prominent in the tendinous insertion of the muscles. The nerves of the cornea are derived from the apices of the loops which connect one penetrating nerve to the next around the limbus.

NUTRITION OF THE SCLERA

Because in the normal eye the blood vessels only traverse the sclera and do not supply it directly, the stroma of the sclera derives its nutrition from a distance and not through intimate contact with the capillary bed. This implies that the sclera must be freely permeable to fluids and metabolites as indeed has been found by Bill (1965) who showed that the high molecular weight substances pass from the suprachoroidal space to the outside. Whether this flow forms part of the normal flow of fluid from the choroidal space is uncertain but very probably it materially assists the removal of subretinal fluid after re-apposition of the retina to pigment epithelium. In response to an inflammatory stimulus in the sclera, cells pass readily from blood vessels of the choroid and episclera to the site of the insult in as short a time as half an hour and yet the choroidal and intraocular tumours seem to have great difficulty in penetrating the scleral coat. They may spread out of the globe through the emissary foramen but usually have to cause a secondary inflammation before the cells can penetrate the scleral barrier (Blatt, Ursu and Popovici, 1958). Inflammatory cells are able to dissolve the intracellular cement substances but tumours are not. The tumours do not appear to be confined by an inflammatory reaction but the cells which are able to migrate may well be dealt with elsewhere provided only a few manage to get outside the globe. Intraocular abscesses are confined by the scleral coat in the same way that any abscess will be restricted by a fibrous envelope. Reactive inflammation of the episclera always accompanies intraocular or intrascleral abscesses so that organisms which pass through the sclera are dealt with in the episclera itself.

EMBRYOLOGY OF THE SCLERA

At about the 20-mm stage of development a subepithelial vascular layer develops in what is to be the outer layer of the optic vesicle in undifferentiated paraxial mesoderm. This vascular layer forms the uveal tract and outside this the mesoderm arranges itself concentrically around the optic vesicle. It has been suggested that the uvea and in particular the pigment epithelium is responsible for the induction of the sclera (Gruenwald, 1944). Certainly if the outer layer of the optic vesicle is destroyed, the sclera does not develop (Giroud, 1957). The choriocapillaris develops at the same time as the pigment epithelium to which it is intimately related, but the relation between the sclera and chorio-capillaris is still far from clear (Mann, 1957). Scleral development starts at the limbus and is contiguous with the cornea, passing backwards to the insertion of the developing muscles by the sixth week and to the equator by the eighth week. The limbus at this stage overlies the ciliary body and moves forwards later. The sclera continues to increase in thickness until five years of age, possibly by progressive laying down of collagen fibrils on its inner aspect. In fact the more mature collagen fibrils are found in the outer part of the sclera and the younger smaller collagen fibrils on its inner aspect. Formation of the posterior sclera is much delayed, possibly because there is no vascular network in this region at this stage. Whatever the cause, the sclera is not obvious at the posterior pole until about the end of the fifth month (von Ammon, 1858; Duke Elder and Cook, 1963). Arrest of fetal development at this stage or the failure to lay down new collagen on the inner aspect of the posterior sclera might well account for some of the changes found in congenital myopia (Mann, 1957; Blach, 1963).

ARTHROLOGY

Because joint disease is so common and most connective tissue diseases also affect the joint, this is the prime site for the study of connective tissue in health and disease. The kinship between diseases of the sclera and joints is possibly because necrosis occurs in relatively avascular tissue which lies close to a very vascular one. Adjacent to the virtually avascular sclera is the episclera and choroid, while avascular cartilage is adjacent to the synovial membrane.

Synovial joints have a capsule to which or through which the tendons of the muscles are inserted. The capsule is continuous with the periosteum covering the bone. The non-articular surfaces within the joint are covered by synovial tissue. Articular cartilage lies on subchondral bone (Figure 2.13).

Joint Capsule

In most joints the capsule is composed of bundles of collagenous fibres which are arranged somewhat irregularly, in contrast to their more regular arrangement in tendons and many ligaments. These bundles tend to spiral which makes them sensitive to tension in most positions that the joint adopts. Thus the slightest movement alters the tension in the bundles and this change stimulates proprioceptive nerve endings in the capsule and ligaments. Most ligaments therefore have both mechanical and proprioceptive functions.

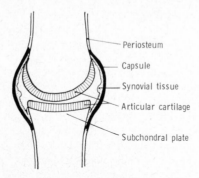

Figure 2.13. Diagram of a diarthrodial joint.

Synovial Tissue

The synovial membrane is a specialised connective tissue lining the capsule of diarthrodial joints, bursae and tendon sheaths. Its main function is to produce synovial fluid which has useful biomechanical properties and in addition provides nutrition for articular cartilage.

The embryonic synovium forms from a mesenchymal tissue interzone between chondrogenic zones which themselves are destined to form the cartilage matrix. In this interzone, clefts appear at eight weeks' gestation which enlarge to form the joint cavity and are lined by synovial cells except at the ends of the cartilaginous precursors of bone. Mesenchymal cells also form the joint capsule and ligaments, and epithelial tissue is not involved. The synovial lining cells have no basement membrane and the joint cavity is therefore separated from blood in the synovial capillaries only by endothelial cells and basement membranes of these capillaries (Barland, Novikoff and Hamerman, 1962), a similar situation to that which pertains in the eye between choroid and sclera and choroid and retina.

Studies carried out in the developing chick synovial membrane (Henrikson and Cohen, 1965) show that the synovial membrane is not a continuous structure. The cells appear to be embedded in the rich collagenous matrix. There are differences between joint tissue and other tissues, the main differences being the lack of epithelial tissue in every part of the joint, the marked vascularity of the synovium and the complete avascularity of articular cartilage. This may explain why, although rheumatoid arthritis is a disease with systemic manifestations, the major site of injury is the joint itself.

The normal synovium, glistening, slightly pebbly and with multiple redundant folds in its gross appearance, has only three to four cell layers lining its surface (Castor, 1960). It is customary to divide the synovial lining cells into those that are macrophage-like and have primarily a phagocytic function (Type A) and those that are secretory and similar to fibroblasts, with a large amount of endoplasmic reticulum (Type B). However, there are many cells which do not fit either of these types (Roy, Ghadially and Crane, 1966) and the classification of specific synovial cells is arbitrary. It has been suggested by Fell (1975, personal communication) that intimal synoviocytes belong to a single cell type which assumes the A or B form according to local environmental conditions and that these cells belong to the mononuclear phagocyte system. Whatever their origin they have counterparts in very similar cells found in the ciliary body, choroid, vitreous and sclera.

The synovium is a specialised connective tissue and the intercellular substance or matrix has an amorphous and a fibrous component. The matrix is composed primarily of glycosaminoglycans, proteoglycans and collagen. With inflammation, both quantitative and qualitative differences occur in the biosynthesis of these components. Increased numbers of collagen fibrils are formed in the intercellular spaces between the intimal lining cells, suggesting synthesis (Wyllie, Haust and More, 1966). It is probable that synovial tissue formation requires the integrated activity of intimal lining cells, stromal cells and vascular tissue (Castor, 1971a).

Neither the structure of the synovium nor the composition of the synovial fluid suggests that there is a major barrier to fluid movement between the synovial capillaries and the synovial cavity. Also fenestrated capillaries have been described in the superficial part of synovium (Schumacher, 1969) and this type of capillary is usually found in tissues where fluid and plasma protein flux between blood and tissues is relatively high, as in the choroid.

Synovial fluid

Normal synovial fluid is essentially a dialysate of blood plasma with the addition of hyaluronic acid which is secreted by synovial lining cells and imparts to the fluid its stickiness and high viscosity. Both the concentration of hyaluronic acid, normally about 3.5 g/l of fluid and its molecular weight are reduced in conditions of inflammatory synovitis, particularly rheumatoid arthritis, with a resulting decrease in fluid viscosity. The concentration of protein is approximately one-third that of serum, with about 70 per cent of albumen, which rises in inflammatory synovitis. Studies indicate that the permeability of the human synovial membrane to plasma proteins is quantitatively related to the molecular size of the proteins and to the degree of inflammation in the synovium (Kushner and Somerville, 1971). It seems likely that molecular sieving is mediated in joints by synovial capillaries and the adjacent interstitial hyaluronate.

The functions of synovial fluid are lubrication (in association with articular cartilage) and nutrition of underlying cartilage cells. It is many times more efficient than the best mechanical lubricant. It is normally present in only small quantities, for example the knee contains less than 3 ml, but the amount is increased in many forms of joint disease.

Vascular tissue

Vascular and lymphatic channels are prominent and they frequently lie in close proximity to synovial lining cells. They are found in parallel layers with an innermost subintimal plexus of net-like vascular loops with many interconnections. Arteriovenular anastomoses, which may act as short-circuit vessels, have been described at the base of synovial villi, and inflammation may lead to shunting of blood away from the villous tips and to promotion of glycolytic metabolism. Monolayer cultures of rheumatoid synovial membrane show that the rate of glucose consumption and lactate formation per cell is greater in rheumatoid cells than in normal control cells (Castor, 1971b). Dick, Pond and Provan (1970) have used the clearance of ^{133}Xe as a measure of synovial perfusion and have suggested that α- and β-adrenergic receptors act to control synovial perfusion both in the normal and diseased state.

Neural components

Synovial membrane is relatively insensitive to pain but, in contrast, capsular and ligamentous structures are usually very sensitive to pain or pressure stimuli. Synovial membrane has an autonomic nerve supply alongside the vessels.

STRUCTURE OF CONNECTIVE TISSUE

Many of the pathological conditions which affect the sclera attack the collagen of which it is composed. This collagen is very similar to that which is found elsewhere in the body and about which a great deal is known, so that certain analogies can be drawn between what is known to be happening elsewhere and what can be seen with the slit-lamp microscope. Conversely, the changes seen on the slit lamp can be used to infer a pathological state of the same type elsewhere.

The conventional functional view which gave rise to the term 'supporting' or 'connective' tissue attracted little interest from pathologists and clinicians. An understanding of its complex and indeed dynamic nature has only come about through the recognition that changes in this tissue are associated with a group of significant diseases (Klemperer, Pollack and Baehr, 1941).

Connective tissue supports and connects the organs of the body, largely by its extracellular fibrous and amorphous components which are produced and maintained by the connective tissue cells. A number of ancillary functions are performed by connective tissue, such as secretion and storage of materials, phagocytosis and antibody formation, and therefore a number of different cell types are found. Prominent among these are the fibroblasts, macrophages, mast cells and plasma cells.

Connective tissue is composed of actively metabolising substances very far removed from Virchow's 1858 definition of collagen as the body's 'excelsior' or inert stuffing. The fundamental structure consists of a network of fibres in a water—gel containing polyanions (protein polysaccharides or proteoglycans).

Where a high tensile strength is required, the number of fibres is increased
and their direction is related to prevailing forces. Resilience is primarily due
to the water content; the large extended proteoglycan molecules which are
entangled with the fibrous network hinder the flow of water outwards (J. H.
Fessler, quoted by Muir, 1973). This impedance to flow is greater the higher
the concentration of proteoglycan.

Fibrous Component

The fibres of connective tissue consist of collagen, reticulin and elastin; these
can be distinguished by histochemical stains and electron microscopy as they
have distinctive physical and chemical properties. The proportions of the various
constituents vary with the different types of connective tissue so that, whilst
in the synovium elastin fibres are rare and usually lie near the surface, in
the sclera they are more obvious near the end of each collagen fibre, are
more frequently found anteriorly than posteriorly and most are found near
the equator. Reticulin fibrils surround capillaries and fat cells.

Collagen is the most abundant protein in the body and makes up 90 per
cent or more of the protein in cartilage, tendons, ligaments, bone and eye,
and 25 per cent of the total body protein. Collagen fibres are responsible
for the functional integrity of tissues and contribute a framework within which
the tissue functions, in which they are closely associated with glycosaminoglycans, the polysaccharides which form the ground substance. The relative
proportion of collagen to ground substance and the exact nature of this composition impart characteristic features to tissues. We are beginning to understand
the significance of particular chemical groupings on the collagen molecule
and the mode by which they may impart tissue specificity; thus collagen
is in its highly polymerised stable form in sclera but in its most soluble
form in vitreous. The collagen of cornea and sclera differ in composition,
particularly mucopolysaccharide content, which in part gives them their different
properties both in health and disease. Tendons differ yet again in being tough
and inelastic.

In its stable form collagen has a high tensile strength but is easily denatured
by heat, acid or alkali. Warming converts the collagen to gelatin. Collagen
is synthesised by fibroblasts (Layman, McGoodwin and Martin, 1971), osteo-
blasts, chondroblasts and other similar cells (Figure 2.14) as single molecules
formed of three polypeptide chains each containing slightly more than 1000
amino acids. These polypeptides (or α-chains) are coiled in a helical configuration about each other to form the triple helical collagen molecule 3000 Å
long and 15 Å in diameter (Figure 2.15). The structure is stabilised by intra-
molecular hydrogen bonds. The major features of the triple helical structure
of the collagen molecule are the occurrence of glycine in every third position
of the amino acid sequence and the high content of the amino acids proline
and hydroxyproline (Traub and Piez, 1971). The chief function of hydroxyproline is stabilisation of the triple helix (Rosenbloom, Harsch and Jiminez,
1973). Hydroxylysine is also prominent and this functions both as a site of
carbohydrate attachment and as a component of cross-links that develop among
collagen molecules (as well as between the polypeptides of each collagen

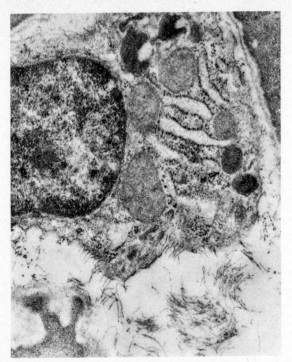

Figure 2.14. Vitreous collagen fibrils being formed at the pars plana of a nine-month-old child. The cells producing the fibrils are very similar to those seen in the synovium of joints. Electron micrograph, × 80 000, uranyl acetate.
Courtesy of Dr Gartner, Basel.

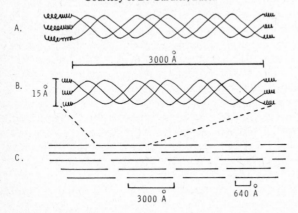

Figure 2.15. Structure of collagen. The organisation of collagen into fibrils. (A) represents pro-collagen with an amino-terminal 'registration peptide' which may facilitate formation of the triple helix within the cell after each α-chain is synthesised. (B) represents the collagen monomer after the 'registration peptide' has been cleared away by procollagen peptidase. There are non-helical portions (represented by three wiggly lines at ends of helical portion) at both amino- and carboxy-terminal ends of the molecule; collagen aggregates readily to form fibrils. (C) The quarter stagger overlay pattern results in the appearance of 640 Å periodicity when fibrils are stained and viewed under the electron microscope (Figure 2.7).

molecule). These cross-links provide stability to collagen and may provide resistance against specific enzymes capable of degrading collagen fibres (Ramachandran, 1967; Traub and Piez, 1971).

The fibres consist of tropocollagen molecules arranged in chains, lying head to tail, their side-to-side alignment being staggered by one-quarter of the molecular length; this arrangement accounts for the characteristic electron-microscope appearance of collagen fibres—cross-banding with a periodicity of 64 nm (640 Å (Perez-Tamayo and Rojkind, 1973).

It has long been considered that fibre formation takes place outside the cell, whilst tropocollagen units are synthesised intracellularly. The biosynthesis of collagen involves a series of sequential steps (Grant and Prockop, 1972):

1. Synthesis of polypeptides on polyribosome aggregates of the endoplasmic reticulum (protocollagen).
2. Post-ribosomal hydroxylation of proline and lysine residues, governed by protocollagen proline hydroxylase and protocollagen lysine hydroxylase, both enzymes requiring oxygen, ferrous iron, and α-ketoglutarate and ascorbic acid as cofactors.
3. Addition of carbohydrate to hydroxylysine.
4. Formation of triple helix, creating a precursor or transport form of collagen (procollagen).
5. Secretion of procollagen.
6. Removal of peptide extensions on NH_2-terminal ends of procollagen by specific peptidases, permitting fibre formation.
7. Collagen fibre formation.
8. Cross-linking of fibres.

Procollagen is larger than the final collagen molecule, is more soluble, and does not have the ability to form fibres. The extra portion at the N-terminal end governs the correct alignment of the three polypeptide chains during helix formation, by means of disulphide linkages between the non-collagenous extra portions. Procollagen passes via the cisternae of the rough-surfaced endoplasmic reticulum to reach the exterior of the cell. Here the molecule is converted to tropocollagen by proteolytic removal of the 'non-collagenous' parts of the polypeptides (Muir, 1973). Spontaneous aggregation into fibrils results from the interaction of charged side-groups on adjacent molecules.

The component polypeptide chains are characteristic for a tissue source, and it is felt that the amino acid composition of the α-chains may be important in determining the physical properties of α-collagen. In the last seven years several genetically different types of collagen have been identified (Miller and Matukas, 1969; Trelstad et al, 1970; Strawich and Nimni, 1971; Chung and Miller, 1974):

Type I   with the chain composition $[(\alpha^1)I]_2\ \alpha^2$ is found in cornea, skin, bone and tendon.

Type II $[(\alpha^1)II]_3$ has been identified in hyaline cartilage.

Type III $[(\alpha^1)III]_3$ is found in several connective tissue diseases, sclera, fetal skin and vascular tissue.

Type IV $[(\alpha^1)IV]_3$ is the name given to basement membrane collagen, including that found in the lens.

Intercellular collagen is actively synthesised by synovial tissue cells (Castor and Muirden, 1964) and both normal and rheumatoid synovial tissue synthesises

Type I and Type III collagen. The collagens of normal and rheumatoid synovia do appear to differ in their susceptibility to dissolution by pepsin treatment, a finding which may be related to an altered level of covalent cross-linking and rate of metabolism in diseased tissue. The distribution of the different types of collagen in the avian eye has been investigated by Trelstad and Kang (1974) who have found several different, and possibly some new types of collagen: cornea and the fibrous portion of the sclera contain Type I, but the latter also appears to have a different type of α^2-chain; the cartilaginous sclera contains Type II collagen while the lens and vitreous body appear to contain an α^1-chain different from any described so far. The final organisation of the collagen in the cornea is particularly interesting, since only in this tissue is Type I collagen transparent. This property depends on the regular layers of parallel sheets of collagen fibres, each layer turned through an angle of 90° from the one below. Thus there are at least five different α-chains, each coded for by a different structural gene, so that heritable defects could occur affecting only one of the collagen types.

Collagen fibrils consist of long branch fibres with banding of average macroperiodicity of 640 Å (range 350 to 750 Å) and microperiodicity of 110 Å (Sakai, 1962). The individual collagen fibrils vary in diameter from 30 to 300 nm even within the same bundle, but the fibrils are relatively parallel to each other. In the early stages of embryonic development the collagen fibrils of both cornea and sclera are equal in diameter and both structures are equally translucent. During the early years of life the diameters of the scleral fibres change in size, contributing to the opaqueness of the sclera, although this is partly a function of the high water content of the sclera (68 per cent). It seems probable that the nature of the proteoglycan in any one tissue may affect the polymerisation and ultimate size of the collagen fibres (Barrett, 1975).

Certainly the fine structure of the collagen fibres of cornea and sclera is not identical, the sclera more closely resembling the structure of tendon. The fibrils of the substantia propria of the cornea are smaller and remain like embryonic connective tissue, whereas those of the sclera take on a more adult form. In addition, apart from the regular arrangement of the bundles, the corneal fibrils are embedded in a thick cement substance, not present around scleral fibrils, which is of similar refractive index to the collagen fibril (Winkelman, 1951; Schwarz, 1953a). The transition from the corneal pattern of collagen fibril and mucopolysaccharide coat to the scleral pattern occurs gradually through the limbal area, which accounts for the gradually decreasing transparency as the sclera is approached (Sakai, 1962).

The structure of the sclera gives protection through the dense aggregation of the fibres of which it is composed. Its shape is preserved by the pattern the collagen fibres take up, the presence of elastic tissue and by the damping effect of the ground substance. The sclera is visco-elastic and when the intra-ocular pressure is raised artificially by injecting fluid into the eye, the pressure will rise rapidly and then gradually fall to its original level. This is caused by an initial lengthening of the fibres followed by slow sliding of the fibres one upon another (Gloster, Perkins and Pommier, 1957; St. Helen and McEwan, 1961); the amount of stretch is not directly proportional to the change in pressure, the stretch of the fibres giving rise to 'increasing rigidity'. The immediate intraocular 'rigidity' is due to the pressure–volume change and is important in Shiotz tonometry. The additional time-dependent ocular 'rigidity' which relates pressure to time is of importance in tonography (Friedenwald, 1937).

Changes in the banding of the collagen and the arrangement of the muco-polysaccharide coat occur with increasing age and rigidity of the scleral fibres. These changes are only complete when the eye reaches its full size so that if the pressure rises before this age, permanent stretching of the fibrils may occur.

Reticulin resembles collagen in amino acid composition, but is made up of fine branching filaments. Reticulin fibres are usually rich in carbohydrate (Perez-Tamayo and Rojkind, 1973) and these profuse polysaccharide side-chains reduce the ability of collagen to aggregate (Muir, 1973) and prevent cross-linking.

Elastic fibres appear to consist of a meshwork of polypeptide chains inter-twined in a substance rich in mucopolysaccharides. The electron microscope has revealed little about the structure of these fibres.

Amorphous Components

Proteoglycans

Proteoglycans are the chief components of the ground substance surrounding collagen fibrils in all connective tissue and form the 'filler' within the fibrous matrix. This material is the product of fibroblasts consisting of:
1. Proteins which are soluble precursors of collagen.
2. Non-collagenous protein, occurring in a protein–polysaccharide complex.

The proteoglycans are of high molecular weight and derive their negative charge from the presence of long-chain acidic polysaccharides, known as glycos-aminoglycans, bound to protein. Both the type of glycosaminoglycan and probably also the nature of protein can vary, leading to a group of proteo-glycans (Muir, 1973). A glycosaminoglycan consists of a number of similar disaccharide repeating units linked end to end. Each disaccharide 'building-block' comprises an N-acetylated amino sugar which may or may not be sulphated, and either a uronic acid, or a simple hexose. Each glycosaminoglycan exhibits a characteristic unit (Figure 2.16), thus hyaluronic acid consists of glucuronic acid and N-acetyl glucosamine, chondroitin sulphate consists of glucuronic acid and N-acetyl galactosamine, and keratan sulphate consists largely of galactose and N-acetyl glucosamine.

In the proteoglycan molecule, glycosaminoglycans form side-chains attached covalently to a central protein core (Figure 2.17). During synthesis the carbo-hydrate and protein moieties are formed in parallel. Assembly of the protein core occurs in the rough-surfaced endoplasmic reticulum together with initiation of the glycosaminoglycan side-chains. More than one type of glycosamino-glycan can be found within the same proteoglycan molecule, the degree of maturation and age of tissue being important factors in determining the size of the molecule and the amount and type of glycosaminoglycan present (Muir, 1973).

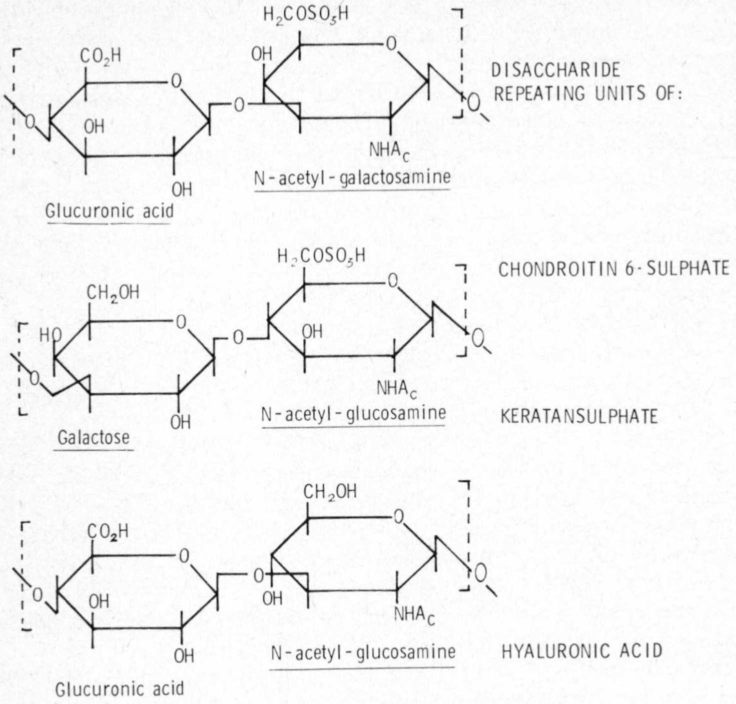

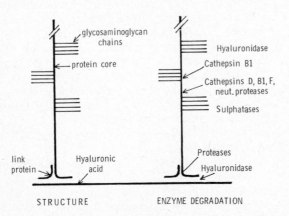

Figure 2.16 Chemical structure of glycosaminoglycans.

Figure 2.17. The glycosaminoglycans are attached to a central protein core which may be broken down by enzyme activity at different points on the core.

Proteoglycans in solution are kept extended by the mutual repulsion of their multiple negative charges. This property has three important physiological actions (Maroudas, 1973):

1. The extended form impedes their motion within a fixed fibrous meshwork: under a compressive load water will flow outwards more slowly the greater the concentration of proteoglycan.
2. The proteoglycan molecule occupies a domain of solvent which is inaccessible to other molecules. In addition, the charge on the proteoglycan molecule exerts a Donnan effect on the distribution of mobile ions. Hence the type and amount of proteoglycan influence the nature of other solutes in the gel.
3. The proteoglycans make a major contribution to the 'swelling pressure' of the tissue. Hence the fibrous meshwork in which the proteoglycan molecules are entangled is kept expanded by them.

The sclera has very little ground substance when compared with other ocular tissues such as the vitreous which is virtually all ground substance and no collagen, and the cornea which contains four times as much as the sclera. Scleral mucopolysaccharides also differ from the corneal ones in that they contain no keratan sulphate. Half the mucopolysaccharide is dermatan sulphate, the other half being made up of chondroitin sulphate similar to that found in cartilage, tendon and aorta. Histochemical staining techniques are revealing further differences between corneal and scleral proteoglycans, the significance of which are not yet clear; for instance, the carboxyl groups of proteoglycans can be stained in sclera but not in cornea (Čejková, 1974) and inactive enzymes can be detected on the surface of the collagen fibril in cornea but not in sclera.

Unlike collagen fibrils which have a slow turnover in tissue once they are formed and cross-linked, proteoglycans have a much more rapid turnover. Proteoglycan synthesis appears to be under some type of 'feedback control' from the extracellular matrix; depletion of proteoglycans, for example, by limited digestion with trypsin stimulates proteoglycan synthesis by the cells. The turnover is much more rapid in sclera than cornea, as judged by the uptake and elimination of ^{35}S (Dohlman and Boström, 1955). Proteoglycans can be destroyed either by agents that break down the protein core or those that degrade the polysaccharide subunits (Figure 2.14). It is believed that cathepsin D, a lysosomal protease active maximally below pH 5, is the enzyme primarily responsible for proteoglycans degradation (Dingle, Barrett and Weston, 1971). Neutral proteases may be released by inflammatory tissue and play a role in early proteoglycan destruction in the extracellular space. The enzymes now known to be capable of degradation are shown in Table 2.1 and are discussed in detail in Chapter 6.

The mucopolysaccharide coating of the scleral collagen fibres in the adult is sparse when compared with that in the cornea, though the coating is different in the fetus to the newborn child. Schwarz (1953) felt that this might in part account for the loss of transparency of the sclera. If the sclera is dehydrated, as can occur in retinal detachment procedures when the sclera is exposed for a prolonged period, then the sclera becomes more transparent, which Maurice (1969) considers to be due to concentration of the mucoprotein near to that reached by cornea. Scleral fibres possess a much higher degree of double refractivity than those of the cornea. When the water content of the sclera rises above 90 per cent or falls below 40 per cent, the sclera becomes more transparent and the double refractivity diminishes (Pau, 1955).

The increase in transparency which follows inflammation is due to the rearrangement of the fibres of the sclera and partly to a physiochemical change which alters the double refractive properties of the sclera; it is only rarely due to true thinning of the scleral coat.

Hyaluronic acid

This is an extracellular glycosaminoglycan secreted by synovial cells and similar cells in the ciliary body and possibly in the retina. It is very viscous because of its high molecular weight and the concentration in normal synovial fluid is 3.5 to 4 mg /ml and in the vitreous 32 to 55 mg /ml.

Hyaluronate binds to cartilage and acts as a boundary lubricant between opposing cartilage surfaces and in the vitreous is largely responsible for the maintenance of viscosity and structural stability.

Collagen—proteoglycan interaction

Collagen interacts with glycosaminoglycans and proteoglycans during fibre formation, influencing eventual fibre numbers and thickness and possibly stabilising the mature fibre. Obrink (1973) has shown that whilst chondroitin sulphate, dermatan sulphate and their proteoglycans accelerate fibre formation, keratan sulphate may have a slight decelerating effect.

Cellular Components

The cells of connective tissue are the fibroblast, macrophage, mast cell and plasma cell. Of these the basic cell and the most important in the less differentiated form of connective tissue (dermis, fascia) is the fibroblast. This is stellate or spindle-shaped with a large nucleus and relatively scanty cytoplasm which contains elongated mitochondria and an endoplasmic reticulum with attached ribosomes. The cells vary in size according to function so that, during secretory activity, the cytoplasm becomes filled with a Golgi zone, vacuoles, vesicles and lysosomes. The fibroblast is responsible for the synthesis of hyaluronic acid and other glycosaminoglycans of the ground substance, as well as the fibrillar proteins of fibro-elastic connective tissue, as tropocollagen is formed in the endoplasmic reticulum. The fibres following secretion lie on the cell surface whilst full maturation occurs. Gusek (1962) considers that fibroblasts may give rise to histiocytes, blast cells or eosinophils. They also give rise to the keratocytes, sclerocytes and hyalocytes which replenish the collagen structures of the eye. It is assumed that their chameleon-like transforming ability must vary inversely with cell maturation.

Histiocytes, blast cells, lymphocytes and plasma cells migrate through connective tissue, the histiocytes acting as macrophages and removing degraded tissue or foreign bodies. These cells contain multiple vesicles, vacuoles and lysosomes.

Mast cells are characterised by their coarse metachromic granulation and resemble eosinophils. They are widely dispersed in the connective tissue. In the eye they are present in large quantities at the limbus, around the vessels of the sclera and choroid, but are sparse in the iris, ciliary body and retina (Smith, 1965). They are frequently seen in synovial membranes and contain heparin, histamine and 5-hydroxytryptamine. Their biological function has not yet been fully defined, but they are active in acute inflammatory states and are often seen at sites of episcleral and scleral inflammation and during the healing of scleral wounds.

Collagen Catabolism

It is very likely that without specific collagenases, collagen cannot be degraded enzymatically. These enzymes have been found in numerous tissues, including rheumatoid synovium and granules of polymorphonuclear leucocytes. They have one main function: to cleave the collagen molecule at one locus through all three polypeptide chains. Once this happens, at physiological pH and temperature, that particular cleaved collagen molecule falls apart and becomes susceptible to multiple tissue proteases. This will be discussed in Chapter 6. Table 2.1 lists the proteinases involved in connective tissue degeneration.

Table 2.1.   *Proteinases which could be involved in connective tissue degradation*

| Enzyme | Active against | | | pH range | Intracellular localisation |
	Collagen	Proteo-glycan	Other proteins		
Cathepsin B1	+	+	+	5.0–6.0	Lysosomes
Cathepsin D	−	+	+	3.5–5.0	Lysosomes
Cathepsin E	−	+	+	3.0–4.0	Lysosomes?
Cathepsin F	n.d.	+	n.d.	4.5–5.0	Not in lysosomes
Collagenase	+	−	−	6.5–8.0	Not stored? (granules in PMN)
Neutral proteinase	−	+	+	7.0–8.0	?
Elastase	+	+	+	7.0–9.0	Granules in PMN

n.d. = not determined.
PMN = polymorphonuclear leucocytes.

Collagenase can be demonstrated on the surface of the corneal collagen fibrils but cannot be demonstrated in sclera or in any other connective tissue. This implies that corneal collagenase can be more easily activated or is activated by different triggers from scleral collagenase, and may in part account for the differences seen in pathological reaction between cornea and sclera.

Regulation of Connective Tissue Metabolism

Included among the factors involved in the normal regulation of connective tissue synthesis in general and collagen in particular are several hormones (growth hormone, thyroxine, androgens, oestrogens and adrenal corticosteroids). When present in excess the corticosteroids suppress formation of granulation tissue and interfere with the production of both hyaluronic acid and collagen.

The role of ascorbic acid as a cofactor in the enzymatic hydroxylation of proline and lysine is believed to explain the faulty connective tissue synthesis that occurs in scurvy. In addition various trace metals appear to be important in the normal metabolism of connective tissue. Copper deficiency in chicks leads to a defect in the production of elastin, and that which is formed is abnormal in its physical properties. It has been suggested that this abnormality is based on a defect in cross-linking and that copper may be a cofactor in enzymes involved in this action.

The defect in cross-linking of collagen found in experimental lathyrism has been traced to the action of β-aminopropionitrile (the active principle in the sweet pea, *Lathyrus odoratus*) which blocks the enzyme involved in the formation of the cross-linkages of collagen and elastin.

The maintenance of the structure and function of connective tissue requires the continual synthesis and destruction of both cellular and extracellular macromolecules. The turnover rate of the various molecules can vary widely, from hours to perhaps hundreds of days; nevertheless, this catabolic activity of cells in organised tissues is as characteristic of life as cell division. It follows that a pathological situation could result from a change in the rate of synthesis or degradation of one or more of the macromolecules. Inflammatory conditions of the eye and joints increase synthesis but the concentration of macromolecules is reduced, leading in the case of hyaluronate to decreased viscosity of synovial fluid and vitreous. The rates of both synthesis and destruction are greatly accelerated under conditions of remodelling, which occur for example in growth or wound healing. The two most important matrix components are collagen and proteoglycan. Both these macromolecules are so large that the formal steps of assembly of the molecules have to take place outside the cell. There is, therefore, a further stage at which control of synthesis could be interfered with in addition to the normal steps of protein–polysaccharide synthesis within the cell.

REFERENCES

Barland, P., Novikoff, A. B. & Hamerman, D. (1962) Electron microscopy of the human synovial membrane. *Journal of Cell Biology*, **14**, 207–220.

Barrett, A. J. (1975) In *Dynamics of Connective Tissue Macromolecules* (Ed.) Burleigh, P. M. & Poole, A. R. Ch. 10. Amsterdam: North Holland.

Bill, A. (1965) Movement of albumin and dextran through the sclera. *Archives of Ophthalmology*, **74**, 248–252.

Blach, R. K. (1963) *The Nature of Degenerative Myopia*. MD thesis, University of Cambridge.

Blatt, N., Ursu, A. & Popovici, V. (1958) Invasion potential of malignant intra-ocular tumours. Resistance power of the sclera. *Klinische Monatsblätter für Augenheilkunde*, **132**, 818–828.

Castor, C. W. (1960) The microscope structures of the normal human synovial tissue. *Arthritis and Rheumatism*, **3**, 140–151.

Castor, C. W. (1971a) Abnormalities of connective tissue cells cultured from patients with rheumatoid arthritis, II. Defective regulation of hyaluronate and collagen formation. *Journal of Laboratory and Clinical Medicine*, **77**, 65–75.

Castor, C. W. (1971b) Connective tissue activation, II. Abnormalities of cultured rheumatoid synovial cells. *Arthritis and Rheumatism*, **14**, 55–66.

Castor, C. W. & Muirden, K. D. (1964) Collagen formation in monolayer cultures of human fibroblasts. The effects of hydrocortisone. *Laboratory Investigation*, **13**, 560–574.

Čejková, J. (1974) Histochemical identification of acid mucopolysaccharide in the sclera. *Československá Oftalmologie*, **30**, 246–249.

Chung, E. & Miller, E. J. (1974) Collagen polymorphism: characterisation of molecules with the chain component [α^1 III]$_3$ in human tissues. *Science*, **183**, 1200–1201.

Dick, W. C., Pond, M. J. & Provan, C. (1970) Adrenergic control of canine synovial perfusion in experimentally induced osteoarthritis and synovitis. *Research in Veterinary Science*, **11**, 587–590.

Dingle, J. T., Barrett, A. J. & Weston, P. D. (1971) Characteristics of immuno-inhibition and the confirmation of a role in cartilage breakdown. *Biochemical Journal*, **123**, 1–13.

Dohlman, C. H. & Boström, H. (1955) Uptake of sulphate by mucopolysaccharide in the rat cornea and sclera. *Acta Ophthalmologica*, **33**, 455–461.

Duke Elder, S. (1958) *System of Ophthalmology*, Vol. 1, p. 450. London: Kimpton.

Duke Elder, S. & Cook, C. (1963) *System of Ophthalmology*, Vol. 3, p. 162. London: Kimpton.

Fessler, J. H. (1960) A structural function of mucopolysaccharide in connective tissue. *Biochemical Journal*, **76**, 124–132.

Friedenwald, J. S. (1937) Contribution to theory and practice of tonometry. *American Journal of Ophthalmology*, **20**, 985–1024.

Giroud, M. (1957) Phénomènes d'induction et leurs perturbations chez les mammifères. *Acta Anatomica*, **30**, 297–306.

Gloster, J., Perkins, E. S. & Pommier, E-L. (1957) Extensibility of strips of sclera and cornea. *British Journal of Ophthalmology*, **41**, 103–110.

Grant, M. E. & Prockop, D. J. (1972) The biosynthesis of collagen. *New England Journal of Medicine*, **286**, 194–199, 242–249, 291–300.

Gruenwald, P. (1944) Studies on developmental pathology, II. Sporadic unilateral microphthalmia and associated malformations in chick embryos. *American Journal of Anatomy*, **74**, 217–257.

Gusek, W. (1962) Submikroskopische Untersuchungen zur Feinstruktur aktiver Binderwebszellen. In *Veroflentlichungen aus der morphologischen Pathologie*. Stuttgart: Fischer.

Henrikson, R. C. & Cohen, A. S. (1965) Light and electron microscope observations on the developing chick interphalangeal joint. *Journal of Ultrastructure Research*, **13**, 129–162.

Hogan, M. J., Alvarado, J. A. & Weddell, J. E. (1971) *Histology of the Human Eye, An Atlas Textbook*, p. 309. Philadelphia: Saunders.

Klemperer, P., Pollack, A. D. & Baehr, G. (1941) Pathology of disseminated lupus erythematosus. *Archives of Pathology*, **32**, 569–631.

Kokott, W. (1934) Das Spaltlinienbild der Sklera. *Klinische Monatsblätter für Augenheilkunde*, **92**, 177–185.

Kushner, I. & Somerville, J. A. (1971) Permeability of human synovial membrane to plasma proteins. Relationship to molecular size and inflammation. *Arthritis and Rheumatism*, **14**, 560–570.

Layman, D. L., McGoodwin, E. B. & Martin, G. R. (1971) The nature of collagen synthesised by cultured human fibroblasts. *Proceedings of the National Academy of Sciences of the U.S.A.*, **68**, 454–458.

Mann, I. (1957) *Developmental Abnormalities of the Human Eye*, 2nd edition, p. 370. London: BMA.

Mann, I. (1964) *The Development of the Human Eye*, 3rd edition, p. 255. London: BMA.

Maroudas, A. (1973) Physicochemical properties of articular cartilage. In *Adult Articular Cartilage* (Ed.) Freeman, M. A. pp. 131. London: Pitman Medical.

Maurice, D. (1969) In *Physiology of the Eye* (Ed.) Davson, H. 2nd edition, p. 489. Boston: Little, Brown.

Miller, E. J. & Matukas, V. J. (1969) Chick cartilage collagen: a new type of α^1 chain not present in bone or skin of the species. *Proceedings of the National Academy of Sciences of the U.S.A.*, **64**, 1264–1268.

Muir, I. H. (1973) Biochemistry. In *Adult Articular Cartilage* (Ed.) Freeman, M. A. p. 100. London: Pitman Medical.

Obrink, B. (1973) The influence of glycosaminoglycans on the formation of fibres from monomeric tropocollagen in vitro. *European Journal of Biochemistry*, **34**, 129–137.

Pau, H. (1955) Die Doppelbrechung von Sklera und Cornea. *Albrecht Graefe's Archiv für Ophthalmologie*, **156**, 415–426.

Perez-Tamaya, R. & Rojkind, M. (1973) *Molecular Pathology of Connective Tissue.* New York: Dekker.

Ramachandran, G. N. (1967) *Treatise on Collagen*, Vol. I. New York: Academic Press.

Rohan, J. (1961) The histological structure of the chamber angle in primates. *American Journal of Ophthalmology*, **52**, 529–539.

Rosenbloom, J., Harsch, M. & Jiminez, S. (1973) Hydroxyproline content determines the denaturation temperature of chick tendon collagen. *Archives of Biochemistry and Biophysics*, **158**, 478–484.

Roy, S., Ghadially, F. N. & Crane, W. A. (1966) Synovial membrane in traumatic effusion. Ultrastructure and autoradiography with tritiated leucine. *Annals of the Rheumatic Diseases*, **25**, 259–271.

Sakai, T. (1962) A comparative study on the collagen fibrils of the sclera by electron microscopy. *Acta Societatis Ophthalmologica Japonica*, **66**, 1145–1156.

Salzmann, M. (1912) *The Anatomy and Histology of the Human Eyeball*, translated Brown, E. V. Chicago: University of Chicago Press.

Schumacher, H. R. (1969) The microvasculature of the synovial membrane of the monkey: ultrastructural studies. *Arthritis and Rheumatism*, **12**, 387–404.

Schwarz, W. (1953a) Electron microscope studies of the structure of the human sclera and cornea. *Zeitschrift für Zellforschung und Mikroskopische Anatomie*, **38**, 26–49.

Schwarz, W. (1953b) Electron microscope studies of the differentiation of human corneal and scleral fibrils. *Zeitschrift für Zellforschung und Mikroskopische Anatomie*, **38**, 78–86.

Smith, R. S. (1965) Mast cells and the eye. *Eye, Ear, Nose and Throat Digest*, **27**, 83–87.

Spitznas, M. (1971) The fine structure of human scleral collagen. *American Journal of Ophthalmology*, **69**, 414–418.

Spitznas, M., Luciano, L. & Reale, E. (1970) Fine structure of rabbit scleral collagen. *American Journal of Ophthalmology*, **71**, 68.

St. Helen, R. & McEwan, W. K. (1961) Rheology of the human sclera. *American Journal of Ophthalmology*, **52**, 539–548.

Strawich, E. & Nimni, M. E. (1971) Properties of a collagen molecule containing three identical components extracted from bovine articular cartilage. *Biochemistry*, **10**, 3905–3911.

Traub, W. & Piez, K. A. (1971) The chemistry and structure of collagen. *Advances in Protein Chemistry*, **25**, 243–352.

Trelstad, R. L. & Kang, A. H. (1974) Collagen heterogeneity in the avian eye: lens, vitreous body, cornea and sclera. *Experimental Eye Research*, **18**, 395–406.

Trelstad, R. L., Kang, A. H., Igarashi, S. et al (1970) Isolation of two distinct collagens from chick cartilage. *Biochemistry*, **9**, 4993–4998.

Virchow, H. (1858) *Die cellular Pathologie in ihre Begründung auf physiologische und pathologische Gewebelehre.* Paris: Hirschwald.

von Ammon, A. (1958) Die Entwicklungsgesichte des Menschlichen Auges. *Albrecht Graefe's Archiv für Ophthalmologie*, **4**, 1–8.

Winkleman, J. E. (1951) The difference between corneal and scleral connective tissue. *Ophthalmologie*, **122**, 107–109.

Wolff, E. (1968) *Eugene Wolff's Anatomy of the Eye and Orbit*, 6th edition revised by Last, R. J., p. 265. London: Lewis.

Wyllie, J. C., Haust, M. D. & More, R. H. (1966) The fine structure of synovial lining cells in rheumatoid arthritis. *Laboratory Investigation*, **15**, 519–529.

CHAPTER THREE

Clinical Examination of the Eye in Scleral Disease and Clinical Examination of the Joints

---

CLINICAL EXAMINATION OF THE EYE

'Eyes have they, but they see not'. Psalms 115, 5.

It is surprising that we can spend years looking at and examining patients and yet we miss particular features until they are pointed out to us. So it is with examining the sclera, partly because the sclera looks uniformly white and featureless in the uninflamed eye and partly because scleral disease is uncommon. Clinicians often fail to recognise the features which indicate underlying pathological changes and yet they are simple enough to detect, provided the eye is examined in a logical sequence and with care. Fortunately for the physician and rheumatologist the important signs which enable one to distinguish the more serious forms of scleral disease can be detected with the naked eye.

It is also fortunate that conjunctival inflammation only rarely leads to changes in the episclera and is always accompanied by some form of discharge. Beware of the red eye without a discharge or which just waters, because it usually hides some more sinister condition. It is also fortunate that inflammation which starts in the episclera only very rarely extends to involve the deeper scleral tissue; however, the converse is not true because in scleral disease the episclera is almost always inflamed. Because the sclera is always swollen in scleral disease we can ignore the more obvious episcleral inflammation and look deeper. The purpose of the clinical examination is therefore to determine the depth of the inflammation in order to detect scleral swelling or necrosis. Episcleral swelling and the red eye it produces lead one to consider the diagnosis of scleral disease, but whether it constitutes a serious menace to the patient and his eyesight depends on whether the stroma of the sclera is involved in the inflammatory process. Scleral swelling can be determined by noting

40

the salient features in the history and by systematic gross and microscopic examination with the slit lamp. Occasionally it is difficult to be sure that the sclera is indeed swollen when the patient first attends the clinic, but as the physical signs in scleral disease change rapidly the diagnosis soon becomes certain, usually within a week of the onset of symptoms.

Knowing how excrutiatingly painful it is to have a foreign body in the eye, it might be reasonable to expect all eye diseases to be painful. In fact, very few are. Pain in the eye is caused either by exposure of the nerve endings, as with corneal abrasions, ulcers and foreign bodies or by stretching of the nerve endings which occurs when the eye is expanded, as in acute glaucoma and

Table 3.1.   *Examination of the eye*

History:	Speed of onset Site, type and severity of pain
Examination of sclera:	
	Gross examination in daylight
	Colour Areas of scleral inflammation Areas of scleral transparency Areas of sequestration
	Microscopic examination

	Red-free light
	Type, distribution and abnormalities of vascular networks
	Avascular areas
	Slit examination
	Examination for depth of inflammation
	   (1/1000 adrenaline may need to be instilled to clear
	   superficial inflammation)

General eye examination:	Visual acuity

	Examination of cornea for keratitis
	   „ „ anterior and posterior chambers for uveitis
	   „ „ ciliary body for ciliary effusion and swelling
	   „ „ retina and choroid for exudative detachment
	Proptosis
	Extraocular movements

Laboratory investigations	
Special investigations:	*Eye* Tests if posterior disease is suspected
	Joint Radiographs
	Biopsy Only if absolutely necessary

iritis. Perhaps the severest pain of all is that which accompanies severe scleritis where both of these factors operate. The pain, which often radiates to the temple and the jaw, is so severe that eyes have occasionally had to be removed for this reason alone. Naturally pain of this severity is accompanied by intolerance to light and watering of the eyes, but pain is the important and predominant symptom. By contrast, if the episclera alone is involved then the sensations described are of hotness, pricking, dryness, discomfort, a slight ache, but never of severe pain. Enquiry as to the type of discomfort experienced by the patient forms a most important part of the examination in scleral disease.

Because scleral disease rarely changes its character and the different clinical entities can be distinguished when the patient is first seen, it is important to follow a strict routine of examination (Table 3.1) so that no important features are missed or forgotten. Using this routine we have found that it has only been necessary to change our initial diagnosis in less than five per cent of our patients.

Gross Examination

Examination of the eye in daylight

Almost as much information can be obtained by close examination of the patient with the naked eye, magnifying glass or a loupe as can be obtained by the use of the slit-lamp microscope, provided this examination can be undertaken in daylight.

There is something in the colour tones of daylight which does not seem to be reproduceable in Tungsten or fluorescent light and which enables one to distinguish the salmon-pink colour of episcleritis from the much deeper purple hue of deep scleral disease. Even coating on windows which is currently so much used in hospitals is enough to destroy this very delicate differentiation. In addition it is possible to see areas of scleral thinning and areas of deep

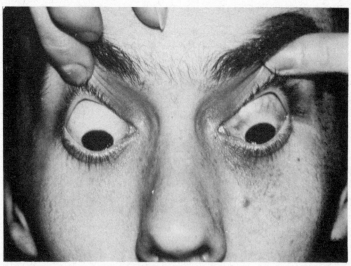

Figure 3.1.   A patient with diffuse scleral pigmentation. Subtle colour changes such as this are often only seen when the eye is examined in daylight.

inflammation and oedema which are impossible to observe by any other method (Figure 3.1). After recurrent attacks of inflammation, the sclera becomes more transparent, taking on a blue-grey colour. If this colour change is observed under an area of active inflammation, it indicates that tissue necrosis is taking place. This most important observation, which directly affects the treatment prescribed, is undetectable by any other method of examination.

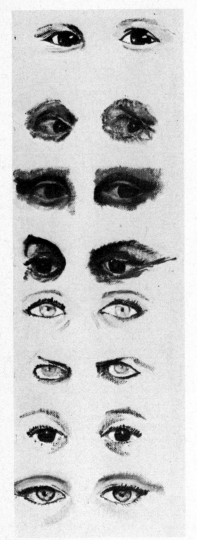

Figure 3.2. A painting of the eyes of people of different age groups to show that the expression comes not only from the configuration of the lids but from the reflectivity of the tear film and the colour and thickness of the episclera.

The thickness of the sclera varies in normal individuals, being thinner in women and under the origin of the muscle. The sclera and the episclera become thinner as age advances and the episclera becomes less vascular. As a result of this and of some reorientation of scleral fibres the sclera can become transparent in places in older people (Figure 3.2). The colour also alters to a more yellow hue because of the deposition of lipid between the fibres. The sclera becomes thinner than normal and more transparent if it is dehydrated. The increased transparency observed from these causes is different from that seen as a result of scleral disease where the area of scleral transparency has a much more defined edge with a dark centre and gradually lightening edges (Figure 3.3). If a sequestrum is about to form, a fine crack first appears in the sclera through which the dark brown choroid can just be seen. The area inside the crack then becomes white as the destruction of the tissue begins (Figure 3.3). These subtle colour changes are first detectable in daylight. As these sequestra can occur with very little, if any, surrounding inflammation and can largely be prevented if detected in time, it is most important to look for them in patients at risk, such as those with long-standing rheumatoid arthritis.

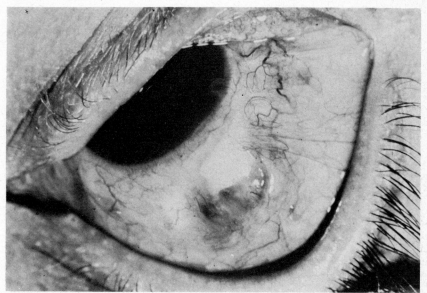

Figure 3.3. A patient with necrotising scleritis without inflammation (see also page 120). A sequestrum is forming in the sclera. When the condition has progressed to this stage the sequestrum will separate, but if detected early this can be prevented. Treatment prevented the pale area below the necrotic area from sequestrating.

Documentation of the gross findings

Because most of the physical signs can be detected on gross examination, it is important to document the findings at this stage. It is imperative that any progression of scleral disease be arrested before it can seriously damage the eye, and thus it is most important to have records showing those areas in which only the episclera is involved, those in which the sclera is involved, and those where scleral transparency or thinning is commencing. Scleral photography is probably the most satisfactory way of documenting the progress of the condition, but this is available to very few and is therefore unsatisfactory for routine clinical use.

We have adopted the system shown in Figures 3.4 and 3.5 and this has stood the test of time. Inspection of past notes which has at times shown progression of disease has enabled us to adopt rigorous methods of treatment in some patients as soon as they returned for treatment rather than adopting a wait-and-see policy. In others we have been able to say that the condition is recurring at the same site, is causing no damage and therefore does not need to be treated with potentially hazardous drugs.

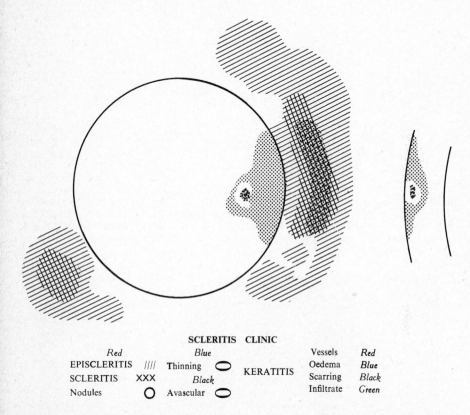

Figure 3.4. The method of documentation of scleral disease used in the scleritis clinic. The diagrams are normally drawn with coloured pencils. This patient with necrotising scleritis has two areas of active scleritis and an associated area of keratitis. The episcleritis is much more extensive in both areas than the scleritis and under the active area at 3.00 o'clock there is an area of scleral transparency (marked with dots in this diagram). The slit section shows that the superficial stroma is infiltrated but not ulcerated.

Microscopic Examination

Determination of the depth of the inflammation and the source of oedema

Oedema is a constant accompaniment of scleral and episcleral inflammation and can be extremely severe in episcleritis with an accompanying conjunctival chemosis and swelling of the lid, but more usually it is confined to one particular

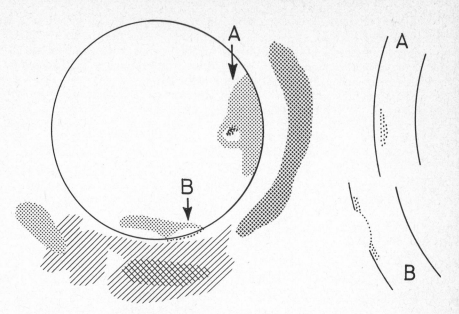

Figure 3.5. The same patient as Figure 3.4 three months later. The scleritis is now inactive at the original sites but has left areas of increased scleral transparency. A new area of activity (B) has appeared at 6.00 o'clock accompanied by keratitis on which an ulcer has formed. Diagrams of this type record progress of the disease and are much more valuable than descriptions.

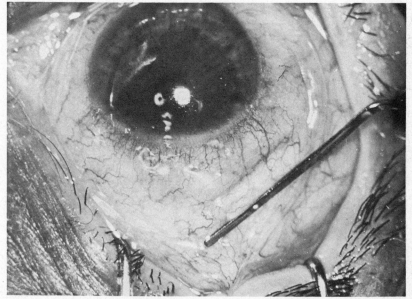

Figure 3.6. Pitting oedema of the conjunctiva and episclera in a patient with diffuse anterior scleritis. The indentation of the superficial tissues left by the iris repositor can easily be seen.

area of the episclera (Figure 3.6). Oedema of the sclera is less easy to detect and usually has to be implied by the displacement of the deep episcleral plexus of vessels. It should not be forgotten that inflammation of the posterior sclera may present with oedema of the conjunctiva and episclera anteriorly. Fortunately, the anterior sclera is almost always inflamed as well, but as this may be at the level of the equator or at the tendon sheath insertions alone, it must be carefully looked for.

As we have seen, there are three vascular networks which are readily distinguished on the slit lamp (Figures 2.9 and 3.7):

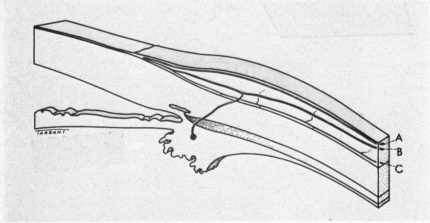

Figure 3.7. A diagrammatic representation of the vascular plexuses overlying the anterior segment of the eye (see also Figure 2.9): (A) conjunctival plexus, (B) superficial episcleral plexus, (C) deep episcleral network.

1. The conjunctival vessels derived from the anterior ciliary arteries supplying the conjunctiva and subconjunctival tissue.
2. The superficial episcleral plexus lying in Tenon's capsule, also derived from the anterior ciliary vessels, containing mostly venous channels and having a radial distribution.
3. A deep arterial episcleral network in the episclera which is intimately applied to the sclera itself. When the eye becomes inflamed, these separate layers of vessels stand out very clearly and are particularly easy to see if red-free light is used. The severity, position and extent of the oedema can be estimated by observation of the vessel layers and by their degree of separation (Figure 3.8 and 3.9).

Examination of the eye in red-free light

The green filter fitted to almost all standard slit lamps enables the eye to be viewed in red-free light. The slit diaphragm is opened to its full aperture to enable as wide an area as possible to be viewed and this brings the vessels into very sharp contrast with the background, enabling the position of maximum

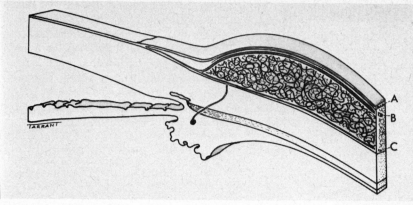

Figure 3.8. Episcleritis. The episclera only is involved. The superficial vascular plexus is very congested and is displaced forwards leaving the slightly congested deep episcleral plexus flat on the sclera.

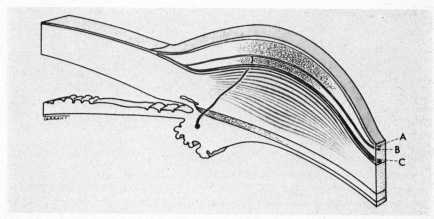

Figure 3.9. Scleritis. The sclera is swollen. The maximum congestion is in the deep episcleral vascular plexus. There is some overlying episcleritis which needs to be ignored when examining the patient.

inflammation to be determined with certainty and the configuration of the vessels to be studied. The red-free light has the additional advantage that infiltration of Tenon's capsule can be distinguished from the infiltration of the more superficial layers of the conjunctiva. Areas of infiltration from whatever cause —and these are usually lymphocytes in episcleritis—appear as deep yellow or yellow-brown patches in Tenon's capsule and the deeper the infiltration the darker the colour. The episclera is rarely infiltrated by these patches in deep scleral disease even though it is much inflamed.

Slit-lamp examination

A narrow slit beam with white light is used to determine whether there is any swelling of the deep scleral tissue. Any changes in the cornea, anterior chamber or posterior segment are noted at this stage.

Slit-lamp examination is directed to detecting scleral oedema if it is present, ignoring the fact that the overlying episclera will be congested and oedematous. In episcleritis there is no oedema of the sclera, all the inflammation being confined to the episclera. If the sclera is involved, the deep edge of the narrow beam of the slit lamp will be displaced forwards by the scleral swelling. This is particularly easy to detect over a nodule in the sclera but can be detected in almost every patient if the normal and abnormal areas are compared. If the congestion of the episcleral vessels is extreme, then the application of 1/1000 adrenaline or other vasoconstrictor to the conjunctival sac will constrict the superficial vessels but will have relatively little effect on the deeper ones. Once the superficial vessels have been blanched it is usually simple to detect any displacement of the underlying sclera.

The deep episcleral vessels overlying an area of scleral swelling will, of course, be displaced forwards by the underlying oedema so that the examination in red-free light and the slit-lamp examination are complementary to each other. This is perhaps best illustrated by reference to a particular example.

Case study. Mrs J.M., aged 27, nursing sister, five months before she was first seen had what she described as chilblains on the calf which were tender and disappeared without trace after four months. Two or three days after the lumps had disappeared, the left eye suddenly became bloodshot and started aching. Over the next three days, the redness and pain increased to such an extent that she had to stay in bed. The pain was relieved by aspirin for about an hour but came back just as severely after the effects had worn off. On the third day, the right eye also became inflamed and painful. She then consulted her doctor who prescribed steroid eye drops without improvement. The pain was now very severe, radiating to the forehead and to the temple and preventing her from sleeping.

This history is very suggestive of scleral inflammation. She was also extremely photophobic and the eyes were very tender. However, there was no inflammation of the anterior segment and the rest of the eye was normal. Superficially the sclera did not appear to be severely involved (Figure 3.10). From this photograph, taken when she was first seen, it is very difficult to decide if there is any deep inflammation or swelling because the episcleral oedema and swelling is the predominant feature. Examination with the red-free light immediately revealed not only the intense congestion of the deep episcleral network of vessels, but also one completely avascular patch, a finding of great significance as it indicated an underlying vasculitis and necrotising disease. When the conjunctival vessels were blanched with 1/1000 adrenaline and the deep sclera inspected with the white-light narrow beam of the slit lamp the area posterior to the avascular patch could be seen to be swollen.

She was at this stage reluctant to take any systemic therapy, so she continued to apply local steroid drops and was seen six days later. The pain had continued throughout this period and both eyes had continued to be extremely inflamed. The appearance in Figure 3.11 shows that the area which had been avascular now contained large tortuous vascular channels and that the sclera underlying

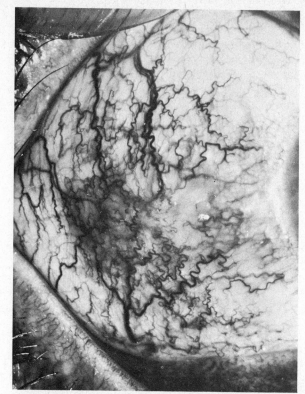

Figure 3.10. Mrs J.M. The eye when first seen. The superficial examination has the appearance of nodular episcleritis but examination in red-free light revealed displacement of the deep episcleral plexus indicating that the sclera is involved. Notice the small avascular patch of episclera at 9.00 o'clock. This is a highly significant finding indicating the presence of an early necrotising scleritis.

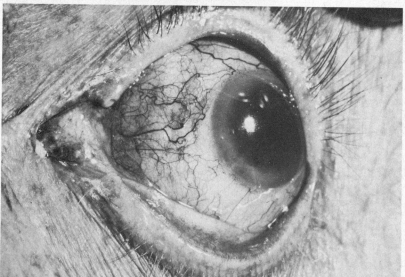

Figure 3.11. Mrs J.M. 14 days later. The early necrotising scleritis is now obvious with some loss of tissue and congested and abnormal vascular channels surrounding the centre of the inflammatory process.

it was swollen and beginning to show the early signs of necrosis. Prompt treatment with systemic medication reversed the process within two weeks and although she has had one recurrent attack four years later, no permanent harm has come to her eyes.

Even if the history had not been suggestive of severe scleral disease, it would have been possible to tell from the start that this patient had severe scleral disease, which, if left untreated, would lead to severe necrosis of the sclera. That she was reluctant to undertake systemic treatment enabled us to confirm our prognostication because within a week necrosis had begun. This is not an isolated case and does illustrate the necessity for a careful and accurate assessment at the very first hospital visit.

Other Vascular Anomalies

Apart from the generalised congestion of all the vascular plexuses, certain other changes occur which can be of importance in determining the cause of the inflammation.

Avascular areas

We have already alluded to the presence of avascular areas in the scleral or episcleral networks of vessels. These areas, which must be diligently searched for, are sometimes very obvious and at other times difficult to find, but they are always of significance, because if left alone they may extend, leaving an area of necrosed, sloughed sclera which may involve the full thickness of the sclera over a very large area.

Anastomotic channels

Another vascular anomaly which indicates the presence of deep underlying scleral disease is the development of anastomotic vascular channels between the larger vessels in the superficial or deep episcleral networks.

When the superficial episclera is simply congested, as in Figure 3.12, all the vessels in both superficial and deep episcleral plexuses are dilated and readily visible but retain their normal relationship to each other. In Figure 3.13 large deep channels have joined up and other abnormal anastomoses have occurred between the deep and superficial networks. These are presumably channels already present but which are not usually used. Whilst these large channels could represent dilatation of the capillary network in order to remove the increased supply of blood from the site of inflammation, as in Figures 3.14 and 3.15 in which the limbal arcade is involved, the explanation seems unlikely in the majority of patients because the new vascular channels appear to form around areas of relative episcleral ischaemia and at the edges of areas of severe scleral necrosis. Vessels not normally present are found histologically surrounding granulomas in the sclera and it is probably that these new vessels, which are sometimes enormous, form on the venous side of the

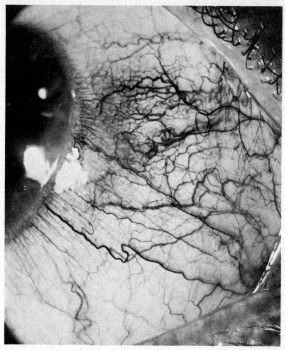

Figure 3.12. Vascular channels in simple episcleritis. In the inflamed area the vessels of all the plexus except the conjunctiva are congested but retain their normal pattern and anatomical relationships.

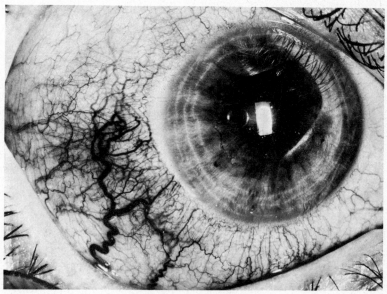

Figure 3.13. Anastomoses between the deep and superficial vascular plexuses in an area of constantly recurring episcleritis.

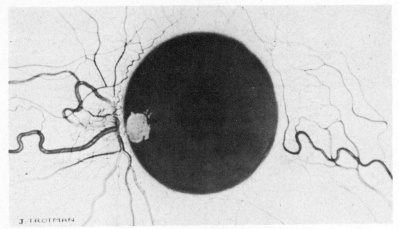

Figure 3.14. Dilatation of the limbal vascular arcade at the site of a scleral nodule and associated sclerokeratitis.

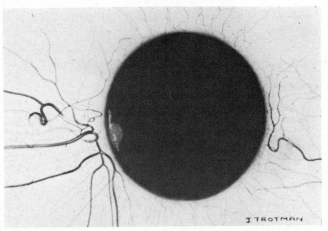

Figure 3.15. The same area as Figure 3.14 three months later after treatment. The sclera is not inflamed and the corneal lesion is very small but the abnormal vasculature remains.

circulation to drain blood away from the granuloma. These channels are an almost universal finding in deep scleritis and sclerokeratitis, and in severe necrotising scleritis sometimes the only area of normal sclera is that underlying these engorged venous channels (Figure 3.16).

Beading and microaneurysm formation

Another vascular abnormality not uncommonly found in these patients is beading of the superficial episcleral vessels with occasional true aneurysm

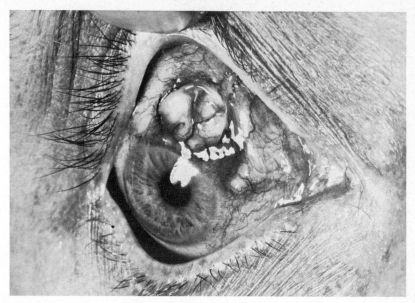

Figure 3.16.   Necrotising scleritis in which there is massive destruction of scleral tissue. Large venous channels traverse the affected area. The sclera, which lies apparently immediately underneath the vessels, is normal.

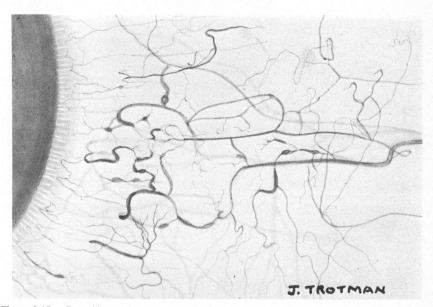

Figure 3.17.   Branching and aneurysmal dilatation of episcleral vessels in a patient with scleritis and temporal arteritis.

formation where the vessels divide (Figure 3.17). These changes do not appear to be confined to either the arterial or venous side of the circulation and may sometimes bleed. If the circulation is observed in these adjacent vessels, it is usually sluggish. Whether these changes are of any significance is uncertain as they can be found in some normal individuals and in others with other types of intraocular inflammation. Beading and aneurysmal changes are not uncommonly found in the conjunctival vessels (Kanagasundaram, 1956; Duke Elder, 1965), but these do not usually affect the deeper vessels. It was thought that the changes were a result of sludging in the circulation associated with a high sedimentation rate and the presence of abnormal globulins in the circulation, and whilst this certainly can be the case, for instance in cryo-globulinaemia and in those patients with temporal arteritis and scleritis, it is by no means always related.

General Eye Examination

Although scleral inflammation can occur as an isolated lesion, it is usually accompanied by other eye signs, and, more important, its presence is often unsuspected because of the severity of the other ocular manifestations. When we investigated eyes which had been removed with a primary histological diagnosis of scleritis, it was found that the diagnosis of scleritis was not even suspected in 40 per cent of these patients, particularly if the primary inflammation of the sclera was at or posterior to the equator. The clinical diagnosis varied from acute congestive glaucoma, malignant glaucoma and Mooren's ulceration to ciliary body malignant melanoma (Fraunfelder and Watson, 1976).

Visual acuity

The visual acuity will be reduced in up to 50 per cent of patients with scleritis even if they are adequately treated. The whole purpose of treatment of scleral disease is to prevent or at least to reduce this fall to a minimum. As the visual acuity is a most accurate assessment of visual function, it must be assessed at each visit as a fall may herald the onset of some further complications. Most commonly the fall in visual acuity is attributable to keratitis, particularly if it is accompanied by uveitis. If cataract formation is the cause, this is usually obvious but involvement of the posterior segment or the optic nerve can lead to a disastrous, permanent and unexpected fall in acuity and should always be considered if no obvious cause can be found.

Change in refraction

Although refraction does not have to be performed as a routine, it is worth remembering that an intense myopia can be induced by simple episcleritis because of ciliary spasm and that hypermetropia may occur as a result of orbital inflammation or posterior scleral inflammation near the posterior pole of the eye because of the increased thickness and oedema of the globe.

Corneal involvement

Corneal changes result either from its direct involvement by the same processes which affect the sclera or from oedema and subsequent vascularisation spreading from an adjacent area of scleritis. In either case, the changes themselves are characteristic, so much so that if a patient is seen when the scleritis is quiescent, the residual corneal changes are highly suggestive that he or she has had scleritis at some time in the past.

As corneal changes occur in almost one-third of those patients who develop scleritis, it is important that changes are carefully documented according to the slit-lamp appearances. Corneal sensation is reduced in certain patients with scleral disease. Lyne (1976, unpublished data) in our clinic has just examined 27 patients with scleritis and found that the corneal sensation was reduced in 26 of them and that unless the necrotising changes were very severe the sensation returned to normal when the scleritis was treated. Only four of the 19 patients with episcleritis had any reduction in corneal sensation.

Involvement of the anterior uveal tract or ciliary body

Anterior uveitis is easy to diagnose by the presence of an aqueous flare and cells in the anterior chamber. Keratic precipitates caused by deposition of these cells on the back of the cornea occur but they are never large enough to be visible with a magnifying glass or with the naked eye. The circum-corneal injection which is so characteristic of a primary anterior uveitis is present but often obscured by the accompanying scleral inflammation.

Much more difficulty is experienced in the diagnosis of a posterior uveitis or a cyclitis in which the ciliary body only is involved in the inflammatory process. Cells can be seen in the posterior chamber behind the lens, the lens iris diaphragm is moved forward so that the anterior chamber depth on the affected side is shallower, and when the pupil is dilated the peripheral retina can be seen, indicating that it is displaced forwards by the swollen ciliary body.

Involvement of the choroid

If the inflammation is behind the ciliary body, then an exudative retinal detachment will occur. This is a fluid retinal detachment in which no retinal tear can be found and, in the early stages, may easily be moved by posturing the patient. Later, if the exudate thickens, the fluid is not so mobile and a demarcation line becomes visible. White spots can usually be seen in the retina, underlying the site of the exudation.

Raised intraocular pressure

This examination should never be omitted in any patient with scleral inflammation as the onset of glaucoma is insidious and not always accompanied by intraocular inflammation. Asymmetry in the depths of the anterior chamber may possibly indicate the presence of angle closure due to forward movement of the lens iris diaphragm because of synechiae, posterior scleritis or annular scleral inflammation with ciliary body oedema.

Orbital involvement

As the posterior sclera and the optic nerve can be involved in granulomatous disease within the orbit, and a granulomatous change within the sclera can extend to involve the extraocular muscles, the vision may fall, the eye become proptosed and its movements limited.

Proptosis

As the proptosis is unilateral it can be assessed clinically in the usual manner by observing the eyes directly from above the head comparing one with the other. The displacement is axial because the inflammation occurs uniformly in the orbit and muscle cone. For comparative purposes this is best measured with the Hertl exophthalmometer, remembering that this instrument is only accurate to $\pm$ 2 mm of displacement of one eye against the other.

Extraocular movements

Generalised reduction of extraocular movements occurs because of infiltration of the muscle or surrounding oedema giving rise to double vision in the affected field of vision. As with infiltrative thyroid myopathy the limitation of movement is best measured with the Lee's screen or Hess chart. By dissociating one eye from the other and by making each eye move through its full range of movements, a map of the limited movement of one eye as against the compensatory over-action of the other can be produced (Figure 3.18). Repeating this test at different stages in the course of the disease can give a very valuable assessment of progress of the condition or lack of it.

Visual field assessment

Visual field assessment is usually unnecessary unless it is suspected that the patient has optic nerve involvement or a chronic form of glaucoma. Although a localised field defect can be picked up related to an area of posterior scleritis and choroiditis, these areas can usually be seen with the ophthalmoscope or fluorescein angiography. We have, however, one patient whose first complaint was of a 'fuzzy area in the field of vision below the centre of the vision'. When the optic nerve is affected, there is a generalised constriction of the peripheral visual field preceded by central and paracentral scotomas to red objects. However, we have seen patients with altitudinal hemianopias, possibly due to occlusion of vessels supplying the optic nerve.

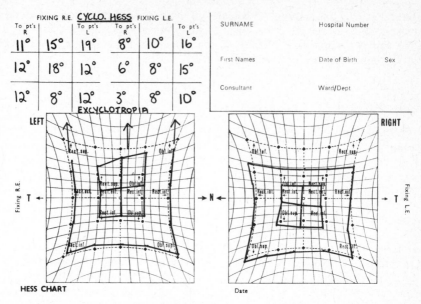

Figure 3.18. Hess chart in a patient with posterior scleritis of the right eye. The movements of the affected right eye were limited in elevation but returned to normal after treatment.

The glaucomatous field defects differ in no way from those found in glaucoma due to other causes, progressing through arcuate scotomas to the final constriction of the visual field. These changes can, however, occur with alarming rapidity, presumably because the pressure can rise to very high levels very fast.

CLINICAL EXAMINATION OF THE JOINTS

'They have hands but they handle not'. Psalms 115, 7.

The combination of joint disease and scleral disease is common enough for it to be important for every ophthalmologist to appreciate the symptoms of joint disease and to know how to examine at least the easily accessible joints in order to be certain that he is dealing with an inflammatory and not a degenerate type of arthritis.

Rheumatoid arthritis and osteoarthrosis are the commonest causes of joint disease and their differentiation is usually simple. However, the separation of rheumatoid arthritis from the less common causes of inflammatory arthritis is often much more difficult because there are no absolutely distinctive physical signs and no definite diagnostic laboratory investigations. The results of all the tests must be considered carefully in the light of the history and clinical findings if they are to be of any value in diagnosis, prognosis and management.

An accurate diagnosis is essential in the care of a patient with joint disease and, as a physician should always look for a cause of 'fever', so he should also seek the cause of arthritis. To achieve this in a patient with polyarthritis, several important steps need to be taken. The first task is to identify the tissue in which a pathological process is at work; the second is to define the nature of the process, be it inflammatory, traumatic, neoplastic or degenerative. There are therefore five important points to note:

Type of pathological change. Is the joint enlarged due to overgrowth of bone or other tissue or is the process erosive, causing joint destruction and deformity? Is there swelling, warmth, pain and redness indicating inflammation?

The pattern of joint involvement. The various forms of arthritis have characteristic patterns of joint involvement and a clinical joint survey will give a helpful lead to diagnosis.

Disease of other connective tissue structures. Disorders of bursae, tendons, skin, heart valves and blood vessels are associated with certain types of arthritis.

Natural history. An accurate history including past history may reveal a characteristic mode of onset and development of the disease.

Radiological and laboratory aids. Radiographs will demonstrate the proliferative and destructive bone changes. The sedimentation rate is a simple and useful index of inflammation. A raised serum uric acid is a strong indicator of gout and a positive test for rheumatoid factor is helpful. Culture of organisms in joint fluid confirms infective arthritis and the demonstration of crystals in joint fluid establishes a crystal synovitis.

History

The history should include information regarding a prodromal illness and a description of the pattern of onset, including the rapidity of progression of symptoms, severity of pain, amount and location of swelling, symmetry of joints involved, extent of limitation of movement, persistence of symptoms and the degree of disability. This information gives a guide to the general pattern of joint involvement since onset.

It is also important to enquire into precipitating or aggravating circumstances and to record the amount, location and duration of morning stiffness; this gives a good guide to the degree of activity of inflammation. The family history may suggest gouty arthritis, ankylosing spondylitis, rheumatoid arthritis, Heberden's nodes. Other important aspects of the history are:

1. Age, sex, race, occupation.
2. Main complaint: When did it start? How did it start (sudden, gradual, time of day)? Precipitating factors, e.g. trauma. Which joints are affected? Morning stiffness. Pattern (continuous, episodic, migratory). Associated symptoms.
3. Ask for skin disease, diarrhoea, venereal disease, drug therapy, recent visits overseas.
4. Past medical history.
5. Family history: gout, diabetes.

General Physical Examination

Physical signs of special import are as follows:
1. General appearance; pallor, pigmentation; posture and gait.
2. Examination of joints:
    (a) Overlying skin: colour, temperature, consistency (smooth, shiny, thick, thin, pitting).
    (b) Swelling: articular or periarticular; effusion (fluctuant), synovial thickening (soft non-fluctuant) or bony swelling (hard).
    (c) Tenderness.
    (d) Position, deformities: range of motion, crepitus.
    (e) Periarticular soft tissues: muscle wasting, tendon involvement, bursae, tender points.
3. Complete physical examination essential. Look particularly for tophi (ears or periarticular), nodules (ulnar surface of forearm), lymph nodes, skin lesions, finger clubbing; record temperature. Routine examination of cardiovascular system, chest, abdomen and central nervous system. Examine penis if suspicious of Reiter's disease.

In addition, the temperature of the skin may be helpful; contrast the cold, moist extremities of rheumatoid arthritis with the marked heat of gouty or infective arthritis. Subcutaneous swellings such as nodules in the elbow area in rheumatoid arthritis or subcutaneous tophi of gout in the ear or elsewhere should be looked for. Lymphadenopathy, splenomegaly and hepatomegaly are seen in juvenile rheumatoid arthritis, in Felty's type of rheumatoid arthritis or in systemic lupus erythematosus.

On examining the musculoskeletal system, inspection, palpation and range of movement are all important and the joint must always be compared with the opposite side. In articular disease, the way a patient moves, sits, walks, bends, uses his hands, dresses and gets on the examination couch may be all important.

Assessment of a joint requires observation concerning swelling, pain, skin changes, muscle wasting, movements, deformity. In most patients the history and a quick survey will reveal which joints are involved so that attention can be focused at these points.

Swelling

In inflammatory joint disease swelling may be due to soft tissue swelling or to fluid. An effusion may occur in an arthropathy from any cause or in a joint close to a focus of inflammation. The contour of the joint may indicate fluid (Figure 3.19) as may the presence of fluctuation within the cavity. Distended bursae or cysts near joints produce localised cystic swellings and they may communicate with the main joint cavity.

Pitting oedema of tissues overlying a joint is an indication of the acuteness of the inflammatory process and is seen in early rheumatoid arthritis. However, apparent swelling of a joint may be produced by overlying oedema due to conditions outside the joint, for instance it is possible to mistake prepatellar bursitis as arthritis of the knee joint. Other para-articular swellings such as ganglia, lymph glands, tophi, and rheumatoid nodules (Figure 3.20) must be differentiated, as must bony enlargement from osteophytes at articular margins in degenerative joint disease. Spur formation at the articular margins of the terminal phalangeal joints of the fingers accounts for much of the enlargement of Heberden's nodes seen in osteoarthrosis (Figure 3.21).

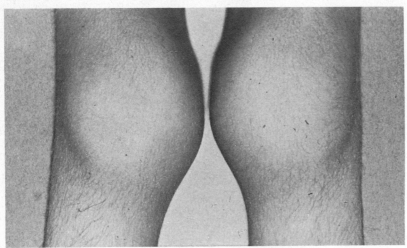

Figure 3.19. Bilateral effusions in both knee joints in a child with Still's disease. Part of the swelling is due to synovial hypertrophy.

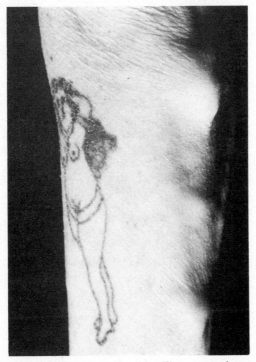

Figure 3.20. Three rheumatoid nodules at the elbow. They commonly occur over pressure points.

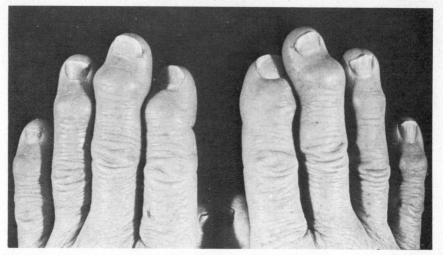

Figure 3.21.   Bony swelling at distal interphalangeal joints in primary osteoarthrosis. These Heberden nodules can be painful in the early stages.

Pain

Pain may be present at rest and also may only be produced by moving a joint or by pressure over it. Again it is important to distinguish whether inflammation lies inside or outside a joint. In degenerative joint disease, localised tender areas can be detected in relationship to ligaments and other structures around a joint.

Skin changes

Increased warmth of the skin overlying an inflamed joint is a good indication of inflammation within a joint. If the skin is red, it indicates an acute inflammatory reaction and is found in septic arthritis, crystal synovitis and rheumatic fever. It is uncommon in rheumatoid arthritis. In gouty arthritis the skin is shiny and dry.

Muscle wasting

Painful and inflamed joints usually cause a reduction in the bulk of adjacent muscles. In the knee in particular, quadriceps wasting occurs rapidly.

Movement

It is wise to test both active and passive movements, for active movements may be impaired by muscle weakness or tendon lesions. Full examination of the joint requires measurement of normal movement and the testing for the presence of abnormal movement. The presence of pain or palpable crepitus should be noted. Soft fine crepitus is found in rheumatoid arthritis, and there is more coarse crepitus in osteoarthrosis and the badly damaged joint. Crepitus may also arise from tendon sheaths.

The hand

Examination of the hand is often as valuable in the differential diagnosis of polyarthritis as the examination of the rest of the patient. It is the patient's 'visiting card'. It is possible to study the distribution of the arthritis, and look for characteristic changes in the skin, nails, and tendon sheaths. In seeking evidence of arthritis it is important to look for slight 'spindling' of the digits produced by early rheumatoid involvement of the proximal interphalangeal joints (Figure 3.22) and to test each of the small joints in turn for discomfort on pressure. Flexor tendon sheaths have linings similar to those of synovial joints and may be involved in the same pathological process. Effusions in the sheaths may produce sausage-shaped swellings in the fingers or in the palms. Palpable nodules may be detected and an area of stenosis may impair movement of a finger—'trigger finger'. Tendons may be weakened by rheumatoid involvement and rupture leading to loss of active movement.

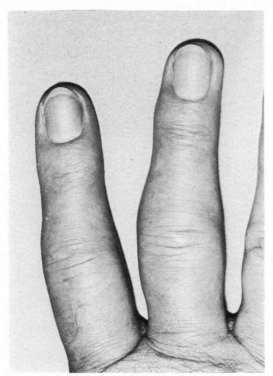

Figure 3.22. Synovial swelling of proximal interphalangeal joint of finger. Symmetrical involvement of these joints is seen in rheumatoid arthritis.

Function of the hand is vulnerable to changes both in the joints and in the tendons and their sheaths; lesions at one point may produce disturbance of more distal joints. Rheumatic disorders may also interfere with peripheral nerve function and assessment of an arthritic hand must include a neurological examination.

In arthritis, when the hand is involved the pattern of joint deformity and other local changes is often highly characteristic of the disease in question. In osteoarthrosis, Heberden's nodes (firm swellings at the base of distal phalanges) (Figure 3.21) are seen. In rheumatoid arthritis, fusiform fingers from interphalangeal joint involvement occur. Later, the boggy swelling of wrist and metacarpophalangeal joints and wasting of the intrinsic muscles complete the picture. If the disease progresses, more gross deformities, due to joint destruction and tendon dysfunction lead to ulnar deviation of the fingers, often with palmar subluxation of the proximal phalanges (Figure 3.23). Characteristic deformities of the fingers in rheumatoid arthritis include boutonnière (due to the proximal interphalangeal joint protruding through the extensor expansion) or swan-neck deformities (due to hyperextension at the proximal interphalangeal joint) (Figure 3.24). In addition to abnormalities of the flexor tendon there may be thin skin or nail-fold lesions indicative of digital arteritis (Figure 3.25).

Psoriatic arthritis typically involves terminal interphalangeal joints, and the swelling of these joints in association with the pitting of nails is characteristic (Figure 3.26). Progressive systemic sclerosis, systemic lupus erythematosus and dermatomyositis may all produce a mild symmetrical polyarthritis affecting the small joints of the hands, with the emphasis usually on the proximal

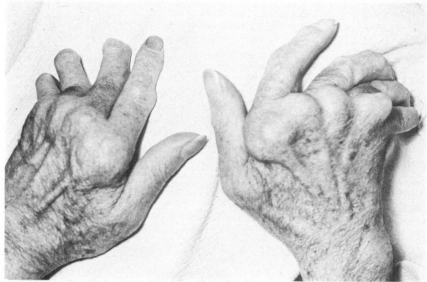

Figure 3.23.   Characteristic deformities in rheumatoid arthritis. Note the synovial swelling of the metacarpophalangeal joints, the ulnar deviation of the fingers, and the subluxation of the metacarpophalangeal joints.

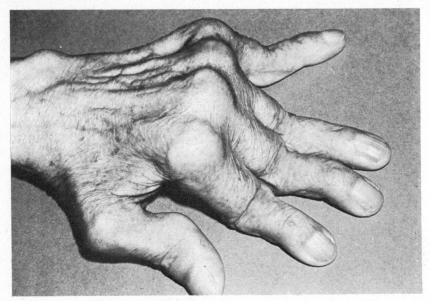

Figure 3.24. Swan-neck deformities of the fingers in rheumatoid arthritis. Notice also the wasting of the small muscles of the hand.

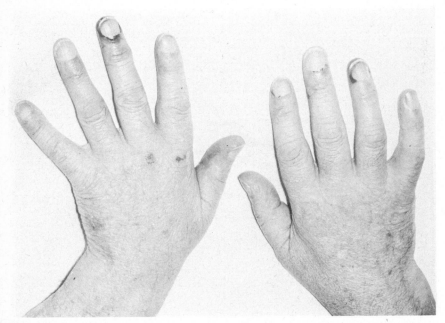

Figure 3.25. Nail-fold lesions due to arthritis. There are also areas of tissue death due to infarction.

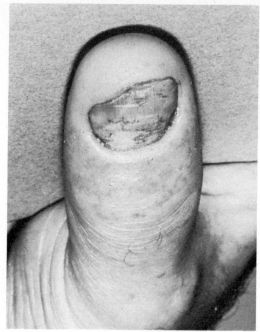

Figure 3.26.   Deformity of nail and inflammation of the distal interphalangeal joint in psoriatic arthritis.

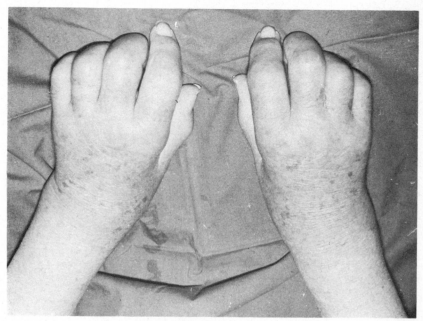

Figure 3.27.   Smooth tight skin and joint inflammation leading to flexion deformities of the fingers in systemic sclerosis.

interphalangeal joints. Each of these conditions has characteristic skin changes; in systemic sclerosis skin oedema and joint swelling combine to produce 'sausage fingers'; the obliteration of cutaneous creases and appendages gives the skin a smooth characterless appearance (Figure 3.27). In polymyositis, the skin changes in the fingers resemble those seen in the former condition, and may vary from slight waxy thickening to gross sclerodactyly with atrophy of the digital pulp. In systemic lupus the skin changes are frequent and variable, the classical erythematous rash across the bridge of the nose and cheeks (butterfly rash) is the commonest change (Figure 3.28). Also there are often hair changes which may lead to total baldness (Figure 3.29).

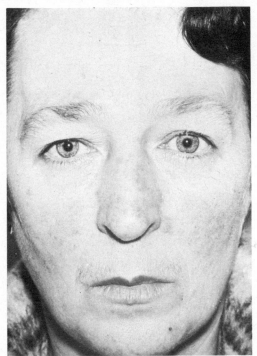

Figure 3.28.   Butterfly rash across nose and cheeks in systemic lupus erythematosus.

Figure 3.30 illustrates the joints usually affected by rheumatoid arthritis and osteoarthrosis. Such involvement is usually symmetrical in the two hands in these conditions, but gout, psoriatic arthritis and infectious arthritis do not usually involve symmetrical finger joints. Distal interphalangeal joint involvement is common to osteoarthrosis, psoriatic arthritis, and occasionally gout. Proximal interphalangeal involvement usually infers rheumatoid arthritis if there is an effusion or soft tender swelling of the joint, but firm non-tender enlargement of these joints characterises the so-called 'Bouchard's nodes' of osteoarthrosis. These are the counterpart of Heberden's nodes of the distal interphalangeal joints. Metacarpal phalangeal joints are rarely involved except in rheumatoid arthritis. Pain and swelling in the ulnar styloid area are highly suggestive of rheumatoid arthritis, and these may occur early in the disease.

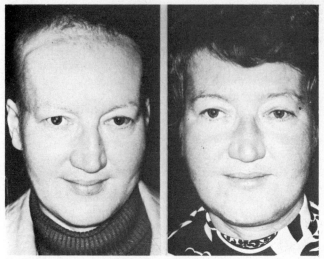

Figure 3.29. Alopecia in active systemic lupus erythematosus, also showing regrowth of hair when the disease is under control.

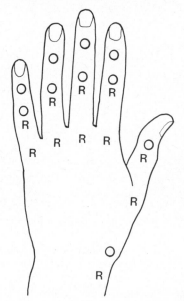

Figure 3.30. Joints of the hands involved in osteoarthrosis (O) and rheumatoid arthritis (R). Note how OA affects the carpometacarpal joint of the thumb, whilst RA affects the wrist.

Fever

A low-grade fever is common, particularly in patients with untreated rheumatoid arthritis and the other connective tissue diseases. Indeed, these diseases may present as a pyrexia of unknown origin.

ANCILLARY INVESTIGATIONS

Laboratory Investigations

Many different conditions give rise to very similar changes in both the sclera and joints, so the purpose of laboratory investigations is to help to differentiate these underlying conditions and to eliminate some conditions or to confirm a clinical diagnosis. Unfortunately, laboratory investigations are often not helpful in the earliest stages of scleritis or inflammatory joint disease. In the early stages of arthritis, chest and joint radiographs are often normal or demonstrate only the soft tissue swelling seen on clinical examination, and this is usually when objective confirmation is most needed.

In view of the common association of connective tissue and chronic granulomatous diseases with scleral disease, the investigations detailed in Table 3.2 are performed as a routine in order to eliminate the former as a cause. If these do not produce a positive result or require confirmation, then further special investigations are undertaken.

Table 3.2. *Laboratory investigations undertaken as a routine in all patients with scleral disease*

Haematological investigations	x-rays
Haemoglobin	Chest x-ray
Total and differential white blood count	x-ray of hands and feet
Erythrocyte sedimentation rate	
Plasma proteins and immunoglobulins including anti-nuclear factor	
Test for rheumatoid factor	
Serum uric acid	
Serological tests for syphilis	

Haemoglobin

A moderate, normocytic, hypochromic anaemia is a common feature of rheumatoid arthritis and the connective tissue diseases, and in rheumatoid arthritis the degree of anaemia correlates with the activity of the disease (Mowat, 1971).

The serum iron is low in the presence of active disease and it may be the best indicator of such activity. The iron binding capacity is normal and this further helps to differentiate the anaemia from true iron deficiency anaemia in which raised values are found.

Iron absorption is normal and gastrointestinal blood loss due to drug therapy is rarely an important contributory cause. It is only in the small group of patients with true iron deficiency that oral iron will have any therapeutic effect. Osteoarthrosis does not cause anaemia.

White cell count

The white cell count and the differential count are usually normal in patients with rheumatoid arthritis. Modest increases occur occasionally, but values over 14 000 /mm³ suggest factors other than the disease itself, but may be due to infectious arthritis due to corticosteroid therapy. A low white count due to hypersplenism (Felty's syndrome) may occur or may be due to drug therapy, e.g. phenylbutazone or gold salts.

Leucopenia is common in systemic lupus erythematosus, although counts of under 2000 are infrequent. Eosinophilia may be a feature of polyarteritis nodosa, particularly in those with pulmonary involvement.

Erythrocyte sedimentation rate (ESR)

This is the most important single laboratory test of inflammatory activity. It is influenced most by plasma fibrinogen, alpha- and gamma-globulins, and any disease which raises the concentration of these components will raise the ESR. The upper limits of normal rise with age and the following normal limits (mm /hour Westergren) have been suggested: below 50 years, 15 for men and 25 for women; above 50 years, 20 for men and 30 for women (Böttiger and Svedberg, 1967).

Serum uric acid

Approximately five per cent of uric acid levels in any normal population will exceed the upper limits of 7 mg /100 ml for men and 6 mg /100 ml for women (Figure 3.31) (Hall et al, 1967). Clinicians must watch for changes in laboratory methods which influence the values for the normal range in different centres. The serum uric acid increases with age, reaching plateau values at the age of 20 to 25 years in men, and after the menopause in women. The combination of hyperuricaemia and acute arthritis does not prove a diagnosis of gout. This is because of the appreciable incidence of essential

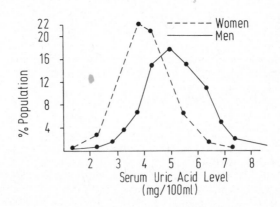

Figure 3.31.   Distribution of serum uric acid in the population.

hyperuricaemia in the population (Figure 3.31) and the chance that such an individual may have another cause for acute arthritis. The probability that the attack is due to gout increases when there is a history of previous acute attacks, or when there are extra-articular manifestations of gout. Nevertheless it has been shown that if the serum uric acid is 9.0 mg/100 ml or more, the chances of developing clinical gout within ten years are 83 per cent (Hall et al, 1967). The diagnosis can only be established conclusively by finding urate crystals in a joint effusion or nodule (Currey, 1968).

Causes of hyperuricaemia

Increased serum uric acid values may be caused by small doses of salicylates (less than 2 g/day), all the commonly used diuretics and pyrazinamide. High values also occur in hypothyroidism, hyperparathyroidism, renal failure, psoriasis and with ketosis from starvation or diabetes. Secondary gout is caused by leukaemia, reticulosis, polycythaemia and myeloma (Table 3.3).

Table 3.3. *Conditions associated with hyperuricaemia and their causes*

1. Essential hyperuricaemia and idiopathic gout
   Increased purine synthesis, decreased uric acid excretion, or a combination, occurring without an obvious cause.

2. Myeloproliferative diseases and reticuloses
   Increased nucleic acid turnover.

3. Chronic haemolytic states
   Increased nucleic acid turnover.

4. Psoriasis
   Increased nucleic acid turnover.

5. Drug treatment: diuretics, pyrazinamide, salicylates in small doses
   Inhibition of the active tubular excretion of uric acid.

6. Starvation ketosis; acute alcoholism
   Inhibition of active renal tubular excretion of uric acid.

7. Type I glycogen storage disease (glucose-6-phosphatase deficiency)
   Increased purine synthesis and decreased renal excretion of uric acid.

8. Lesch—Nyhan syndrome and its incomplete clinical variants
   Complete or partial deficiency of hypoxanthine—guanine phosphoribosyl transferase. This leads to a decreased feedback inhibition of the first stage of purine biosynthesis and causes an increase in the rate of uric acid production.

9. Chronic glomerulonephritis and pyelonephritis
   Decreased renal clearance of uric acid caused by a combination of glomerular and tubular damage.

10. Hypothyroidism

11. Hypoparathyroidism and hyperparathyroidism.

Serological tests for syphilis

Both the VDRL (Venereal Disease Research Laboratory) slide test and the WR (Wassermann reaction) are the usual routine hospital tests, but neither is specific for syphilis and false positive reactions may occur, particularly in connective tissue disease (Tuffanelli, 1968). Although both tests usually become positive soon after the appearance of the primary sore, this may be delayed for several weeks. In an untreated patient, the tests remain strongly positive for one or two years and then decline gradually. It is important to remember that serology may be misleading. About 25 per cent of patients become seronegative, sometimes even in the presence of late active lesions; patients treated before the tests who become positive may never develop a positive test. Conversely, if treatment is delayed, positive serology continues and is not an indication for further treatment.

Three further tests are useful in diagnosis, but tend to be more expensive and more complex. The commonly used Reiter protein complement fixation test (RPCFT) has the advantage of greater specificity and of becoming positive earlier than the WR and VDRL.

The fluorescent treponemal antibody test and its newer modification (FTA ABS) use virulent but dead treponema as antigen and the *Treponema pallidum* immobilisation test uses living treponema. Both are specific for antibodies against syphilis, and the former has the advantages of being fairly simple to do and of becoming positive well before other tests. A characteristic pattern may be seen with FTA ABS in connective tissue disease (McKenna et al, 1973).

Biological false positive

The WR and VDRL are nonspecific tests and may become positive in patients who have never had syphilis. They become transiently positive in many infections such as glandular fever, infectious hepatitis and chicken pox. False reactions also occur in pregnancy and in leprosy and tend to persist a longer time. Positive tests may sometimes persist for life in some patients: this is commoner in women, a few of whom develop one of the connective tissue diseases, sometimes years later.

Immunological tests

These include tests for rheumatoid factor, antinuclear factor, LE cells, immunoglobulins and complement levels. Although of great value, these tests tend to be abused as too much reliance is placed upon positive results and they should not be used in isolation.

Plasma proteins and immunoglobulins

The total protein content of the serum is not altered in connective tissue disease but electrophoresis (Figure 3.32) shows fairly nonspecific changes in

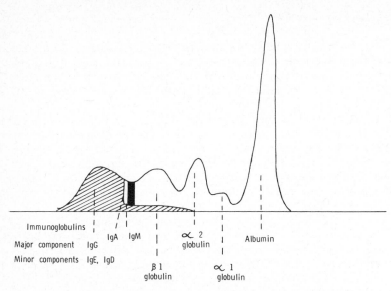

Figure 3.32. Electrophoretic strip showing position of protein fractions.

patients with almost all types of inflammatory joint disease. These include a reduction in serum albumin due to an increased rate of catabolism and a rise in alpha-2 and the gammaglobulin fractions (Bonomo, 1957). The immunoglobulins (Ig) which can be separated by ultracentrifugation consist of three major classes and two minor classes. Their different molecular weights cause them to sediment at different rates in the ultracentrifuge and these constants are termed Svedberg units (S units) (see Chapter 6).

Seventy per cent of the immunoglobulins consist of immunoglobulin G (IgG, 7S), and 25 per cent immunoglobulin A (IgA) (7S, 85 per cent). The rest consists of immunoglobulins M (IgM, 19S), E (IgE, 8S) and D (IgD, 7S). Immunoglobulin M has a high molecular weight of approximately 1 000 000 (19S) but like IgG and IgA has smaller components. The size of the circulating components may be important in determining the clinical manifestations of the disease produced.

Immunoglobulin levels show rises in IgA, IgG and IgM in most patients with connective tissue disorders (Cass et al, 1968). However, these measurements are of little value in routine management or diagnosis. In particular the IgM levels are only slightly higher in patients with positive tests for rheumatoid factor than in those with negative tests (Mongan et al, 1969) because rheumatoid factor comprises only a part of this immunoglobulin.

Serum protein electrophoresis and immunoglobulin values are most useful in diagnosing the monoclonal peaks of myeloma and the macroglobulinaemias. The normal range of values in most laboratories is:

IgG	1240 ± 220 mg/dl	Total protein 6.8–8.2 g/dl
IgA	390 ± 90 mg/dl	Albumin 4.2–5.4 g/dl
IgM	120 ± 35 mg/dl	Globulin 2.3–3.1 g/dl

Serum rheumatoid factors

The most consistent serological feature of rheumatoid arthritis is the presence of circulating antibodies ('rheumatoid factors') which react with human or heterologous IgG. Antiglobulin factors in rheumatoid arthritis were first described by Waaler (1940) and Rose et al (1948) who showed independently that sheep erythrocytes sensitised with a subagglutinating dose of rabbit antibody were agglutinated by a high proportion of sera from rheumatoid subjects. It is now known that classical rheumatoid factor is an IgM antibody to antigenic determinants on the heavy chains of IgG immunoglobulins. It is thought that the antigenic determinants are actually present in the individual's own IgG molecules, although some configurational alteration from the native state occurs before their reactivity and the appropriate rheumatoid factors become detectable (McCormick, 1975).

The latex test is widely used as a diagnostic screening measure, as polystyrene latex particles readily absorb purified IgG in solution. There are differences in sensitivity between the screening tests due to differences in the kind of particles and the source of IgG used to coat them. Those using human IgG as reactant (Latex) are more sensitive, but this is at the expense of specificity. About 20 per cent of patients with rheumatoid arthritis are seronegative and their disease tends to run a milder course than those with strongly seropositive disease (Alexander and McCarthy, 1966). The incidence of a positive test is four per cent in the normal population (Lawrence et al, 1970). The presence of rheumatoid factor in the serum does not necessarily lead to the development of rheumatoid arthritis, even in those with a positive family history of the disease.

Recently the discovery of IgG rheumatoid factors has narrowed the difference formerly thought to exist between seropositive and seronegative rheumatoid arthritis (Torrigiani and Roitt, 1970). These serum IgG antiglobulins are the counterpart of IgM rheumatoid factor, but appear to be more widely distributed because raised levels have been found in patients with ankylosing spondylitis, psoriatic arthritis and gout, all conventionally seronegative groups. It seems therefore that most arthritic subjects have raised levels of antiglobulins, though not necessarily the classical IgM rheumatoid factors detected by the Rose–Waaler sheep cell agglutination test (SCAT). These levels of antiglobulins may have significance for the pathogenesis of rheumatoid disease, but for the sake of clarity should not be termed rheumatoid factor.

Although some seronegative rheumatoid arthritis patients will become seropositive in the course of time, in the majority, once the serological status is established, little change can be expected. It follows that it is important to search for diagnoses other than rheumatic arthritis in seronegative patients, particularly if tests for rheumatoid factor are persistently negative throughout the first year of symptoms (Dixon, 1960).

Patients with ankylosing spondylitis do not have rheumatoid factor in the serum but the factor can be detected in 20 per cent of these patients if the peripheral joints are involved. In all other forms of inflammatory joint disease and in osteoarthrosis the incidence of positive tests is normal. However, up to 40 per cent of patients with other connective tissue diseases will have positive tests and in Sjögren's syndrome the incidence approaches 100 per cent (Hill and Greenburg, 1965). Table 3.4 lists other conditions in which an incidence of positive tests of more than ten per cent in one or other test system has been found. Therefore the results of these tests must be interpreted with caution. In chronic infective states, the rheumatoid factors virtually disappear when the infection is overcome. The characteristic persistence of rheumatoid factor in arthritis may therefore be taken as evidence of persistent infection or alternatively of the persistence of some antigens whose combination with IgG constitutes an adequate stimulus (McCormick, 1975).

Table 3.4. *Diseases in which an incidence of positive results for rheumatoid factor is found*

	Positive Rose–Waaler SCAT (per cent)	Positive latex test (per cent)
Subacute bacterial endocarditis	27	23
Infective hepatitis	20	24
Myeloma	4	13
Virus infections	14	16
Sarcoidosis	18	10
Syphilis	4	13
Cancer	11	11

Antinuclear antibodies (ANA)

This is a useful screening test. Although it is positive in nearly all patients with active systemic lupus erythematosus (SLE), the test may be positive in 30 per cent of patients with rheumatoid arthritis and the other connective tissue diseases (Hijmans, 1966). In juvenile chronic polyarthritis 90 per cent of those that develop chronic iridocyclitis have positive antinuclear antibodies (Schaller et al, 1974). As this may precede the onset of eye signs, it is useful in identifying patients at risk from this serious complication.

In addition positive tests are also found in many conditions which have in common some alteration in immune mechanisms (Table 3.5). It is therefore less specific than the LE cell test.

In SLE, a range of serum antibodies may be present which are directed against various nuclear, cytoplasmic and membrane antigens of cells. The first classic 'LE cell factor' to be discovered was an IgG antinucleoprotein antibody which is able to opsonise naked cell nuclei in vitro for phagocytosis. The various other antibodies are detected by immunofluorescence, complement fixation, haemagglutinin or precipitin tests. They react specifically with mitochondria, microsomes, whole nuclei, nuclear extract, nucleoprotein, DNA or histone. Any SLE patient's serum will give positive reactions with one or more of these antigens. Some autoantibodies which react with nuclear constituents are diagnostically significant. Others, such as anti-DNA antibody, have a clearly defined role in pathogenesis (Hughes, 1975).

Table 3.5.   *Diseases in which antinuclear factor is positive*

Polymyositis
Chronic hepatitis
Polyarteritis nodosa
Thyroiditis
Interstitial pulmonary fibrosis
Progressive systemic sclerosis
Pernicious anaemia
Ulcerative colitis

Methods of immunofluorescence

Frozen sections of normal tissue (rat liver) or peripheral blood smears are incubated with the patient's serum and the preparation washed in saline. A second treatment with fluorescein-labelled antihuman immunoglobulin antibody, followed by inspection under a fluorescent microscope, shows whether immuno-globulin from the patient's serum has been bound to nuclei in the section or smear.

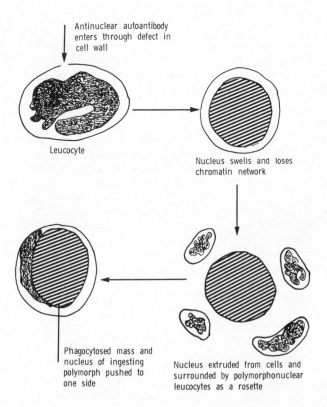

Antinuclear autoantibody enters through defect in cell wall

Leucocyte

Nucleus swells and loses chromatin network

Nucleus extruded from cells and surrounded by polymorphonuclear leucocytes as a rosette

Phagocytosed mass and nucleus of ingesting polymorph pushed to one side

Figure 3.33.   Formation of LE cell following damage of nucleus of leucocyte by antibody. The extruded nucleus is ingested by a polymorph producing an LE cell.

LE cell test (Figure 3.33)

This is time-consuming and requires an experienced observer to examine the material. Although occasionally these cells can be found on direct examination of joint or pleural fluid or in the bone marrow (Hunder and Pierre, 1970) they are usually found after the in vitro incubation of peripheral blood. There is little correlation between the number of LE cells and disease activity, although LE cells tend to disappear with treatment. LE cells are found in:
1. 80 per cent of patients with SLE.
2. Occasionally in chronic discoid lupus erythematosus.
3. Up to 10 per cent of patients with severe RA.
4. Occasionally in scleroderma, dermatomyositis and the other connective tissue diseases.
5. 10 per cent of chronic active (lupoid) hepatitis.
6. Drug sensitivity. A long list of drugs can cause a syndrome resembling SLE (Alarçon-Segovia, 1975).

Complement and anti-DNA antibodies

The nine-stage complement system is activated in immunological reactions and a number of tests using antisera diffusion techniques are useful (Schur, 1975). At the moment, they have most value in SLE when the serum values provide an indicator of disease activity—alterations towards or away from normal values often preceding changes in symptoms and signs.

Immunofluorescent studies of renal biopsy tissue in SLE suggest that immune complexes cause nephritis. Both DNA and anti-DNA have been identified in these deposits.

In patients with active disease, low serum complement and raised serum anti-DNA antibody levels are often found and their measurements are valuable in monitoring activity, especially in patients with renal disease (Hughes, 1975). C3 estimations by the Mancini radial immunodiffusion method provide a ready means of following serum complement levels. Anti-DNA antibodies may be measured by several methods. The most commonly used is Farr's ammonium sulphate precipitation assay with radiolabelled native (double-stranded) DNA as antigen (Hughes, Cohen and Christian, 1971). Normal values were obtained in the majority of patients with Sjögren's syndrome, rheumatoid arthritis, fibrosing alveolitis, drug-induced lupus and chronic active hepatitis (Hughes, 1973). The exact relationship of drug-induced lupus to true SLE is not known, but it tends to affect older people and both sexes equally. It usually spares the kidneys and has a better prognosis than true SLE.

Antistreptolysin-O titre (ASO titre)

A single estimation is of little value. A rising or falling titre is required to diagnose a recent streptococcal infection and therefore one has to consider rheumatic fever, Henoch–Schönlein purpura or erythema nodosum as a possible cause of joint symptoms.

Urine examination

Proteinuria is the commonest abnormality and is of no diagnostic value. It may well be a direct result of drug therapy. Routine tests for proteinuria should be undertaken in patients receiving gold or penicillamine, and analgesics can cause nephropathy (Murray, Lawson and Linton, 1971). More serious proteinuria as part of the nephrotic syndrome may be the result of secondary amyloidosis. Proteinuria occurs in patients with chronic gout since renal lesions are common in this disease and renal failure is a frequent cause of death.

Urethritis

This feature of Reiter's syndrome and gonococcal arthritis is usually found on waking, and examination of the urethral discharge reveals numerous pus cells.

Radiographs

The skeletal system can react to disease in a limited number of ways and it is therefore not surprising that different pathological conditions may, to some extent, exhibit similar radiological features, and as a consequence radiological investigation complements the clinical findings. The features which should be looked for are: the pattern of the skeletal lesions particularly the symmetry of the changes; the particular sites known to be affected in certain conditions. As a general rule, therefore, radiographs of the joints most affected should be requested, but in widespread joint disease a few carefully selected films may be of more value than those of a variety of joints. Attention to these details should enable one to distinguish between inflammatory and degenerative joint disease.

Hands and feet

These are usually the most valuable films, for the bones and joints of the hand and wrist are involved in many types of arthritis, the connective tissue diseases and some metabolic diseases. Films of both hands and both feet should be taken since they may demonstrate diagnostic features despite the absence of symptoms and signs in these joints. This is particularly so in rheumatoid arthritis, juvenile rheumatoid arthritis and psoriatic arthropathy.

Large joints

Lateral as well as anterior-posterior films should be taken because additional features may be demonstrated; in particular, artificial narrowing of the joint space due to joint flexion may be seen. Radiographs of the legs, particularly of the knees, should be taken standing and may provide useful information regarding deformity and subluxation.

Diagnostic changes in rheumatoid arthritis

Early radiological changes are more likely to be seen on films of hands and wrists than of larger joints (knees, ankles, hips) even if the latter hurt more, because of multiple joints in the hands and wrists, relatively thin cortices of bone and minimal soft tissue. The most important of the radiological signs of rheumatoid arthritis for diagnostic purposes are the early ones. However these are often missed:

1. Soft tissue changes. An increase in soft tissue shadows due to an effusion is probably the very earliest sign of rheumatoid arthritis, although this is best appreciated clinically. It should alert the radiologist to look for small bone changes.
2. Juxta-articular osteoporosis. Rarefaction of bone due to decreased use caused by pain is a useful localising sign when comparing bilateral symmetrical regions.
3. Uniform narrowing of joint space. This implies loss of cartilage.
4. Erosions at margins of joints (near origin of synovium and capsule). This is the most definitive radiological change and implies removal of bone substance (Figure 3.34).

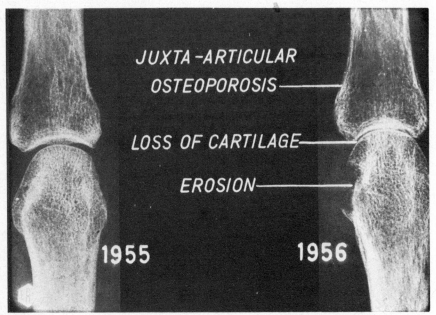

Figure 3.34. Radiograph of metacarpophalangeal joint showing development of erosion one year after onset of rheumatoid arthritis.

Asymmetrical joint changes, particulary if they occur in larger joints, should cast doubt upon the diagnosis since such changes do not reflect the usual pattern of the disease. However, asymmetrical lesions may occur in a patient who is hemiplegic.

In most patients, it takes at least three months for irreversible joint changes to appear (e.g. cartilage thinning or bone erosion). Occasionally, these may not be evident for six months or longer; it is unusual to see them within weeks of clinical onset.

Bone erosion occurs near the attachments of the joint capsule. The most conspicuous sites of erosion correspond to those parts of the bone within the joint which are not covered with articular cartilage. Thus in the metacarpophalangeal joints the erosions tend to occur earliest and most extensively on the radial-volar aspect of the metacarpal heads and they are larger on the proximal than the distal side of the proximal interphalangeal joints of the hands. The ulnar styloid is commonly eroded. Although the bone never returns to normal at the site of erosion, the margins may become sclerotic in long-standing lesions when there is reconstitution of bone.

Radiology is helpful in the diagnosis of conditions mimicking rheumatoid arthritis. In the case of gout, tophi may erode bone outside the joint capsule (unusual in rheumatoid arthritis) and frequently tophi have greater density than surrounding soft tissue. In degenerative arthritis, reactive bone formation is prominent, distal interphalangeal joint involvement is common and osteopenia around joints and metacarpophalangeal joint damage are rare. It should be remembered that degenerative changes in joints are a natural feature of ageing and such features should not be used indiscriminately to explain musculoskeletal symptoms in the elderly. Whereas the radiocarpal and distal radioulnar joints are commonly damaged in rheumatoid arthritis, they are rarely affected in osteoarthrosis. Chondrocalcinosis is a radiological diagnosis of the condition responsible for 'pseudogout' or calcium pyrophosphate arthropathy. This is characterised by attacks of acute arthritis and the finding of crystals

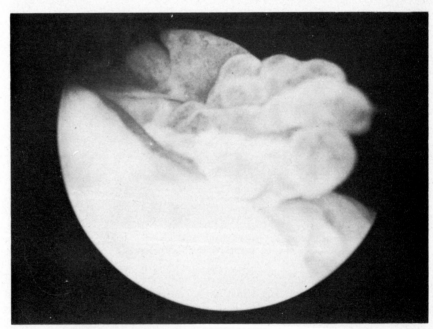

Figure 3.35. Synovial hypertrophy as seen through an arthroscope.

in synovial fluid. Calcification involves fibrocartilage, particularly the menisci of the knee, the triangular cartilage of the wrist, the acetabular and glenoid labra, symphysis pubis and the intravertebral discs. Calcification also appears in the hyaline articular cartilage of synovial joints. Films of the pelvis, knees and wrists therefore constitute an effective screening procedure.

Reiter's syndrome and psoriatic arthritis

Virtually any joint may be involved, but in psoriasis there is commonly terminal interphalangeal joint involvement, particularly of the hands. Persistently asymmetrical joint involvement is much more common than in rheumatoid arthritis and severe destruction of some joints with complete sparing of adjacent ones is common, especially in Reiter's syndrome. Resorption of the ungual tips of the fingers occurs in psoriasis. The pattern of bone erosion and reaction differ from rheumatoid arthritis in that there is extensive destruction of bone ends with little selectivity for marginal areas and bone resorption extends along the shaft. This results in a 'pencil-in-cup' deformity which is characteristic but not pathognomonic. An exuberant subperiosteal reaction is common and is a major distinction between these conditions and rheumatoid arthritis. It is seen particularly in the metacarpals, metatarsals and calcaneus. Spondylitis is common and may be indistinguishable from ankylosing spondylitis (Riley, Ansell and Bywaters, 1971).

There are certain differences between the radiological changes of psoriasis and Reiter's syndrome. Widespread involvement of the hands and wrist is common in psoriasis but unusual in Reiter's syndrome, whereas the latter usually involves the feet. The combination of severe, selective destruction of the pedal joints and sacroiliac arthritis should suggest this diagnosis.

Juvenile rheumatoid arthritis

Abnormalities of bone growth are common, particularly in the fingers and jaw as a result of the disease, altered vascularity and corticosteroid therapy. Single joint involvement is commoner than in adult rheumatoid arthritis and radiological changes may be delayed due to greater cartilage thickness. Later ankylosis is common, affecting particularly the cervical spine.

Ankylosing spondylitis

Evidence of bilateral sacroiliitis is essential for a firm diagnosis, but the interpretation of sacroiliac films can be very difficult in young patients (Macrae, Haslock and Wright, 1971). Indeed the interpretation of early radiological changes at any age is subject to a high degree of observer error and only later changes of bone sclerosis, erosion and fusion are of real diagnostic value. As the disease extends up the intervertebral joints there is 'squaring' of the vertebral bodies and calcification of the annulus fibrosus, giving the characteristic syndesmophytes which fuse to form the classic 'bamboo spine'.

Special Investigations

Ocular electrodiagnostic tests

Three types of electrophysiological measurements are available for clinical use: the electroretinogram, the electro-oculogram and the visually evoked response.

The electroretinogram (ERG) measures the resting current which flows from the outer layers of the retina to the cornea and its modification when the retina is stimulated by a light. The electrical changes are recorded by placing an electrode on the cornea with a contact lens and electrodes on adjacent areas of skin. The normal light-adapted ERG has three components, the a, b, and c waves. The c wave behaves independently of the a and b waves and is derived from the pigment epithelium (Pi). Most of the b wave arises from the inner nuclear layers of the retina (Pii) and the a wave probably arises from the inner segments of the retinal receptors (Piii). The summation of Pi, Pii and Piii gives rise to the ERG.

The electro-oculogram (EOG) measures the modification of the resting potential of the eye when it is moved. Electrodes placed on medial and lateral canthi pick up the current when the eye is moved from left to right as if the eye were a magnet being moved in a magnetic field. The standing potential varies according to the state of dark adaptation so the test is performed first in darkness and then in the light. The lowest potential recorded in the dark is compared with the highest in the light and the result expressed as the Arden index, the normal value of which is 180 per cent. The EOG probably reflects changes in the regeneration of photo-pigment and although the changes in the ERG and EOG parallel each other in pathological conditions, the EOG appears more valuable in conditions where the choroid is affected; certainly the EOG falls very rapidly in patients with necrotising scleral disease before the ERG is much affected.

The visually evoked responses (VER) are the responses recorded over the occipital cortex when a light is repeatedly flashed in the eye, by observation of a chequer-board pattern in which the white and black squares are inter-changed (pattern reversal stimuli). The VER is a foveal response and reflects not only the retinal function in this area but also the integrity of the visual pathway throughout its course, and is markedly reduced in patients with optic nerve or orbital involvement in posterior scleritis.

Ultrasonography

High-frequency sound waves are reflected by interfaces between bodily tissues (echography). Three methods are now available for detailing changes in and around the eye and it seems that the best results are obtained by using a combination of these. A-scan echograms show reflections of ultrasonic energy as vertical lines rising from a horizontal zero line; in B-scan echograms (scanned intensity modulated ultrasound) the scanner is passed across the eye repeatedly, cutting further backwards at each excision. The reflected sound is converted to electrical energy and is portrayed as an oscillograph. As there is a long delay in the fading of the image, a picture of the eye and its contents can be obtained at any particular cross section.

Kinetic A-scan combines the sensitivity of the A-scan with the visual advantages of the B-scan and its sensitivity is such that deficiences and excrescences of the ocular coat of 2 mm or more in size can be portrayed (Ossoinig, 1975, personal communication).

Ultrasonography is now being combined with holography in an attempt to produce three-dimensional views of the eye and orbit.

B-scan ultrasonography can be of great assistance in the detection of posterior swellings of the sclera and intraorbital granulomas. Williamson has used this method to distinguish true deficiences in the sclera from apparent defects where the sclera has become transparent because of repeated attacks of inflammation.

Fluorescein angiography

As a general rule fluorescein angiography of the anterior segment (Bron and Easty, 1970; Amalric and Rebiere, 1971) gives no additional information that cannot be detected by careful slit-lamp examination using red-free light. It had been hoped that in addition to detecting and confirming the presence of avascular areas in the episcleral network of vessels, it would indicate the presence of new vessels and the vessels associated with granulomas, particularly in the early stage of their formation in necrotising scleritis. Unfortunately the leakage from these vessels is so profuse and occurs so early in the arterial phase of dye transit that it has proved impossible to distinguish between congested normal vessels and newly formed or newly opened channels. Fundus fluorescein angiography is also of value in detecting and confirming the early lesions and complications of posterior scleritis.

Ohmic resistance

Oksala and Lehtinen (1960) described a method of measuring the ohmic resistance of the eye and found that it fell in scleral disease. We have not attempted to use this method but it could be useful if there is any doubt as to whether the condition is inflammatory or not. The change in resistance is probably due to the changes occurring in the proteoglycans of the sclera as a result of inflammation.

Skin Testing

Skin testing is often used to screen for specific allergy as the skin is a mirror of immunological changes brought about in the body as a result of exposure to antigens from many different sources. There are three types of hypersensitivity skin test reactions: I, III, and IV, as defined by Coombs and Gell (1975) (Figure 3.36).

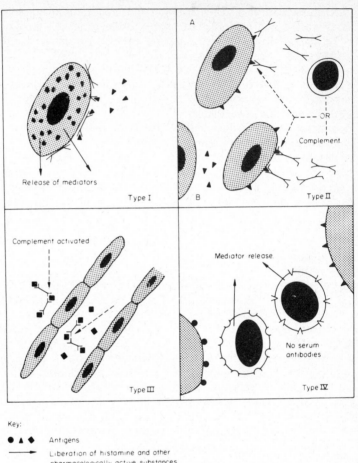

Key:

● ▲ ◆   Antigens

———   Liberation of histamine and other
           pharmacologically active substances

⟩
⟩<⟩ ⟩<⟩   Antibody

- - - - ▶   Sites of involvement of complement or
           non-allergized lymphocytes

⟩ ⟨   Specific antigen-combining receptors on
           membrane of specifically allergized lymphocytes

Figure 3.36.   The different types of hypersensitivity responses.

Type I (immediate) allergy. The reaction develops within minutes as an urticarial weal and resolves within one to two hours. It is attributed to the release of histamine from mast cells sensitised mainly with reaginic IgE antibody, although certain IgG antibodies can also sensitise mast cells. This type of allergic reaction is essentially reversible and not tissue damaging. Type I allergy is tested for by the prick test in which a hypodermic needle is introduced almost horizontally into the superficial epidermis through a drop of allergen extract on the skin. This is particularly useful for many extrinsic allergens, such as pollens, danders and organic materials, but it is not particularly useful in the assessment of drug hypersensitivity. Positive reactions therefore are of practical value in confirming allergens suggested by the history, in suggesting causes otherwise unsuspected and in providing knowledge about the atopic status of the patient. It cannot be used in isolation to identify causes. It must be remembered that negative reactions may be due to inappropriate or inadequate extracts.

Type III (Arthus, late) allergy. This reaction develops over several hours as an oedematous ill-defined swelling. It is maximal at five to seven hours and resolves within 24 to 36 hours. It is mediated by soluble immune complexes formed by the combination of precipitating antibody with a moderate excess of antigen, which then fix and activate the C_3 component of complement. Polymorphonuclear neutrophils are essential for the development of this reaction, and this is potentially tissue damaging. This reaction is utilised particularly in allergic bronchopulmonary conditions, for prick tests give positive reactions in only a small proportion of patients who tend to lack specific IgE antibody (Pepys, 1969).

Type IV (delayed) allergy. This takes 24 to 48 hours to develop and may persist for several days. It consists of a firm induration, possibly with necrosis and surrounding oedema. The reaction is mediated by sensitised lymphocytes. The classic examples of type IV allergy are the reactions to tuberculin introduced into the skin by scratch or prick tests (multiple puncture test), or by an intracutaneous (Mantoux) test and the reactions in contact dermatitis when the allergens are introduced by patch tests. This skin test is taken as evidence of the capacity of the T-cell lymphocyte system of the body to react, and of the body to resist infection. It should not be used to investigate drug hypersensitivity because it is potentially dangerous and a negative test does not exclude possible systemic hypersensitivity. Patch testing is also used to assess contact dermatitis—a cell-mediated response.

Sensitisation with dinitrochlorobenzene is a useful way of screening for defects of cellular responses. In this test 0.1 ml of a two per cent solution in acetone is applied to the skin of the forearm and allowed to evaporate. After a fortnight, challenge is performed by applying 0.1 ml of a 0.05 per cent solution to the opposite arm. This is covered with a sealed dressing for a period of 48 hours and then the degree of induration is measured.

The Kveim test

Sarcoidosis is most reliably confirmed either by histology or biopsy or by a Kveim test reaction. This test is made by injecting intradermally an antigen consisting of a suspension of human sarcoid tissue. The site of injection is marked and biopsy carried out a month later. This reveals a characteristic granuloma in about 80 per cent of active cases but is less often positive in older fibrotic cases (Siltzbach, 1961). False positive reactions occur with some antigens, and it is difficult to obtain validated material for testing.

The tuberculin test

A delayed (type IV) skin reaction in response to purified protein derivative of tuberculin (PPD) may be specific or nonspecific. The former results from previous infection with the tubercle bacillus, the latter from infection with a non-tuberculous organism. The cause of the nonspecific reaction varies in different countries, but in England is often due to infection by avian myco-bacteria (Sutherland, Miller and Hart, 1964). These two responses can usually be distinguished, as those with previous tubercle infection develop a positive skin test to small doses of tuberculin, whereas the nonspecific reaction usually is elicited by larger doses. Positive reactions to the intracutaneous Mantoux test are now taken, for conventional purposes, to consist of an area of induration at least 10 mm diameter.

Examination of Synovial Fluid

In cases of suspected infection or crystal synovitis, culture and examination of the synovial fluid can confirm the diagnosis; joint fluid analysis is not very helpful. Skill in joint aspiration is easily acquired and it is virtually a painless procedure; in fact, removal of fluid often relieves pain. It is important not to introduce infection and scrupulous attention to asepsis is required. The need for local anaesthetic depends on the doctor's skill and the joint to be aspirated.

Fluid for a differential cell count should be placed in anticoagulant. Fluid for crystal examination and for culture should be placed in a sterile container without anticoagulant or preservative and examined within a few hours. It can be kept overnight in a refrigerator at 0 to 4°C for crystal examination.

The characteristics of synovial fluid are listed in Table 3.6. Normal results have been omitted but are essentially those of non-inflammatory joint disease. However, these findings must be interpreted in the light of clinical and other laboratory features because considerable overlapping of the groups can occur.

Table 3.6. *Synovial fluid changes in joint diseases*

	Non-inflammatory degenerative joint diseases, etc.	Inflammatory rheumatoid arthritis, crystal synovitis	Septic bacterial infection
Colour	Clear	Turbid	Turbid
Viscosity	High	Low	Low
WBC (per mm³)	< 2000	2000–50 000	> 50 000
Polymorphs (%)	< 25	< 50	> 75
Protein	< 5 g/100 ml	< 5 g/100 ml	> 5 g/100 ml
Glucose	= to blood	Decreased	Decreased

Histological examination

There are several features to look for:

1. In rubella arthritis, mononuclear cells predominate.

2. In Reiter's syndrome mononuclear cells containing polymorphonuclear inclusions are often a feature (Pekin cells) (Pekin, Malinin and Zvaifler, 1967).
3. Rhagocytes (polymorphonuclear cells containing particulate inclusions which often include rheumatoid factor) are characteristic, but not specific for rheumatoid arthritis.

Identification of pathological crystals

In practice urates and calcium pyrophosphate crystals are the only crystals of significance to be identified in synovial fluid. Other crystals which may be seen are cholesterol and corticosteroid esters after intra-articular therapy. Urates and calcium pyrophosphate can be accurately identified by utilising the concept of polarising light as there are differences in crystal lattice structure. Urate crystals show strong negative birefringence; calcium pyrophosphate crystals show weak positive birefringence when viewed under the compensated polarised light microscope (Currey, 1968).

Arthroscopy

The arthroscope is being used more frequently as a diagnostic tool. It is particularly useful in aiding the diagnosis in persistent arthritis of the knees and helps to distinguish between inflammatory (Figure 3.35) and degenerative disease.

Arthroscopy can be carried out using local anaesthetic under aseptic conditions. It is possible to examine the appearances of the synovium, articular cartilage, menisci and cruciate ligaments and allow a biopsy to be taken under direct vision. In gout highly refractile white deposits may be seen, whereas calcium pyrophosphate crystals do not have the same qualities.

Unfortunately, synovial biopsy material rarely provides diagnostic evidence. Although the differences between osteoarthritis and inflammatory joint disease are usually clear enough, there is little to distinguish one inflammatory arthritis from another. The finding of crystals, the granulomas of sarcoid and tuberculosis, tumour tissue or amyloid deposits is helpful.

Muscle Biopsy

Biopsy of the most obviously involved muscle will usually provide diagnostic evidence of a myositic process which is most common in dermatomyositis or polymyositis but which may be a feature of any connective tissue disease.

The serum levels of aldolase and transaminases are useful in suspected myositis (Pearson, 1966). The creatine phosphokinase estimation is the most valuable but is not a routine procedure in all laboratories. The values generally correlate well with the activity of the myositis but in chronic cases there may be insufficient muscle bulk remaining to cause elevated values.

Scleral and Episcleral Biopsy

Whilst this method of obtaining a diagnosis can sometimes be of great help in the difficult case, it should be avoided if at all possible because of the very considerable likelihood of perforating the globe if a necrotic scleral nodule is attacked. In the past the operation has usually been performed under local anaesthetic which, combined with the unavoidable trauma in handling the episcleral tissue leads to a massive and immediate outpouring of cells making the histological appearances difficult to interpret. If possible therefore the procedure should be undertaken in theatre with full precautions, under general anaesthetic with the absolute minimal handling of the tissues (see Chapter 10).

REFERENCES

Alarçon Segovia, D. (1975) Drug induced systemic lupus erythematosus and related syndromes. In *Clinics in Rheumatic Diseases*, Vol. 1, pp. 573–583. London: W.B. Saunders.

Alexander, W. R. & McCarthy, D. D. (1966) The significance of the rheumatoid factor. In *Modern Trends in Rheumatology* (Ed.) Hill, A. G. p. 153. London: Butterworth.

Amalric, P. & Rebiere, P. (1971) Fluorescein angiography of anterior segment of the eye: examples of corneal and scleral pathology. *Annales d'Oculistique*, **204**, 731.

Bonomo, L. (1957) Hyperglobulinaemia in rheumatoid arthritis, its relationship with disease activity and its changes under adrenocortical treatment. *Annals of the Rheumatic Diseases*, **16**, 340–351.

Böttiger, L. E. & Svedberg, C. A. (1967) Normal erythrocyte sedimentation rate and age. *British Medical Journal*, **ii**, 85–87.

Bron, A. J. (1973) A simple scheme for documenting corneal disease. *British Journal of Ophthalmology*, **57**, 629–634.

Bron, A. J. & Easty, D. L. (1970) Fluorescein angiography of the globe and anterior segment. *Transactions of the Ophthalmological Societies of the United Kingdom*, **90**, 339–367.

Cass, R. M., Mongan, E. S., Jacox, R. F. et al (1968) Immunoglobulins G, A and M in systemic lupus erythematosus. Relationship to serum complement titer, latex titer, antinuclear antibody, and manifestations of clinical disease. *Annals of Internal Medicine*, **69**, 749–756.

Coombs, R. R. & Gell, P. G. (1975) In *Clinical Aspects of Immunology* (Ed.) Gell, P. G., Coombs, R. R. & Lachmann, P.J. 3rd edition. Oxford: Blackwell Scientific Publications.

Currey, H. L. F. (1968) Examination of joint fluids for crystals. *Proceedings of the Royal Society of Medicine*, **61**, 969–971.

Dixon, A. St J. (1960) Rheumatoid arthritis with negative serological reaction. *Annals of the Rheumatic Diseases*, **19**, 209–228.

Duke Elder, S. (1965) *System of Ophthalmology*, Vol. 8, p. 24. London: Kimpton.

Fraunfelder, F. T. & Watson, P. G. (1976) Evaluation of eyes enucleated for scleritis. *British Journal of Ophthalmology*, **60**, 227–230.

Hall, A. P., Barry, P. E., Dawber, T. R. et al (1967) Epidemiology of gout and hyperuricaemia. *American Journal of Medicine*, **42**, 27–37.

Hijmans, W. (1966) The L.E. cell phenomenon and the antinuclear factors. In *Modern Trends in Rheumatology* (Ed.) Hill, A. G. p. 175 London: Butterworth.

Hill, A. & Greenburg, C. L. (1965) Clinical interpretation of serological tests in rheumatoid arthritis. In *Progress in Clinical Rheumatology* (Ed.) Dixon A. St. J. p. 42. London: Churchill.

Hughes, G. R. (1973) Immunological factors in systemic lupus erythematosus. In *9th Symposium of Advanced Medicine* (Ed.) Walker, J. C. p. 67. London: Pitman.

Hughes, G. R. (1975) Antinucleic acid antibodies in S.L.E.: clinical and pathological significance. In *Clinics in Rheumatic Diseases*, Vol. 1. pp. 545–561. London: W. B. Saunders.

Hughes, G. R., Cohen, S. A. & Christian, C. L. (1971) Anti DNA activity in systemic lupus erythematosus: a diagnostic and therapeutic guide. *Annals of the Rheumatic Diseases*, **30**, 259–264.

Hunder, G. G. & Pierre, R. V. (1970) In vivo L.E. cell formation in synovial fluid. *Arthritis and Rheumatism*, **13**, 448–454.

Kanagasundaram, C. R. (1956) Episcleral microaneurysms. *British Journal of Ophthalmology*, **40**, 568–570.

Lawrence, J. S., Valkenburg, H. A., Bremner, J. M. et al (1970) Rheumatoid factor in families. *Annals of the Rheumatic Diseases*, **29**, 269–274.

Macrae, I. F., Haslock, D. I. & Wright, V. (1971) Grading for films for sacro-iliitis in population studies. *Annals of the Rheumatic Diseases*, **30**, 58–66.

McCormick, J. N. (1975) Rheumatoid factor—its significance in the pathogenesis of disease. In *Current Topics in Connective Tissue Disease* (Ed.) Holt, P. London: Churchill.

McKenna, C. H., Schroeter, A. L., Kierland, R. R. et al (1973) The fluorescent treponemal antibody absorbed (FTA ABS) test beading phenomenon in connective tissue diseases. *Proceeding of the Mayo Clinic*, **48**, 545–548.

Mongan, E. S., Cass, R. M., Jacox, R. F. et al (1969) A study of the relation of sero-negative and seropositive rheumatoid arthritis to each other and to necrotising vasculitis. *American Journal of Medicine*, **47**, 23–35.

Mowat, A. G. (1971) Anaemia in rheumatoid arthritis. In *Modern Trends in Rheumatology* (Ed.) Hill, A. G. pp. 106–116. London: Butterworth.

Murray, R. M., Lawson, D. H. & Linton, A. L. (1971) Analgesic nephropathy; clinical syndrome and prognosis. *British Medical Journal*, **i**, 479–482.

Oksala, A. & Lehtinen, A. (1960) Experimental and clinical study on the ohmic resistance of the cornea and sclera. *Acta Ophthalmologica*, **38**, 153–162.

Pearson, C. M. (1966) Polymyositis. *Annual Review of Medicine*, **17**, 63–82.

Pekin, T. J., Malinin, T. I. & Zvaifler, N. J. (1967) Unusual synovial fluid findings in Reiter's syndrome. *Annals of Internal Medicine*, **66**, 677–684.

Pepys, J. (1969) *Hypersensitivity Diseases due to Inhaled Fungi and Organic Dusts.* Basle: Karger.

Riley, M. J., Ansell, B. M. & Bywaters, E. G. (1971) Radiological manifestations of ankylosing spondylitis according to age at onset. *Annals of the Rheumatic Diseases*, **30**, 138–148.

Rose, H. M., Ragan, C., Pearce, E. et al (1948) Differential agglutination of normal and sensitised sheep erythrocyte by sera of patients with rheumatoid arthritis. *Proceedings of the Society for Experimental Biology,* **68**, 1–6.

Schaller, J. G., Johnson, G. D., Holborow, E. J. et al (1974) The association of antinuclear antibodies with the chronic iridocyclitis of juvenile rheumatoid arthritis (Still's disease). *Arthritis and Rheumatism*, **17**, 409–416.

Siltzbach, L. E. (1961) The Kveim test in sarcoidosis; a study of 750 patients. *Journal of the American Medical Association*, **178**, 476–482.

Sutherland, I., Miller, C. L. & Hart, P. D. (1964) Further studies of sensitivity to avian and human old tuberculin in man. *Tubercle*, **45**, 110–113.

Torrigiani, G., Roitt, I. M., Lloyd, K. N. et al (1970) Elevated IgG antiglobulins in patients with seronegative rheumatoid arthritis. *Lancet*, **i**, 14–16.

Tuffanelli, D. L. (1968) False positive reactions for syphilis. Serological abnormalities in relatives of chronic reactors. *Archives of Dermatology*, **98**, 606–611.

Waaler, E. (1940) On the occurrence of a factor in human serum activating the specific agglutination of sheep blood corpuscles. *Acta Pathologica et Microbiologica Scandinavica*, **17**, 172–188.

CHAPTER FOUR

Clinical Presentation of Inflammatory Episcleral and Scleral Disease

'Yet with toil all that I can attain
By long experience, and in learned schools,
Is for to know that my knowledge is but vain,
And those who think them wise are greatest fools.'
Tragedy of Croesus, II, i (William Alexander, 1567–1640).

Clinical examination of the patient when he is first seen will determine whether the inflammation is confined to the episclera or whether the underlying scleral tissue is also involved. Although certain neoplastic, degenerative and specific inflammatory conditions can be distinguished by clinical examination alone, the majority of patients present with inflammatory signs only. Fortunately, further subdivision of scleritis and episcleritis is both possible, because their clinical appearances differ, and useful because the different types follow different courses and have different prognostic significance.

The differentiation between episcleritis and scleritis has been, and still is, considered by some to be of little importance. Nothing could be further from the truth. Episcleritis is a benign recurrent disease, only rarely being anything but of nuisance value to the patient, whereas scleritis not only causes great pain, misery and discomfort to the patient, but often portends more serious underlying systemic disease. This is not a new problem: Campbell in 1903, in his article on episcleritis, says that considering 'the pathology of the various lesions grouped under this term, one will immediately see that the term episcleritis is not only insufficient but that it is positively misleading; that it is, in short, a term which has by usage, or rather by insufficient detail in classification, been made to do duty for various lesions which are pathologically quite divergent and that they manifest a wide variety of clinical manifestation'. He also says, 'I have never known an acute episcleritis to be complicated by an acute scleritis'. This indeed is the case. It is an extreme rarity for a true episcleritis to progress to involve the deep scleral tissue; we have known it to occur for certain three or four times in the patients with episcleritis we have studied (this excludes three patients with herpes zoster, see page 95). We have even seen one patient who had an episcleritis in one area and a deep scleritis in another area of the same eye, and even though he has had many recurrences over the several years we have been observing him, the inflammation has remained true to type, confined to the areas originally affected.

Detection of scleral disease is important, not only because 46 per cent of these patients have other systemic diseases, but also, if in addition they develop necrotising scleral disease, the chances of them being dead within eight years are about one in five. Early diagnosis leads to early treatment, and if this is adequate and correctly applied both sight and life may be preserved or prolonged.

Many classifications of scleral disease have been proposed: Wolfe (1882), Holthouse (1893), Campbell (1903), van der Hoeve (1934), Franceschetti and Bischler (1950), Duke Elder and Leigh (1965a), Sevel (1967). These have been based on a mixture of clinical and pathological observations and none could be made to correspond with the changes which we had observed clinically.

With some reluctance we have opted for an entirely clinical classification which has the merit that one can detect the various types at the first examination:

Episcleritis
    Simple
    Nodular
Anterior scleritis
    Diffuse scleritis
    Nodular scleritis
    Necrotising scleritis
        (a) with inflammation
        (b) without inflammation (scleromalacia perforans)
Posterior scleritis

There is some overlap between the groups, particularly between the different types of necrotising scleritis, but we have found over the past 12 years that we have been able to assign almost all of our patients to their correct category at the initial examination.

INCIDENCE

It is extremely difficult to arrive at any estimate of the incidence of these conditions, for all the series published are biased in some form or another. Judging from the casualty outpatient attendances at Moorfields Eye Hospital, London, patients are seen with episcleritis about twice as frequently as scleritis, but because episcleritis is not serious and is evanescent, most patients put up with it or are treated by themselves or by general practitioners. They only attend hospital if the recurrences are severe and persistent or they themselves are unduly anxious about them. Williamson (1974) found that only eight cases of scleritis presented at the Eye Department of the Southern General Hospital and Victoria Infirmary, Glasgow out of 9600 new patient referrals (0.08 per cent). Our own series of 220 patients (299 eyes) with episcleritis and 320 cases (464 eyes) of scleritis seen at the Scleritis Clinic at Moorfields Eye Hospital, London is from highly selected patients, all being referred from other departments in the hospital or from elsewhere, either because of intractable recurrent disease, or because there was some difficulty in diagnosis, or because they had an unusual problem. This is reflected in the fact that 90 per cent of the patients who had rheumatoid arthritis were seen within a year of the start of the special clinic.

Even though it is recognised that the figures will be biased in favour of the more serious diseases, the incidence of the various clinically recognised types is given in Table 4.1. Only those patients where the diagnosis of necrotising anterior scleritis is absolutely certain have been included in this category. The incidence may well have been greater than this since active treatment has certainly prevented some patients from developing necrotic lesions. The appearance of necrotising lesions often coincides with a change in the patient's associated systemic condition, and although necrotising scleritis is sometimes obvious when the patient first presents, it may well start as a diffuse or nodular anterior scleritis.

Table 4.1. *Incidence of episcleritis and scleritis*

Diagnosis	Further subdivisions	
Episcleritis	Simple	78.3
	Nodular	21.7
Scleritis	Diffuse anterior	39.6
	Nodular anterior	44.5
	Necrotising	13.9
	with inflammation	9.6
	without inflammation	4.3
	Posterior	2.0

EPISCLERITIS

Simple Episcleritis

The usual sufferer from this type of episcleritis is a young woman who complains that from time to time, and for no particular reason, one eye or the other becomes red, uncomfortable and prickly. There is no discharge and, if nothing is done, the discomfort reaches its peak in 24 hours and gradually subsides during the next ten days. When the inflammation has disappeared, the eye looks and feels perfectly normal whilst she waits for the recurrence which will inevitably occur either in the same place or in another part of the same or opposite eye within the next two months.

The condition, which is twice as common in women as in men, has its peak incidence in the fourth decade. The onset is usually sudden, the eye becoming red, swollen and painful within half an hour of the attack starting. Sometimes, however, there are no symptoms, the redness of the eye being noticed only by accident, whilst looking in the mirror or because attention is drawn to it by another person. The commonest sensations complained of are 'hotness', 'sharpness', 'pricking' and 'discomfort'. Of the 51 per cent who describe the eye as painful, this pain is localised to the eye itself, rather than radiating around the eye as in classic scleral disease.

The redness is often intense and in one-third of the patients congestion covers the whole of the white of the eye but in two-thirds it remains localised to one segment. If the eye becomes tender the tenderness is localised to the site of the inflammation. Although the eyes may water, there is no discharge, but in a severe attack the inflammatory response may be so intense that the lids may swell and the conjunctiva and episclera become chemosed, this reaction being accompanied by miosis, temporary myopia and occasionally severe photophobia (Figure 4.1).

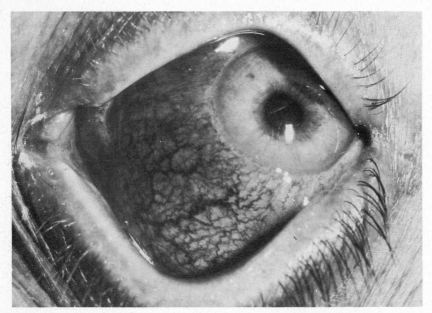

Figure 4.1.   Intense congestion of the episcleral vessels with chemosis of the conjunctiva and miosis of the pupil in a patient with a severe attack of simple episcleritis. These signs resolved within 72 hours leaving a white apparently completely normal eye.

The episclera is diffusely oedematous in the region of the congestion but remains normal elsewhere; the episcleral vessels, although they are engorged, retain their normal radial position and architecture (Figure 4.2). Depending on the intensity of this engorgement the colour of the eye can vary from fiery redness to a mild red flush. The diffuse infiltration of the episcleral tissue which sometimes occurs in this condition shows up as yellow subconjunctival discolouration when viewed with a red-free light. Histologically this infiltration has been shown to be due to masses of lymphocytes, occasional eosinophils and mast cells but no polymorphs.

Episcleritis is most common in the interpalpebral region, often flitting from one side to the other with each attack and even affecting both eyes together. However, some patients always develop the inflammation at the same site. One of our patients who received no treatment over a period of two years

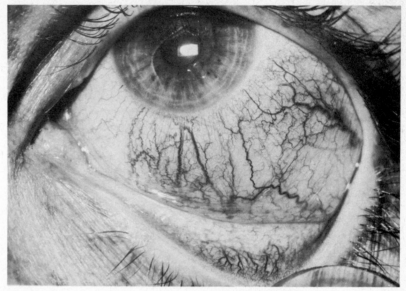

Figure 4.2.   The more usual type of simple episcleritis in which the congestion is segmental
and the vessels retain their normal radial architecture.

kept a careful record of the duration and intensity of his attacks of simple
episcleritis. They varied from the evanescent to as long as one month, and
in intensity from the very mild to the very severe, but there was no predictable
pattern. The majority of the attacks lasted between five and ten days. That
this is indeed the normal pattern in episcleritis was confirmed by a double-
blind controlled study, in the course of which one group of patients was
given a placebo (Watson et al, 1973) (Figure 10.1).

Although the duration of the disease varies a great deal, several patterns
of behaviour have emerged. In over 60 per cent of patients the condition
lasts for three to six years. In those who have the condition for longer—this
can be as long as 30 years—the attacks reduce in frequency after the first
three to four years so that attacks which have been at monthly intervals
occur only after intervals of more than two years. Those who develop the
episcleritis before puberty cease to develop further attacks at puberty and
those who develop attacks at puberty no longer have them at the menopause.
This implies a hormonal mechanism in the progress of the condition and
Alt (1903), Benedict (1924), Moench (1927), Villard (1930), Paufique and
Etienne (1949) and Drouet and Thomas (1952) have suggested that simple
episcleritis is associated with the disturbance of menstruation. We have noticed
this in only one patient whose attacks always occurred two days before her
period was due. Unfortunately, treatment with the contraceptive pill did not
make any difference to the recurrence of her attacks, except that the attacks
then occurred with the onset of the withdrawal bleeding.

Simple episcleritis with its transient character and a strong tendency to
recur with regular periodicity has been recognised for over a century and
has been called many different names: subconjunctivitis by von Graefe, sub-

conjunctival phlegma or simple or phlegmatous conjunctivitis by Mackenzie (1830), and episcleritis periodica fugax by Fuchs (1895), the term adopted by Duke Elder and Leigh (1965b). Judging from the histological appearances and from the sudden onset and its tendency to be worse in spring and autumn, this should be a type I (immediate) hypersensitivity reaction. Very occasionally a clear history of exogenous sensitisation is given, e.g. contact with printing inks; in one instance the patient had only to be inside the printing works for his eyes to flare up. Exposure to the vapours of the ink also produced an attack under hospital conditions but skin testing gave negative results. Skin testing does not suggest increased incidence of atopic disease in any of our patients. Ten of 23 patients investigated by McGavin et al (1976) reacted to some antigen, usually house dust mites. Three of the four who had positive tests to multiple antigens gave a clear history of either hay fever or asthma, very similar to our own series. Two of our patients developed their episcleritis whilst undergoing a course of desensitisation vaccinations for hay fever. As with duodenal ulceration and many other complaints, it is very noticeable that if there are family upsets and worry at work the inflammation will flare up. Sometimes there is a definite psychogenic background, as in the case of a childless woman who developed attacks of episcleritis every nine months until she had an infant, when all trouble ceased (Inman, 1955).

Eleven per cent of our patients had a persistently high serum uric acid level (more than 7.5 mg/100 ml on three readings) and seven per cent had clinical gout. Sometimes patients who have gout will recognise that it is becoming out of control, by noticing the pricking sensation of the eye. If they do not take the appropriate systemic medication they develop either an attack of episcleritis or a full-blown attack of gout.

Heinonen (1923, 1927) suggested that this condition was transmitted as a mendelian dominant characteristic. We have certainly not found this; only seven patients out of the 220 records analysed gave any suggestion of a family history, and in only one of these patients did the attacks seem to resemble the parent's attacks in any detail. We have never seen the type of simple episcleritis which starts suddenly and has frequent recurrences to involve the sclera, nor have we seen any permanent corneal changes following the inflammation, although on several occasions the conjunctiva has been quite grossly oedematous and the lids swollen (Fuchs, 1895).

There is a less well-defined group of patients with simple episcleritis who gave no history of periodicity but rather of mild, prolonged attacks of inflammation. Into this category come almost all those patients who had some other inter-current disease. Five patients had a positive Wassermann reaction, four patients had mild seropositive rheumatoid arthritis with only a few joint symptoms, and one each had erythema multiforme, active tuberculosis, Henoch–Schönlein purpura and rosacea. Herpes simplex had grown from one lesion. Pal (1953) described a patient with ariboflavinosis and amoebic hepatitis who developed a periodic episcleritis which disappeared after treatment of the general condition. McGavin et al (1976) found that all their nine patients with rheumatoid arthritis and episcleritis fell into this category. Even though the history was different, the appearances of the episcleritis did not differ in the two groups and in neither did the episcleritis progress to a scleritis, except in three patients with herpes zoster. In these patients the episcleritis appeared with the vesicular phase of the rash and disappeared completely when the rash had subsided. The scleritis appeared at the same site some three months later but did not progress from one to the other. It could be suggested that the group of patients with this mild prolonged type of episcleritis may represent the earlier stages of a benign form of scleritis. If this were so, one would expect a significant number of cases to progress from episcleritis to scleritis. This is very rare and it seems more likely that episcleritis and scleritis are two different types of reaction to similar antigen within the different tissues.

Nodular Episcleritis

The symptoms of nodular episcleritis are similar to those of simple episcleritis but the course of the condition is much more protracted. Contrary to the traditionally accepted view (Duke Elder and Leigh, 1965) we have found the age and sex incidence to be the same as that for simple episcleritis, with females being affected more than males in a ratio of 2:1. The males almost all developed the disease between 20 and 50 and although women developed the condition most commonly in the forties the distribution is very even from 20 to 70.

The inflammatory signs usually start with slight redness or discomfort in the eye. Over a period of two to three days the area of redness remains localised but increases in size. The episclera becomes infiltrated and oedematous, forming a tender nodule in 40 per cent of the patients (Figure 4.3). The conjunctiva can be moved over the nodule which is firm to the touch and

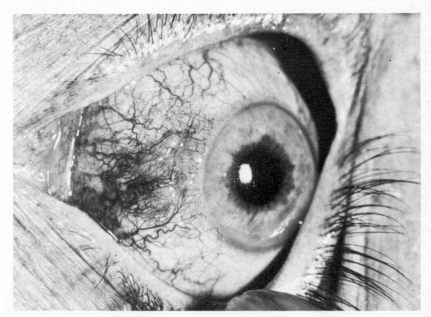

Figure 4.3.   Nodular episcleritis. Oedema and infiltration of the episcleral tissue have caused several small nodules to form. The deep episcleral plexus can be seen deep to the nodules on the sclera which has a normal contour and is not swollen.

only moves very slightly on the underlying sclera. The inflammation, although intense, is confined to the episclera. By careful examination on the slit lamp, particularly with a red-free light, the underlying scleral vessels can be seen lying flat on the sclera which retains its normal contour (Figure 4.4). It is sometimes necessary to decongest the episcleral blood vessels using adrenalin 1/1000 or phenylephrine 10 per cent so that the underlying sclera can be seen clearly. It is very important to determine the depth of the inflammation as soon as the patient is first seen for the most severe form of scleritis, necrotising scleritis, may start with nodular *scleral* disease. If an episcleritis is diagnosed when it is a scleritis, inadequate treatment will be given, but if necrotising nodular scleritis is diagnosed and it is only a nodular episcleritis, far too many potentially hazardous drugs will be given. The episcleral nodule itself is usually very well defined. It is unusual for the surrounding episclera to be inflamed but in some cases, particularly when multiple nodules appear, the rest of the episclera can become congested.

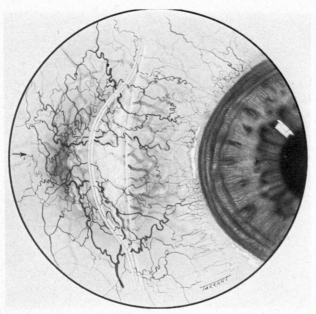

Figure 4.4.   A drawing of the slit-lamp appearances in nodular episcleritis. Although the deep episcleral plexus is congested, the normal curvature of the sclera is maintained.

The purple colour of the nodules is due to the intense vascular congestion of the capillary network, the oedema and the inflammatory exudate which can be seen with the red-free light as a yellow patch (Figure 4.5). The inflammation seems to allow new venous channels to open up so that sometimes the vessels appear to radiate from the nodule. The size of the nodules varies considerably: most are about 2 to 3 mm in size, sometimes multiple and occasionally confluent, but they can be much larger. Campbell (1903) described a nodule which increased in size to one-quarter of the globe before it regressed.

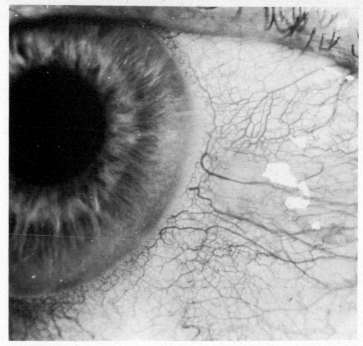

Figure 4.5.   Nodular episcleritis in which there is a marked inflammatory exudate. In red-free light this exudate becomes very easy to see as it is yellow in colour in contrast with the rest of the episclera which is green.

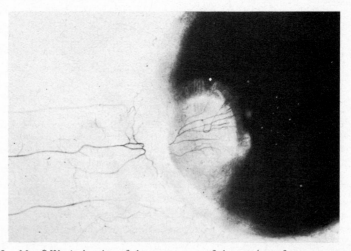

Figure 4.6.   Mrs S.W. A drawing of the appearance of the eye just after a severe recurrence of nodular episcleritis which had occurred at the same site eight times in the preceding two years. The episclera and cornea are still oedematous. Some keratic precipitates can be seen adjacent to the oedematous cornea.

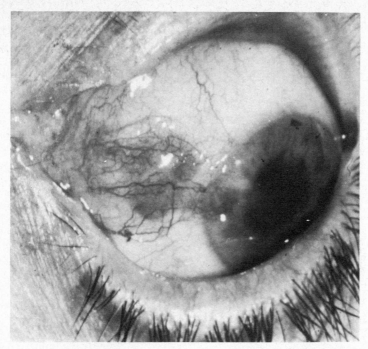

Figure 4.7.   Mrs S.W. Photograph of the same eye one week later. At the site of the episcleral nodule the sclera has become grey and translucent. This alteration in the sclera and cornea is unusual in purely episcleral disease, but can occur after repeated attacks at the same site.

As with simple episcleritis, recurrences occur either in the same place in the same eye, elsewhere in the same eye, or bilaterally. Each attack is self-limiting and usually clears without treatment, but because of the size of the nodule each attack lasts longer than in simple episcleritis, often four to five weeks, but when it disappears the sclera appears as before the attack.

Increased scleral translucency is regarded as evidence that there has been deep scleral disease at some time. Indeed, if translucency is seen there should always be a suspicion that this is indeed an attack of scleritis and not episcleritis which is being investigated. However, if episcleritis recurs constantly at one site over several years, particularly if the initial attack followed herpes zoster, the structure of the underlying sclera will become altered and it will become translucent (Figures 4.6 and 4.7). The same is true of the cornea. As a rule, no changes occur in the cornea in episcleritis, but repeated attacks of episcleritis in the same position, adjacent to the limbus, often lead to diffuse stromal corneal changes (Figure 4.8).

Duke Elder and Leigh (1965d) described a rheumatic nodular episcleritis but we have been unable to recognise this as a separate entity. In fact, most of the episcleritis occurring with rheumatoid arthritis is of the diffuse variety. In 1939 Suganuma in Japan described a condition in which multiple nodules appeared near the limbus and were associated with conjunctival hyperaemia, discharge and sometimes iritis. The nodules were shown histologically to consist of mononuclear cells and eosinophils. This condition was said to be associated with rheumatoid arthritis, but we have never seen it. We have, however, seen an episcleral nodule with sarcoidosis as described by Klein et al (1955) and Donaldson (1964) and on several occasions others which have been an expression of erythema nodosum. It has also been suggested that these episcleral nodules are more common in connective tissue disease but this has not been our experience.

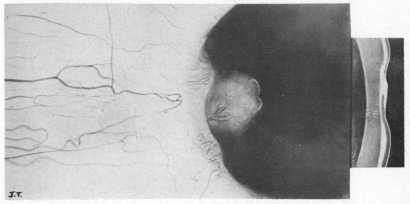

Figure 4.8. Mrs S.W. Drawing—two weeks later the corneal changes have regressed but an area of permanent opacity remains.

SCLERITIS

Inflammation involving the sclera anterior to the equator accounts for about 95 per cent of clinically diagnosed scleritis. Even allowing for the fact that posterior scleritis is underdiagnosed, most cases of scleritis involve the anterior segment. The reason for this is obscure. It is certainly true that the anterior sclera has very many more perforating vessels, but the posterior segment is equally and perhaps even better supplied with extracellular nutriment than the anterior segment, as it is derived from the choroidal plexus of vessels. It does not appear to be necessary for blood vessels to be present for granulomas to form and when granulomas do form in the posterior sclera they are identical to those found in anterior scleritis.

The symptoms of scleral disease, as might be expected from the swelling and destructive changes which take place, are very much more severe in scleritis than episcleritis, pain being the most dominant feature (Figure 4.9). Scleritis is one of the very few severely painful eye conditions, presumably because of direct destruction of the nerve fibres in the sclera and the distension of the organ itself. The pain can be so severe that physicians have doubted whether the pain comes from the eye at all; one of our patients was fully investigated by neurosurgeons as it was thought that he had a cerebral tumour. Wardrop in 1818 described the pain thus:

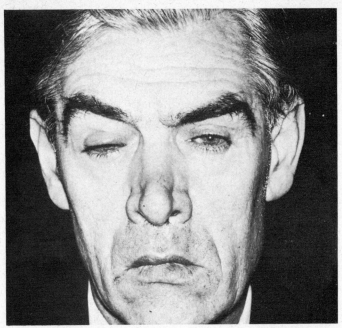

Figure 4.9. The appearance of a patient with severe anterior diffuse scleritis. There is a marked ptosis and some watering of both eyes. The pain, which was felt mainly in the temple and jaw prevented him from sleeping and he preferred not to move the right side of his face because this hurt the eye.

'The seat as well as the kind of pain affords striking characters of this peculiar affection. Generally the chief seat of pain at the commencement of the disease is in the head, though it sometimes also affects the eyeball itself. The pain is usually most severe in the temple of the affected side, but it is often seated in the brow, the cheekbone, the teeth, or the lower jaw. Sometimes the pain is precisely confined to one half of the head, and sometimes there is a severe pain in the cavity of the nose or in the ear. These pains are more of a dull agonizing kind than acute; and though in this disease the pain may be unceasing, yet it varies much in degree, coming on at times in very severe paroxysms, and recurring with great violence when the head is bent downwards. Sometimes the pain is excited by merely touching the scalp, and the patient is unable to rest his head on the affected side or even lean it on a pillow. The pain in most cases is remittent, the paroxysm coming on at four, six or eight o'clock in the evening, continuing during the night, being most severe about midnight, and suffering an abatement towards morning'.

Mackenzie's description (1830) was as 'pulsative, deep-seated; the chief pain, however, is not so much in the eyeball as around the orbit, under the eyebrow and in the temple, cheek, and the side of the nose and is severely aggravated from sunset to sunrise'.

These descriptions cannot be bettered. The pain which increases in the night is one of the worst features, because it is unrelieved by analgesics and narcotics. As a consequence, two patients who were referred to us had had so little sleep and had lost so much weight that they were almost suicidal, begging for the eye to be removed. Their improvement when the pain was relieved by medical treatment had to be seen to be believed. Sixty per cent of our patients with scleritis complained of pain of this severity, but although many others suffered less discomfort, only those with scleromalacia perforans had no pain at all. In his description of scleritis, Wardrop (1818) wrote:

'In the eyeball the patient generally complains more of a sense of fulness and distention than of pain; and though there is a great degree of external redness in this disease, the eye does not seem to suffer from exposure to light, for the eyelids are kept open without appearing to create uneasiness; whereas in most other inflammatory affections of this organ even a very moderate quantity of light cannot be endured'.

We are able to confirm this statement: although 70 per cent of our patients did have some photophobia, it was rarely severe nor was the watering which accompanied it. The photophobia was not made worse by a keratitis, by involvement of the posterior segment, or by the presence of uveitis. We had thought that a reduction of corneal sensitivity might be the reason for so little photophobia, but this has not proved to be the case. The lid contraction which accompanies photophobia is reinforced by a retinal reflex and is possibly the reason that dark glasses help some individuals, but patients with the severest forms of scleritis do not even feel they need this simple aid.

The onset of scleritis is usually insidious, but it is almost always possible to detect the more severe necrotising disease from the more benign diffuse and nodular anterior scleritis, and, although the divisions we have adopted may be somewhat artificial, because we may have prevented necrotising disease from developing in some patients who presented with an anterior diffuse or nodular scleritis, we feel that they are distinct enough to be worthy of separate descriptions. Furthermore, although scleritis is one and a half times as common in women, in all the types, the age and sex distributions vary within the different clinical types. In all the types, about half the cases are bilateral, the second eye becoming involved either within three months of the onset of the disease or a very long time afterwards—in our series over six years. Surprisingly, we found no exceptions to this. Scleritis like episcleritis is a recurrent condition; 69 per cent of patients with scleritis can be expected to have recurrences, some for as long as 30 years or more.

If the scleritis seen in the initial attack is treated fully and effectively, only 20 per cent develop recurrences. The recurrence rate rises rapidly with delay in treatment of the initial attack; if this has been left untreated for three months, the recurrence rate rises to 60 per cent. It is therefore most important to deal effectively with the first attack. Once the disease has advanced to the necrotising stage, patients need very careful follow-up because the disease may continue to progress, even though they are symptom-free and seem to have entered the quiescent stage.

Anterior diffuse and nodular scleritis last about five to six years as compared to four years with episcleral disease, the frequency of recurrence diminishing after the first 18 months. Once necrotising scleritis occurs, however, the disease is progressive with induced or spontaneous remission but never total resolution. A family history was only elicited in three per cent of 207 of our patients with scleritis and in only one of these patients was the similarity of the type of disease remarkable. Marquand (1956) described two sisters with scleromalacia perforans.

The mortality of patients with scleritis is high, particularly if they have necrotising scleritis and connective tissue disease, nearly 30 per cent of our series being dead within eight years of the onset of the disease. McGavin et al (1976) found that their patients with rheumatoid arthritis and scleritis had a very poor prognosis, 45 per cent dying within the period of follow-up. Both series showed that death was largely due to vascular disease (82 per cent in each) which probably resulted from the generalised systemic vasculitis of which the scleritis was just a part.

Anterior Scleritis

Diffuse anterior scleritis

Diffuse anterior scleritis is the most benign form of anterior scleritis. It is also the variety which leads to the most difficulty in diagnosis and because in the early stages the symptoms and signs are not severe it tends not to be taken seriously and is under-treated.

The condition is commonest in females in the fourth to seventh decades but when men are affected, they are between the third and sixth decade, the majority presenting in the fourth decade. The course of the condition is illustrated by the following case:

Case study. A young married woman aged 34 developed what she thought was toothache or sinusitis, having been woken at night with an ache in the right side of her face. She saw her dentist who pronounced her mouth healthy and confirmed with x-rays that she did not have a root abscess. The ache continued for a week so she consulted her general practitioner who could not find anything amiss in the sinuses but did notice that the right eye was congested inside the lower lid. As the patient had not complained of the eye and the eye was not tender, he had the sinuses x-rayed to eliminate an ethmoid or sphenoidal sinusitis and treated the patient with simple analgesics and a narcotic for the night. She slept better on this and was symptomatically improved for a further week, but the eye was becoming redder and the lower lid a little more swollen so the doctor referred her to the hospital, where she was found to have a diffuse anterior scleritis (Figure 4.10).

The insidious onset, with symptoms referred to other parts of the head, is quite typical of this condition. Every now and then the onset can be acute, and if the scleritis is left inadequately treated or not treated at all the patients may present with an eye in which the sclera is entirely obscured by diffuse redness and swollen episclera. The involvement of the sclera itself can only be detected by the use of adrenalin to clear the episcleral inflammation.

In 24 per cent of patients with diffuse anterior scleritis, some other systemic disease can be found, the commonest of which is rheumatoid arthritis (Table 4.2) but in no patient was the accompanying disease severe. Progression from a diffuse scleritis to the necrotising variety has occurred in some of those patients who have presented with the severe anterior scleritis and in some

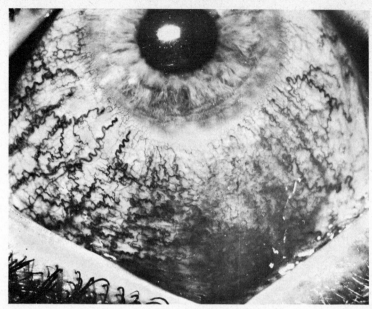

Figure 4.10. Diffuse anterior scleritis. The whole of the lower half of the globe is intensely congested and the sclera swollen between 7 and 3 o'clock. The maximum congestion is in the deep episcleral plexus which is pushed forwards by the swollen underlying sclera.

of those patients who have developed vasculitis or other extra-articular manifestations of rheumatoid arthritis. Equally, patients who seem to be developing necrotising scleritis have remained as diffuse anterior scleritis on treatment and the disease does not appear to have progressed.

Table 4.2 *Systemic diseases found in patients with diffuse anterior scleritis (total 119 eyes)*

Systemic disease	Eyes	Systemic disease	Eyes
Rheumatoid arthritis	8	Herpes zoster	2
Ankylosing spondylitis	2	Clinical gout	2
Systemic vasculitis	1	Essential hypertension	3
Orbital granuloma	1	Onset followed irradiation to opposite	
Active rheumatic heart disease	1	eye	1
Severe asthma or hay fever	2	Fragilitas ossium	1
Active tuberculosis	1	Thyrotoxicosis	1
Active syphilis	1	Degenerative arthritis	1

Adapted from Watson and Hayreh (1976).

Examination of the eye reveals a striking change in the vascular pattern of the superficial episcleral and deep episcleral vessels. Critchett (1854) described the early changes thus:

'On examining the eye it is found highly injected, and on looking more minutely the vessels are found to be situated in the sclerotic coat; they are deep-seated, numerous, but small, and finely pencilled, of a pink colour, and pursuing a straight course towards the cornea, around which they form a capillary plexus; the conjunctiva is usually but slightly involved, a few large loose returning veins being chiefly visible, and being readily distinguishable from the sclerotic vascularity which is a main feature of the disease'.

The extent of the involvement varies from a small area to the whole of the anterior segment. If the inflammation persists for any period of time, the radial pattern of the superficial episcleral network becomes totally lost and is replaced by the normal vascular loops which appear to be derived from the capillary network. New abnormal vascular channels also appear to open up to feed and drain the affected area (Figure 4.11). The underlying sclera is always swollen and the vessels on its surface are greatly congested but the surface of the sclera never breaks down to form an ulcer.

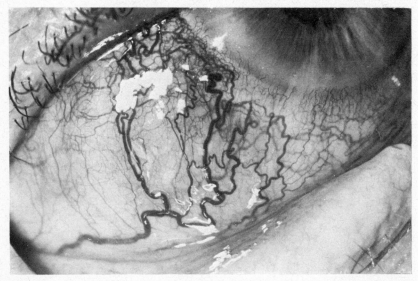

Figure 4.11. Abnormal and newly formed anastomotic vessels overlying a diffuse anterior scleritis. Both the sclera and the overlying episclera are oedematous.

When the inflammation regresses and the sclera is visible again, the colour is often seen to be altered to a slate-blue colour (Figure 4.12, Plate I). This increased transparency, or translucency, is not accompanied by scleral thinning or loss of tissue and is simply due to the rearrangement of the collagen fibres after the inflammation has subsided. Although the vessels may return to a normal size, their configuration remains distorted as a result of the previous inflammation (Figure 4.13). If in doubt, ultrasonics can be used to detect true scleral thinning, A-scan being used to estimate the thickness and B-scan the position of the lesion.

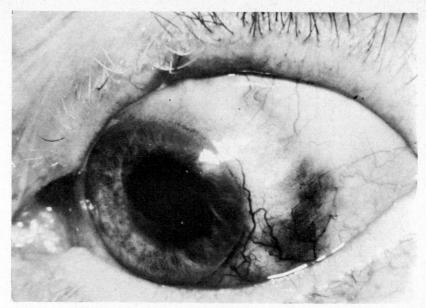

Figure 4.12.   Increased scleral transparency which followed recurrent attacks of diffuse anterior scleritis. The dark grey areas on the sclera appear slate-blue in daylight.

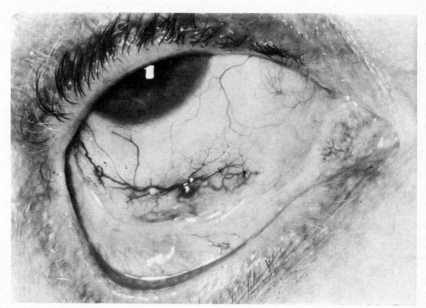

Figure 4.13.   The abnormal vascular channels which remain after the scleritis has regressed or has been treated.

Nodular anterior scleritis

Once it is recognised that nodular scleritis exists and differs from nodular episcleritis, the diagnosis is rarely difficult. Nodular scleritis is intensely painful and the nodule extremely tender, firm to the touch, totally immobile and quite separate from the overlying congested episcleral tissues, which are themselves infiltrated with cells. It is easy to see the swollen sclera beneath these superficial nodules (Figures 4.14 and 4.15, Plate II). The nodule itself has a deep red or violaceous colour which is due to the intense vascular congestion. The vascular pattern is always abnormal, bypass channels opening up in the venous episcleral plexus overlying the area of scleral congestion.

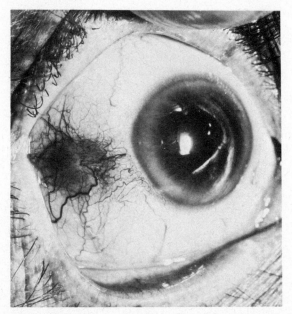

Figure 4.14. Nodular scleritis. The nodule, which is sharply demarcated, is intensely congested and the abnormal vascular channels have opened up over it.

The conjunctival vessels are, however, so little congested that they have to be consciously looked for and moved over the nodule to be certain of their presence. Multiple nodules which may be confluent or discrete occur in about 40 per cent of patients and sometimes reach an enormous size (Figure 4.16). The nodules are found most commonly in the interpalpebral region about 3 to 4 mm from the limbus. However, solitary large nodules tend to be found closer to the equator and the smaller confluent ones close to the limbus. There is one ill-defined, but possibly separate group of patients with nodular scleritis who develop confluent nodules within 2 mm of the limbus. If these nodules occupy more than half the circumference of the globe, an open angle glaucoma develops, presumably due to oedema of the trabecular meshwork (Figure 4.17). As some of these patients go on to develop necrotising scleritis,

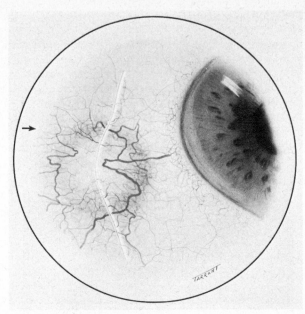

Figure 4.15.   A drawing of the same eye as in Figure 4.14, showing the slit-lamp appearance with displacement of the deep episcleral plexus by the underlying scleral oedema.

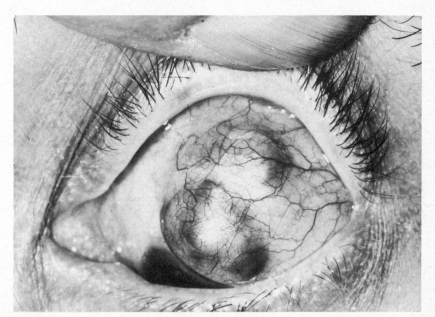

Figure 4.16.   A very large scleral nodule which overlaps the corneal edge, giving rise to a localised anterior staphyloma. The intraocular pressure was 50 in the acute stage of the inflammation.

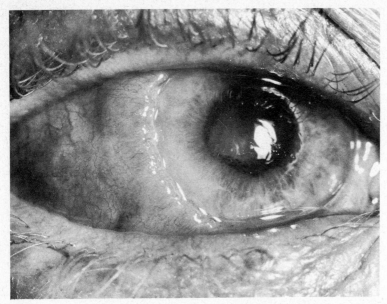

Figure 4.17. Multiple scleral nodules occurring at the limbus which was associated with a marked rise in intraocular pressure and an anterior uveitis.

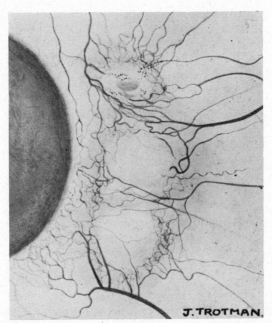

Figure 4.18. Multiple scleral nodules adjacent to the limbus. The centre of each nodule is avascular. This could have been due to capillary occlusion caused by oedema, but the upper one has broken down, indicating that the avascularity is preceding frank necrosis of the tissue.

they must be watched and treated with great care. The two physical signs which indicate that necrotising changes are occurring are the presence of an avascular centre to the nodule which then breaks down, and circumferential progression of the nodular scleritis away from the original site of inflammation (Figure 4.18). Apparently avascular areas can occur in the centre of an intensely inflamed nodule without necrosis following, presumably because the oedema shuts off the capillary network, but this is unusual. Progression of the nodule outwards is always significant. The area adjacent to a nodule is always congested and this inflammation always disappears rapidly with treatment long before the nodule itself disappears. As the inflammation in the nodule subsides, the increased translucency which is left in the sclera becomes apparent. The thickness is not often affected, but occasionally a slight depression can be seen in the surface where the nodule has been. Nodular and diffuse anterior scleritis occurs in almost exactly the same number of patients but by far the largest number with the nodular disease have had a previous attack of herpes zoster (Table 4.3).

Table 4.3.   *Systemic diseases found in association with nodular anterior scleritis*

Systemic diseases	Eyes
Rheumatoid arthritis	4
Psoriatic arthritis	3
Systemic lupus erythematosus	1
Cogan's syndrome	3
Active rheumatic heart disease	1
Erythema nodosum	2
Rosacea	2
Active syphilis	3
Herpes zoster	14
Herpes simplex	2
Clinical gout	3
Thyrotoxicosis	2
Ophthalmia nodosa	1
Systemic hypertension	1

Scleral nodules look as if they should be easy to biopsy. Beware, they often contain only a yellow fluid (an experience first noted by Critchett, 1854). If left alone, the contents become converted to scar tissue, but, if released, leave bare uncovered choroid (see Figure 5.2).

Nodular scleritis is most prevalent from the fourth to the sixth decade but most common in the sixth decade. As in diffuse anterior scleritis, the onset is insidious, gradually reaching its peak after five to ten days. If untreated, the nodules may subside after several months, but may remain until treated and recur when the general condition of the patient deteriorates. Alt (1903) described the natural history at a time when no effective treatment was available:

'During its springing up, growth and disappearance such a nodule never shows any signs of superficial or deeper necrosis and no ulcer results from it. When the affection heals, with or without treatment, the swelling becomes gradually reduced in size, till it finally disappears and usually together with it the congestion which had accompanied it. In other cases the congestion remains behind and new abortive attacks can still be recognized by a sudden localized increase of congestion, although no swelling appears, till finally, like distant lightning after the storm, even this fades out.'

Necrotising anterior scleritis

Necrotising scleritis is the most serious and the most destructive form of scleral disease and has in consequence occupied the lion's share of the literature. It is, fortunately, a comparatively rare disease accounting for only 14 per cent of the known cases of scleritis. When it occurs, however, it is such a dramatic and disastrous condition that every effort must be directed to prevent its development in susceptible individuals, to make an early diagnosis and then to treat it vigorously in those who have the misfortune to suffer from it. Just how serious this condition is can be judged from the fact that 60 per cent of these patients developed ocular or systemic complications, 40 per cent had a significant loss of visual acuity and 29 per cent died within five years of the onset of the disease.

The literature on this condition is extensive and confusing, but our experience has been similar to that of Franceschetti and Bischler (1950) who stated that, although histologically very similar, clinically two types of necrotising scleritis are distinguishable. In one group of patients the inflammatory reaction is fierce and they have much discomfort and pain and develop multiple complications; in the other group the inflammatory reaction is minimal and they have little or no discomfort, but nevertheless develop sequestra of the sclera and the complications associated with this. Both these types need to be distinguished from spontaneous intercalary perforation which does not have necrotising scleritis as its basis.

Necrotising scleritis with signs of adjacent inflammation

The majority of these patients are female, present between the ages of 30 and 60, but of those patients of ours who have presented during the fourth decade, all except one have been male. In sixty per cent involvement was bilateral.

Whilst there has been nothing in the aetiology, the progression or prognosis to justify further subdivision within this group, the clinical appearances at the time of presentation do differ from patient to patient. The commonest presentation in those patients who do not already have some recognised systemic disease is that for no recognisable reason, or about a week after recovering from a 'flue-like illness, the eye becomes red and painful. Both the pain and the redness increase in intensity over a period of three to four days until help is sought. The local medications almost always given at that time fail to give anything but the slightest symptomatic relief, so that specialist advice is sought within three weeks of the onset of the condition. The obvious feature at this stage is very intense pain and discomfort which sometimes appears to be out of proportion to the physical signs, because although the sclera

is obviously swollen and inflamed it does not look too bad. Unlike nodular
and diffuse anterior scleritis, however, the edges of the lesion are much more
intensely inflamed than the centre, and if the condition is observed without
treatment, the areas of inflammation will be found to extend outward up
to but not beyond the equator and circumferentially around the globe (Figures
4.19 to 4.22). The limbal area is rarely affected. As the area of inflammation
advances, the area which was originally affected gradually gets whiter, but
it can be seen that the underlying sclera has been damaged and has become
translucent. The progression around the globe may occur within a few weeks
when the inflammation is florid, or may take many months if the inflammation
is less intense, the area behind the advancing edge becoming extremely thin
and sometimes disappearing altogether (Figure 4.23, Plate III). It is certain
that unless its progression is halted by treatment intraocular complications
will occur. These usually become manifest when the inflammatory process
has passed through 360°. Sym (1896) noted, 'Yet another peculiarity is that
having occurred, recurred again and again, and having perhaps "circum-
navigated" the cornea, scleritis ceases, and in a large proportion of cases
never again troubles the patient'. Unfortunately this is not before the eye
has been seriously damaged by the corneal and intraocular complications.
We have found that in many ways this type of necrotising scleritis is the
most dangerous because of the insidious nature of the destructive process.
Everyone is alarmed by the acute onset of a red eye and destructive process
but many are lulled into a sense of false security by the apparently benign
nature of this type of necrotising process, termed annular scleritis by Parsons
(1902).

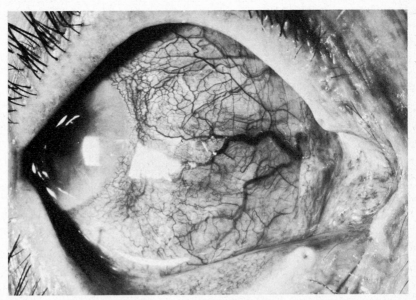

Figure 4.19.   Mrs L.B. Progression of anterior necrotising scleritis in a patient who was unable to
tolerate steroid therapy and in whom no other therapy was effective. Shortly after the onset of the
scleritis, the sclera is swollen and the anterior ciliary veins very congested.

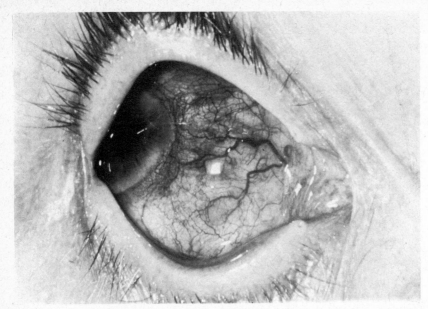

Figure 4.20. Mrs L.B. Two months later. The scleritis has progressed upwards and has left an area of transparent sclera in its wake.

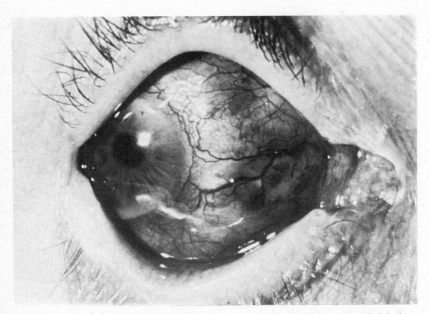

Figure 4.21. Mrs L.B. Four months after the onset of the condition; the scleritis is now extending towards 6 o'clock from the original site of the scleritis which is now very dark in colour.

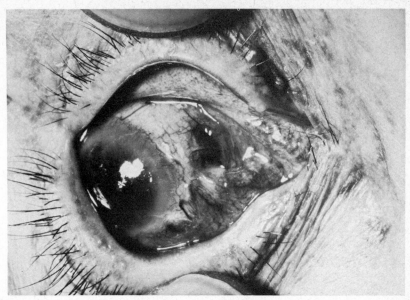

Figure 4.22.   Mrs L.B. Six months after onset. Necrosis is now taking place at the site of the original lesion and the sclera is deficient in this area. Shortly after this the eye was removed because of the intolerable pain.

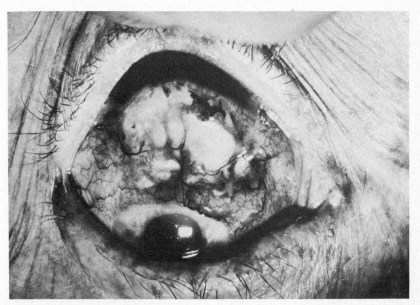

Figure 4.23.   Necrotising scleritis. When the process is more rapid and violent than in Figures 4.19 to 4.22, an area of sclera may become totally avascular and acellular. The slough is gradually removed by the granulation tissue. (The single large vessel which traverses this area has a thin strip of normal sclera on either side of it.)

The more dramatic onset is less usual, but none the less horrific. Over a period of 48 hours the patient, who is often, but by no means always, suffering from some other connective tissue disease such as a systemic vasculitis of one type or another, develops an acutely red, excessively painful eye. Sometimes the oedema which accompanies the inflammation is so severe as to merit the term 'brawny' (Schlodtmann, 1897). The whole of the interior segment rapidly becomes congested and inflamed and the anterior chamber shallows considerably (Figure 4.24), presumably because the inflammation has spread beyond the equator. Most of the cases are bilateral, the onset being almost simultaneous in both eyes.

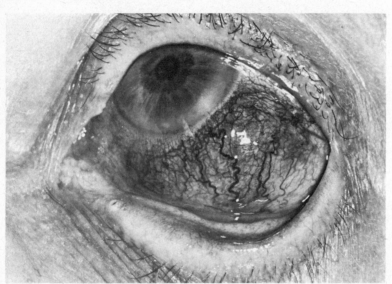

Figure 4.24. Necrotising scleritis. The scleritis in this patient was of dramatic onset of an acute red swollen eye with chemotic conjunctiva. The anterior chamber rapidly became shallow, presumably because the posterior segment was also involved.

Because of the dramatic nature of the condition, treatment given promptly can bring the scleritis under control rapidly, but often not before much permanent change has occurred within the underlying sclera. If the process is allowed to continue, large areas of sclera may slough away, eventually leaving the choroid bare or covered only by a thin layer of conjunctiva. A few vessels cross these areas on bridges of relatively normal sclera to supply the limbal area (Figure 4.23, Plate IV). The choroid does not bulge through these areas unless the intraocular pressure rises.

Midway between the gradually progressive insidious type and the florid 'brawny' type lies a group of patients who present with pain and redness of the eye of gradually increasing severity. The episclera is congested over the whole of the anterior segment and, underlying this, many areas of sclera are oedematous. The scleral oedema is at first patchy, occupying more than one segment of the globe. If left untreated these areas will coalesce (Figure 4.25).

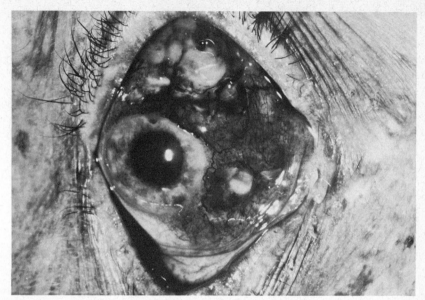

Figure 4.25. Areas of necrosis occurring simultaneously in different segments of the globe. If untreated these areas will coalesce.

Careful examination of the vascular pattern at the areas of maximum congestion and inflammation may reveal avascularity of a patch of episcleral tissue overlying or adjacent to the area of scleral oedema (Figures 4.18, 4.26, 4.27). This sign, found in 27 per cent of patients with necrotising scleritis, is of the greatest possible significance for not only does it reveal the presence of an underlying necrotising process which is so severe that capillary closure has occurred, but also it is a very early sign of severe disease. If treated at this stage, the vessels open up again and the structures return to normal. If this sign is ignored or the patient treated inadequately, deep scleral destruction will take place which leads to the loss of scleral tissue (Figure 4.25, see also Figures 10.3 to 10.8). Rarely, the inflammation can remain localised to one area and, if left unchecked by treatment, will result in almost total loss of scleral tissue there.

Spontaneous perforation can occur (Figure 4.28) but more usually follows surgical or accidental trauma. Thirty-seven per cent of eyes examined histologically have scleral perforation but many of these occur at the time of enucleation and in only one eye was perforation given as the reason for enucleation (Fraunfelder and Watson, 1976).

Even when, in any of these types of necrotising disease, the condition has been allowed to progress too far so that destruction of the collagen structure has taken place, it is still not too late to treat it. Treatment will not only reverse the inflammatory signs but may allow the new collagen to restore completely the integrity of the globe because, provided the damaged collagen has not been sloughed off or absorbed, new collagen can be laid down on the tissue which remains in the defect. All that then remains is to deal with the complications which have occurred during the period of intense activity.

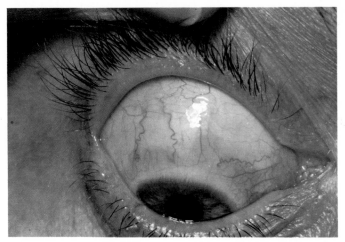

Plate I. Translucent sclera. The blue-grey appearance of the sclera which follows recurrent or severe attacks of scleral inflammation.

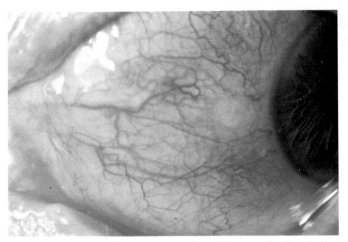

Plate II. Nodular scleritis. The central avascular episclera overlies the scleral nodule.

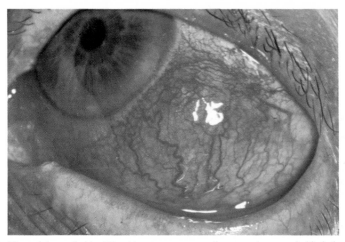

Plate III. Necrotising scleritis. The blue transparent sclera can be seen behind the advancing inflammation.

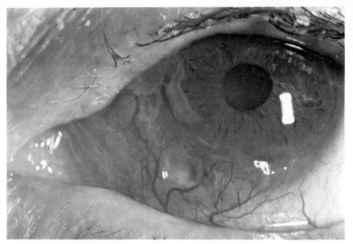

Plate IV. Necrotising sclero-kerato-uveitis. Notice the large bypass vascular channels.

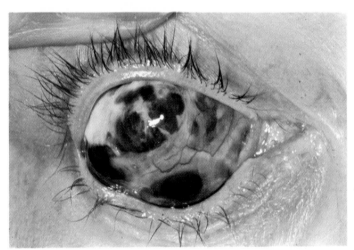

Plate V. Necrotising scleritis without inflammation (scleromalacia perforans). Chalky white avascular sclera in areas of sequestration.

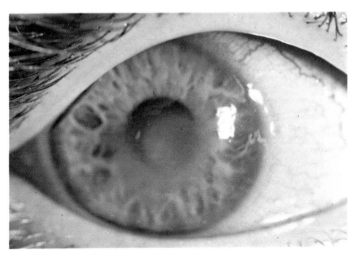

Plate VI. Corneal opacification and calcification following scleritis in a patient with juvenile rheumatoid arthritis.

Plates reproduced by kind permission of Hospital Update.

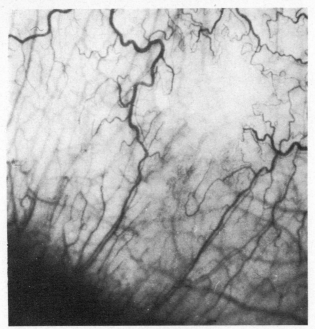

Figure 4.26. An area of diffuse scleral congestion in what appeared to be a diffuse anterior scleritis.
Courtesy of A. Bron, Oxford.

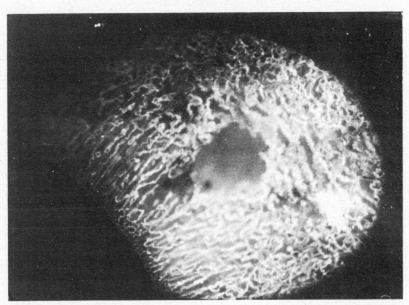

Figure 4.27. Fluorescence angiogram showing an avascular area which later underwent necrosis, proving that this was indeed a necrotising scleritis.
Courtesy of A. Bron, Oxford.

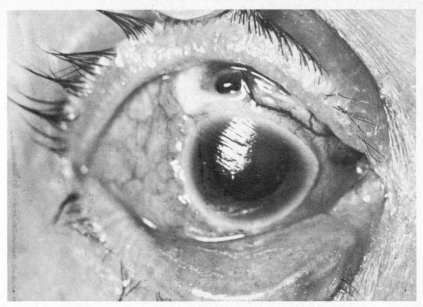

Figure 4.28. Spontaneous perforation (a very rare event) in a patient with severe, untreated, necrotising scleritis.

Necrotising scleritis without inflammation (scleromalacia perforans)

The term 'scleromalacia perforans' was coined by van der Hoeve in 1931. Partly because of its dramatic presentation and partly because it is known to be associated with rheumatoid arthritis, this is the best known of all scleral conditions. It is singularly unfortunate that the term 'perforans' was used originally by van der Hoeve because any eye in which there is loss of tissue of the sclera incorrectly attracts this label. The condition described by van der Hoeve, although histologically indistinguishable from other types of necrotising scleritis, is a rare but precisely defined clinical entity and we feel that the diagnosis of scleromalacia perforans should be reserved for these patients.

van der Hoeve's first case (1931) was of 'a woman, aged 55, who complained that for many years her vision had been diminishing. She was brought to my clinic with some difficulty as she could scarcely move on account of the total or partial ankylosis and swelling of a great many of her joints. Small and large holes in the sclera of both eyes were seen. The conjunctiva, as a whole, seemed to be rather atrophic. Over some of the gaps it was still present, covering the uvea completely; over other holes there were only some rags of conjunctiva, and over still others it was gone, so that the uvea lay bare. Dr van Hoorn told me that sometimes when a hole was being formed, he had seen first a yellowish excrescence below the conjunctiva, appearing like an abscess. However, when this was punctured no pus came out, but only a kind of detritus. Unluckily, this detritus has not been examined. There were no symptoms of inflammation; the corneas and crystalline lenses were clear. It was remarkable that in these cases the uvea did not bulge out of the holes. This was probably caused by the fact that the tension of the eyes was normal, and proves that under certain conditions the uvea can bear the pressure of the eye without the help of the sclera, or that the bare choroid allows enough fluid to pass out to prevent bulging'. In his discussion he says, 'In this disease inflammation plays no role, or at least a very secondary one'.

Of the patients we have seen with this condition, 46 per cent have had long-standing rheumatoid arthritis with severe ankylosing changes and extra-articular manifestations. This is the feature common to practically all the reported cases. The relatively low frequency of severe rheumatoid disease in the 16 patients we have seen with this condition is because the patients were referred because they did not fit into the classical pattern.

The age range of the patients with scleromalacia perforans is from 35 to 75, most cases occurring within the fifth decade. All the patients who had long-standing rheumatoid arthritis were female. Whether or not they have long-standing rheumatoid arthritis, all the patients presented without any sub-jective symptoms, the doctor or patient having noticed a grey or yellow patch on the sclera or, in more severe cases, a complete loss of tissue (Figures 4.29 and 4.30, Plate V). It is said that scleromalacia perforans is almost always bilateral, but we have only found it to be so in 55 per cent.

We have had the opportunity to watch the progression of this condition in a patient who refused to take any medication. She had, at the age of 60, had rheumatoid arthritis for 18 years, and by the time we saw her had developed such deformities that she was confined to bed or to her chair

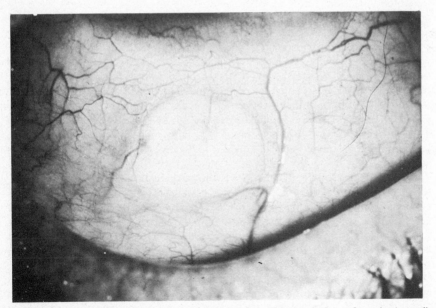

Figure 4.29. Necrotising scleritis without inflammation (scleromalacia perforans). A totally avascular and acellular patch of sclera appearing without any surrounding inflammatory reaction. The episcleral tissue is thin and poorly vascularised.

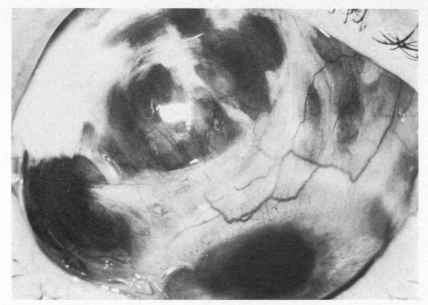

Figure 4.30.   Necrotising scleritis without inflammation (scleromalacia perforans); the opposite eye of the same patient as in Figure 4.29. The sclera has become sequestrated. No staphyloma has occurred because the intraocular pressure remains normal.

to which she was lifted as if a solid piece of wood. She was first seen at home because of difficulty in reading. Her eyes were apparently perfectly normal except that the episclera was very thin and the sclera was noted to be 'like fine old English bone china' with a slight over-all blue tinge. The vision corrected to 6/6 in both eyes and N5 for reading. She was seen again two years later. The appearances of the sclera were unchanged, but she had developed a slight cuneiform lens opacity and the vision could now be corrected to 6/9 in both eyes and N5 for reading. Eighteen months later she remarked to her doctor that she had noticed that her eye 'seems to be changing colour'. This indeed was the case for an area of the sclera in the superotemporal quadrant had changed from blue-white to yellow-grey. There was no redness of the eye.

Examining her on the slit lamp was no easy task, but was well worthwhile for it revealed that the episclera in the affected area was extremely thin and contained practically no vessels. In the area surrounding this, the vessels were very slightly congested but sparse in number. The normal linear striation of the scleral fibres in the affected area had practically disappeared; where this abutted on the normal tissue a faint crack was apparent. Treatment was suggested but politely and steadfastly refused. Over the next few weeks the gap widened between normal and abnormal; the colour of the sequestrum, as it now was apparently becoming, changed from grey to yellow to white (see Figure 3.3). The conjunctiva over the surface virtually disappeared and over the next four months the centre of the white area gradually sloughed away until the underlying choroid became visible and separated from the outside world by only a few scleral fibres (Figure 4.31). All the time the area surrounding the slough remained very slightly congested. The cataracts increased a little reducing the vision to 6/18. Three years after the first eye had begun to be affected, and for no apparent reason, a demarcation line then developed in the sclera of the opposite eye (Figure 4.32). A circular crack appeared and the area inside this took on a yellow-grey appearance which eventually separated both from the adjacent sclera and from the overlying episclera. At this stage there was very mild inflammatory response with a general suffusion of the episcleral tissue and a little increase in redness around the area of the sequestrum.

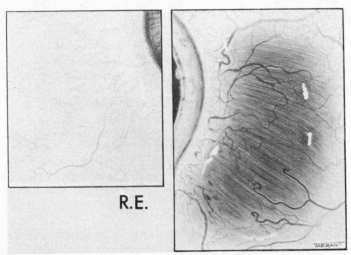

Figure 4.31. Mrs F. Necrotising scleritis without inflammation. The sequestrum in Figure 3.3 has separated and has been absorbed. At 8 o'clock in the same eye the scleral fibres have become radially arranged under their sclera. Left untreated this area would also sequestrate.

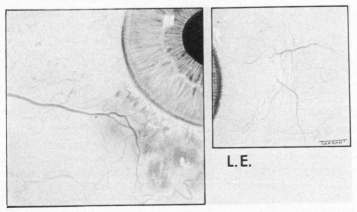

Figure 4.32. Mrs F., the opposite eye. The episclera is extremely thin so that the muscle fibres can be seen easily. The vessels terminate in whorls, leaving an avascular area in the episclera.

Two months later she died suddenly from what was presumed to be a coronary infarct and no postmortem was obtained.

The change in the vascular networks of the anterior sclera seems to be critical in the production of these lesions. Whether the loss of the episcleral coat, the connective tissue of the orbit (Kiehle, 1946) and the underlying scleral changes result from the vascular changes or the other way round is uncertain, but certainly in our experience the first thing which can be detected clinically is a reduction in the number and size of the vessels in the episclera which eventually progresses in some individuals to its complete disappearance (Figures 4.31 and 4.32). The capillary networks close to the sequestrating area anastomose with each other and much larger vessels than normal surround the abnormal area and sometimes cross it to join up with the perilimbal vascular plexus. These vessels have a bridge of tissue on either side of them which sometimes is normal sclera and at other times seems to be newly laid down collagen. Histologically a pannus of vessels can be seen close to the area of collagen destruction. This pannus cannot be detected on the slit lamp, but must be derived either from the choroidal circulation or from the large abnormal vessels as no episcleral vessels can be distinguished. Although the conjunctiva does sometimes disappear completely, as in Anderson and Margolis' patient (1952), this is unusual. If this happens, the remaining conjunctival tissue heaps up at the edge of the defect. More often, as the centre of the sequestrum is resorbed, a very thin layer of connective tissue, which might very well be derived from conjunctiva, remains over the area of the tissue loss. In spite of the fact that very large areas of uveal tissue are exposed, staphylomas do not occur nor, surprisingly, does any alteration in intraocular pressure follow this sequestration.

These eyes are vulnerable to slight trauma. One patient had to have a patch placed over one area which had perforated after he knocked it on the edge of a table.

Spontaneous perforation is rare. One of Roca's (1974) patients noticed 'a heavy tear-drop' rolling down his cheek whilst watching television. It certainly occurred in one of our patients and this was confirmed histologically (Fraunfelder and Watson, 1976). Sevel (1967) has pointed out that clinically apparent perforation is not always confirmed histologically since the thin residual layer of collagen tissue may become dehydrated and consequently transparent. If the eye does perforate and the sclera is not repaired phthisis bulbi will result (Roca, 1974).

Posterior scleritis

Posterior scleritis is undoubtedly an under-diagnosed condition. Reviewing 30 eyes which have been enucleated in the past ten years with a histological primary diagnosis of scleritis, posterior scleritis was found to be present in 43 per cent of the patients and was diagnosed in none of them (Fraunfelder and Watson, 1976). In all these eyes the anterior sclera was also affected. However, Uhthoff (1900) had a histological drawing which shows no inflammation anterior to the equator; Wagenmann (1906) and Coats (1907) had well documented clinical histories with histological confirmation. We have two patients who have presented with the signs of posterior scleritis alone, developing the changes in the anterior segment later. It is quite certain therefore that posterior scleritis can occur alone, but it is an extremely difficult diagnosis to make without some signs of anterior scleral inflammation. It must enter the differential diagnosis of patients with proptosis, limitation of movement or solid or exudative retinal detachments with or without swelling of the optic discs (Boylan, 1964; Goder, 1969).

The physical signs with which the patient presents are dependent on the site and intensity of the scleral inflammation, but it can be said that all have:

1. Pain.
2. Reduction of visual acuity.
3. One or more of the following features:
   (a) Fundus changes:
       (1) exudative retinal detachments
       (2) annular choroidal detachments
       (3) subretinal mass
       (4) choroidoretinal changes
       (5) optic nerve oedema
       (6) macular oedema
   (b) Shallowing of the anterior chamber
   (c) Constriction of the peripheral visual field or central or isolated scotomas
   (d) Proptosis
   (e) Limitation of extraocular movement
   (f) Retraction of the lower lid

Primary posterior scleritis was not found by us to be associated with the connective tissue diseases, but Leira (1975) found that eight of his 20 patients with sclerokeratitis and posterior scleritis had either rheumatoid arthritis, systemic lupus erythematosus, cranial arteritis or systemic vasculitis. Intraocular exudation and detachment in periarteritis nodosa have been reported by Böck (1929), Sampson (1945), Lasco and Nicolesco (1960) and are also known to occur in systemic lupus and with giant cell arteritis. The sclera is often involved by infiltration of granulomatous invasion of the orbit in the necrotising vasculitis (Maumenee, 1956) and has been reported in rheumatoid arthritis (Kennedy and McGavin, 1975), systemic lupus erythematosus (Brenner and Shock, 1974) and polychondritis (Rucker and Ferguson, 1964).

Pain

Pain is a universal accompaniment of posterior scleritis; the further forward the inflammation is in the globe the more intense the pain appears to be. The intensity of the pain is also related to the severity of the necrotic process. As with most scleral pain it is often referred from the eye to the brow, teeth, face or temple and in consequence the eye may not be suspected as the cause of it, particularly as it is sometimes only described as a constant ache or headache.

Visual acuity

Some reduction of visual acuity is almost universal and obviously depends on the site of the inflammation, its severity and the complications produced. It is only permanent and severe if there is long-standing macular oedema. Sometimes the reduction in vision only reflects a transient induced refractive change. Wagenmann (1906) described a case in which a myopia of 2.5D was induced by bulging of the sclera adjacent to the equator and Fuchs (1902) reported an induced hypermetropia of between 3 to 4D from a lesion above the macular. A transitory myopia is not uncommon (Dellaporta, 1950) in both scleritis and episcleritis if the inflammatory process is intense, and results from oedema and spasm of the ciliary muscle. This myopia can occur without any evidence of uveitis.

Fundus changes

Of a total of 12 patients studied by Cleary et al (1975), five developed retinal detachments, two of whom also had annular choroidal detachments and in three (four eyes) a raised yellow-brown subretinal mass was seen. Two patients presented with optic disc oedema only and five had optic disc oedema and macular oedema.

Choroidoretinal changes and exudative retinal detachments

The posterior sclera can become involved either by extension of an orbital granuloma through the sclera or more commonly by a necrotising process taking place within it, which in turn simulates an inflammatory reaction in the adjacent choroid.

From whatever cause, the choroidal inflammatory reaction allows exudation of fluid through to the subretinal space which detaches the retina. If, in addition, a granulomatous mass forms, this becomes visible through the overlying serous detachment and, when it resolves, leaves its mark as choroidal and retinal scars (Figures 4.33 and 4.34).

Exudative detachments caused by posterior scleritis were first described by Purtscher (1891) and Kamocki (1892) and seem to be characteristic of the condition. The patients present with blurring of vision, pain and a mild anterior diffuse scleritis in which the whole anterior segment is involved. (In one patient only one segment was involved and the inflammation extended out of sight posteriorly.) The blurring of vision is usually due to a mobile inferior exudative detachment and a slight or moderate anterior and posterior uveitis. In those who have presented in this way the vision has been 6/18 or better. Areas of exudation occurring beneath the retina appear as pale grey-white spots with a surrounding dark grey line which can be seen through the overlying serous detachment. The lesions can be seen better by posturing the patient to disperse the overlying fluid. In some patients a yellowish-brown elevated mass can be seen, the surface of which is covered with scattered yellow-white circumscribed lesions. Coats (1907) described a similar lesion thus:

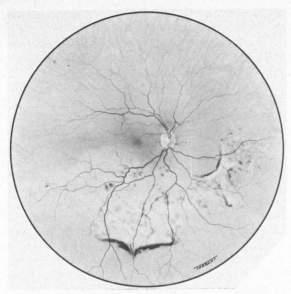

Figure 4.33. The pepper-and-salt pigmentary change in the fundus left after the resolution of posterior scleritis.

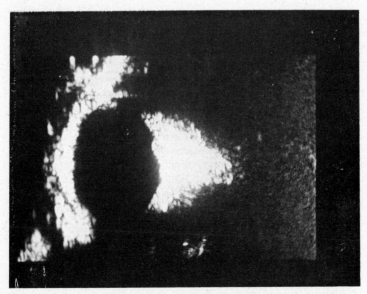

Figure 4.34. Ultrasonogram. The sclera is thickened posteriorly and the retina is seen to be pushed forwards 3 mm and folded.

'It commences 4.5 mm above the disc, and is about 10 mm in diameter. It has the form of a brown island somewhat paler than the fundus elsewhere, surrounded by a moat or gutter of a mottled yellow appearance. The island is bounded towards the moat by a sharply defined darker line. The outer circumference of the moat is equally sharply limited except that between the papilla and the left-hand lower corner there is an area of slightly discoloured atrophic choroid.'

The mass does not obviously involve the overlying retina but scattered intraretinal haemorrhages have been seen in the area of the detachment.

If the scleral involvement is far forward, the ciliary body also becomes involved, giving rise to an annular choroidal detachment which in one patient was so large that the lens iris diaphragm was pushed forwards and precipitated an acute closed angle glaucoma attack (see Figure 10.21).

Whilst this effusion may in some patients represent the presence of choroidal nodules (Hurd, Snyder and Ziff, 1970) the signs produced conform with the description of the uveal effusion syndrome as described by Schepens and Brockhurst (1960). In six of the 13 eyes operated on by them the sclera was excessively thick. A thickened sclera in patients with very similar physical signs had been noted previously by Stallard (1954) and Davenport (1958). Graham (1958) considered scleritis to be the cause of this syndrome: this was later confirmed histologically in a report on an enucleated eye by Rosen and Lyne (1968). Scleritis is undoubtedly a cause of the uveal effusion syndrome with annular choroidal detachments and retinal detachments, differing only from those other cases described by Schepens and Brockhurst in that uveal effusion is nearly always bilateral, whereas posterior scleritis is more frequently unilateral (Kimura and Hogan, 1964).

There appears to be yet another group, so far ill-defined, of patients of West Indian origin who have presented with diffuse choroidal leakage and disc oedema similar to those just described. None of them had any associated systemic disease that we have so far detected and only one has had an anterior scleritis.

Treatment gives prompt relief of pain and resolution of the scleritis. The fundus lesions, however, are considerably more resistant to treatment. Although the retinal detachment in one patient disappeared within five hours of starting treatment, these detachments often extend initially, then are absorbed slowly after an interval of several months. In one of our patients in whom the condition recurred, the retinal detachment became total, and the eye developed a complicated cataract with secondary glaucoma and was eventually enucleated.

When the inflammation has been suppressed, the subretinal fluid becomes absorbed and, provided no complications such as cataract or macular oedema have occurred, the vision returns to normal. All that remains is a slightly raised white subretinal scar in the equatorial fundus, corresponding with the previous yellowish-brown mass. In the patients with annular choroidal detachments, a residual pigmentary speckling of the peripheral retina was evident.

Optic nerve oedema

Posterior scleritis can present with only pain, a slight change in vision and optic disc oedema. Of the three patients we have seen with this condition, one had three episodes of disc swelling without visual loss over a period of three years. An anterior scleritis was identified in this patient at the first examination, and during a subsequent episode, when the anterior scleritis had resolved, a mild proptosis with vertical diplopia was observed. Another developed the swollen disc first and later developed the scleritis. She showed evidence of optic nerve fibre loss, an afferent pupillary defect, and an arcuate scotoma. The visual acuity, nevertheless, was maintained at 6/6. We have seen a patient monthly who first developed optic disc oedema then two months later developed an exudative retinal lesion and finally after another month developed anterior and necrotising scleritis. The optic disc oedema was confirmed in all the patients by fluorescein fundus angiography which showed dilatation of the prepapillary and peripapillary retinal capillaries. Retinal haemorrhages or exudates were not associated with the disc swelling. The visual acuity was 6/6 in the first two patients and 6/9 in the last, a slight reduction on their previous acuities. The disc oedema seems to be due to an extension of the granulomatous inflammation into the optic nerve and its sheath (Gass, 1974).

Macular oedema

Macular oedema can accompany the exudative retinal detachments but in the patients we have seen with this condition it has been much more commonly seen with optic disc oedema. The type of macular oedema is that commonly found either following iritis and cyclitis, or cataract, glaucoma and detachment surgery.

Seven of 12 patients with posterior scleritis recently reported by us (Cleary et al, 1975) developed retinal and optic disc oedema. In five the oedema affected both the optic disc and macula and at the initial examination the visual acuity was 6/24 or worse. All five patients had a moderate to severe cellular response in the vitreous but no evidence of inflammation in the anterior chamber. In one patient the macular oedema was bilateral and exudates were present inferiorly in the vitreous base and on the pars plana. This patient developed a rhegmatogenous retinal detachment in one eye which was successfully treated by a scleral buckling procedure. The macular oedema follows a chronic course and does not resolve completely, despite treatment with systemic or intraorbital steroids. The visual acuity, however, improves with treatment (Figures 4.35 and 4.36).

None of the patients that we have examined with scleritis and macular oedema has shown any evidence of anterior uveitis, although their scleritis was long-standing. In the only patient with diffuse scleral involvement, exudates were noted at the vitreous base and pars plana inferiorly, which in chronic cyclitis Kimura and Hogan (1964) have related to the duration and severity of the inflammation. It is probable that in patients with scleritis, macular oedema is most likely to be related to a similar infiltration of the ciliary body and choroid.

Proptosis, limitation of ocular movements and lid signs

About half the patients with posterior scleritis have some degree of proptosis,

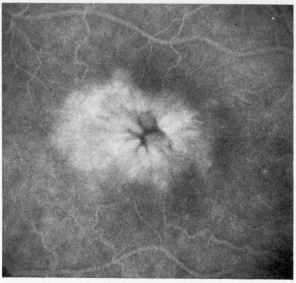

Figure 4.35. Fluorescence angiogram of the macular at the time of active anterior and posterior scleritis. Visual acuity 6 /36.
Courtesy of Philip Cleary, London.

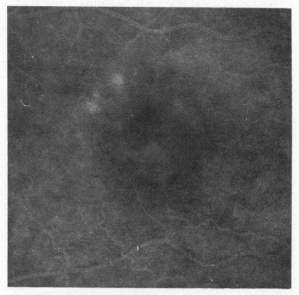

Figure 4.36. Fluorescence angiogram of the same macular after 14 days' treatment with oxyphenbutazone. Visual acuity 6 /9.
Courtesy of Philip Cleary, London.

limitation of ocular movement (with consequent diplopia) and retraction of the lower lid when attempting to look upwards (Figure 4.37). Equally about half of those who present with proptosis and limitation of extraocular movements later develop severe retinal detachment and optic nerve changes (Leira, 1975).

The protrusion of the eye associated with severe orbital pain, chemosis of the conjunctiva and limitation of ocular movement were first described by Birsch-Hirschfeld in 1910 under the title of 'serous tetonitis'. Bertelsen in 1960 showed histologically that the proptosis and limitation of ocular movements were due to muscular involvement by granulation tissue and the

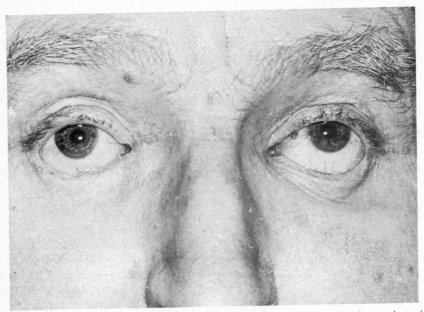

Figure 4.37. Retraction of the left lower lid on attempting to elevate the eye in a patient with posterior scleritis.

proptosis to a diffuse infiltration of all the connective tissue of the orbit. The extent and severity of the signs and symptoms depend on the degree and site of the inflammation, thus if the inflammation is severe and involves the whole of the sclera—as in what has been termed massive granuloma of the sclera (Derby and Verhoeff, 1916)—then there will be much chemosis and gross limitation of movement of the globe because of involvement of the tendon sheaths, slight to moderate proptosis and the intraocular complications of retinal detachment and optic nerve lesions and glaucoma. If, however, the mass as in Figure 5.6, starts in the outer lamellae of the sclera and remains fairly localised there, the proptosis may still be considerable, but the limitation of movement is restricted to the muscle that is involved, and diplopia in one direction of gaze results. There is little or no chemosis of the conjunctiva and no intraocular complications.

Unless a large mass forms in relationship to the outer aspect of the sclera, the proptosis is almost always axial as the maximum infiltration of tissue occurs inside the muscle cone. Retraction of the upper or lower lid is not unusual with inflammatory masses in the orbit. The lid retraction can sometimes be very dramatic, can last a very long time and is thought to be due to involvement of the sympathetic supply at the orbital apex or beyond by the inflammatory process (Rundle, 1941; Eden and Trotter, 1942). More commonly, however, the granulation tissue simply tethers the orbital septum so that the lower lid dimples when the patient attempts to look up (Figure 4.37). The diffuse infiltration of the orbit also leads to the 'pop around' sign, i.e. when the periocular tissues are compressed above, they are so rigid that they push the soft tissues of the lower lid forward.

Because these physical signs seem to be specific for this condition, if they are discovered in conjunction with an anterior scleritis, it can be assumed that the posterior sclera is involved and this must be carefully looked for with fundus examination which includes scleral indentation after full dilatation of the pupil.

OTHER COMPLICATIONS OF SCLERITIS

Corneal Changes

Although corneal changes occur in 29 per cent of patients with scleritis and in 15 per cent of patients with episcleritis, and are highly characteristic for the different types of the condition, they have been given scant attention.

Whilst there is inevitably some overlap, as there is between various types of corneal change found in scleral and episcleral disease, the changes tend to be specific to the different types of scleritis, so much so that it is often possible when looking at an eye which is otherwise apparently normal and uninflamed to tell from the corneal changes not only that the eye has suffered from scleritis in the past but also from which type of scleral disease. Whilst keratitis, particularly of the sclerosing type, can be serious, permanent changes in the central cornea can reduce vision to such an extent that corneal grafting becomes necessary. More often the corneal changes are peripheral and have remarkably little effect on vision. The predominance of these peripheral corneal changes is what would be expected from a condition which is usually an extension of a disease process arising in the adjacent sclera. Dalrymple in 1852 described this extension from the adjacent scleral inflammation:

'Still later in the disease the cornea itself becomes opaque in the vicinity of the subconjunctival swelling and its tissue seems to become softened and swelled, and the opacity assumes a pale buff colour, without, however, distinct vessels pervading it. This degeneration of tissue is apt to spread, and in some cases almost surrrounds the cornea. The vision is much less disturbed for a considerable time than might have been expected.'

Episcleritis

Although minimal corneal changes are seen in 15 per cent of the patients with simple episcleritis and in 15 per cent of those with nodular disease, they are never severe and rarely permanent. The changes seen are dependent on the type and position of the episcleral disease. Those who have severe conjunctival and episcleral oedema develop changes in the cornea adjacent to the oedematous area. The superficial and midstromal tissue becomes infiltrated, swollen and opaque whilst the eye is inflamed and if attacks are repeated in the same position, as is particularly the case in nodular episcleritis, then the corneal changes may become permanent (Figures 4.6, 4.7 and 4.8). This is the only occasion on which the cornea will vascularise and even then the vessels are only found at the extreme periphery of the cornea. Dellen formation is not uncommon when a nodule forms close to the limbus or the conjunctival oedema is very intense, and has been suggested by Barraquer (1965) to be due to a discontinuity of the tear film caused by elevation of the lid by the limbal swelling leading to desiccation of the cornea. It could just as well be due to stagnation of the film at the same site, but whatever the reason the epithelium remains intact and only stromal tissue is lost (Figure 4.8). The corneal gutter usually fills in when the nodular episcleritis is treated or disperses spontaneously but remains if it is the result of or part of active scleritis. Permanent peripheral corneal guttering of a similar type to that found in scleritis has however occurred in three of our patients who had had recurrent attacks in the same area over many months.

Scleritis

Keratitis associated with anterior diffuse and nodular scleritis

Scleritis is associated with four patterns of keratitis seen either separately or in association: diffuse stromal keratitis, sclerosing stromal keratitis, deep keratitis, and limbal guttering. The changes are usually in relation to, or in the same quadrant as the scleral change, and therefore the keratitis seen in nodular scleritis is usually less extensive than in the diffuse disease. When vascularisation occurs, this follows the corneal lesions, and after recurrence there may be a further ingrowth of vessels.

Diffuse stromal keratitis. Diffuse stromal keratitis may come on suddenly or slowly. The single or multiple midstromal opacities expand slowly in size without treatment and may become surrounded by a dense white ring, rather like the 'precipitin ring' seen on agar immunodiffusion. This type of reaction was originally described by von Szily (1913) and results from the localisation of antigen within the cornea. Keratic precipitates conglomerate on the posterior corneal surface in relation to the precipitin ring (Figures 4.38 and 4.39). If untreated or inadequately treated, the opacities eventually coalesce until the whole cornea becomes opaque and swollen. An anterior uveitis usually accompanies these changes but is rarely severe. If the scleritis is treated vigorously with full doses of steroids, these opacities can disappear without trace; more usually, however, linear opacities within the stroma remain and, if central, can impair vision.

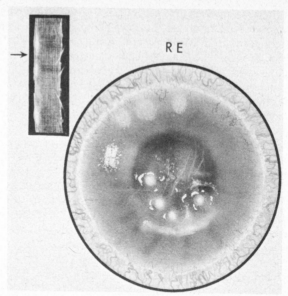

Figure 4.38. Stromal keratitis of acute onset which accompanied a generalised anterior necrotising scleritis. The cornea is infiltrated throughout. The opacities agglomerate as nummular opacities at the periphery and as dense grey spots centrally, around which 'precipitin rings' can be seen.

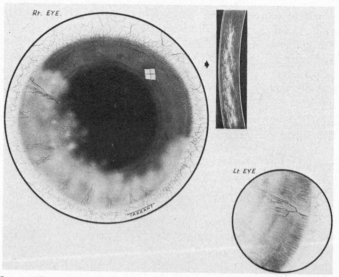

Figure 4.39. A diffuse stromal keratitis of gradual onset in which the scleritis was in the adjacent quadrant to the opacity. The vessels appeared after the opacities.

Sclerosing keratitis. The diffuse changes can progress to a sclerosing keratitis or the sclerosing keratitis may arise de novo. This descriptive appearance is of a change in the corneal stroma which makes it resemble sclera, probably due to irreversible collagen change and reorientation of the collagen fibres. The corneal opacities usually appear gradually, adjacent to the swollen sclera. If the cornea is slightly oedematous, then vessels may infiltrate from the periphery, but although this vascularisation appears to be a passive phenomenon, the presence of these vessels probably determines the extent of resolution and the progression of the opacification of the cornea should the scleritis recur (Figure 4.40). When this happens the cornea swells again and the opacity advances towards the centre of the cornea. Suppression of the inflammation allows partial regression, but eventually the whole cornea becomes opaque because opacities once formed never disappear (Figure 4.41 and 4.42, Plate VI). Corneal grafting is extremely successful in restoring vision.

When the corneal oedema regresses, the corneal lamellae coalesce and, perhaps because lipid is deposited on them, the fibres can reflect the light to look exactly like the sugar crystals of 'candy floss'. Similar changes have been seen following chemical burns, but in the absence of a history of injury, the 'candy floss' can be regarded as the hallmark of sclerosing keratitis (Figure 4.42). There seems to be no particular correlation between the aetiology of the scleritis and the presence of this type of corneal change which can be progressive even in the absence of active scleral disease.

Deep stromal keratitis. This change is unusual, but in long-standing cases of scleritis a white opaque sheet spreads over the cornea at the level of

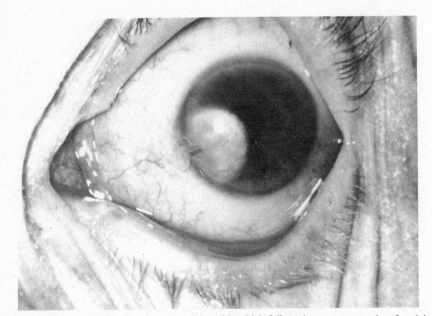

Figure 4.40. Localised sclerosing stromal keratitis which followed recurrent attacks of nodular scleritis which always recurred at the same site. Crystalline deposits are appearing at the central edge of the opacity.

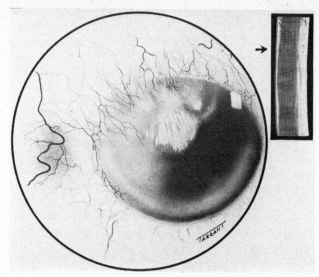

Figure 4.41. Progressive sclerosing stromal keratitis, 'crystalline' deposits in deep stroma, and a 'precipitin ring' around the infiltrate at 12 o'clock. Vascularisation is passive following the advancing edge. Acute diffuse stromal keratitis will progress to this if untreated.

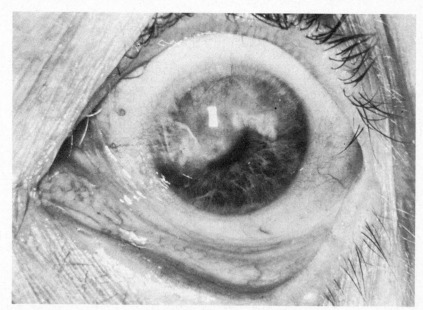

Figure 4.42. The same eye as Figure 4.41 two years later after several more recurrences of the scleritis. The extent of the opacity has increased, the precipitin ring has disappeared and the 'candy floss' opacities have moved closer to the edge of the opacified cornea. The cornea at 8 o'clock which was oedematous but not greatly infiltrated, has cleared completely.

Descemet's membrane with or without some local vascularisation. This may be simply a similar change to that found in sclerosing keratitis but we have seen several patients in whom this type of deep stromal opacification together with a nummular corneal opacity has preceded the onset of scleritis (Holt Wilson and Watson, 1974) (Figure 4.43). All of these patients were under 30 and the deep interstitial keratitis which they developed looked exactly like that seen in the keratitis of congenital syphilis, tuberculosis, leprosy, brucellosis and onchocerciasis. None of the patients, however, had any evidence of these conditions.

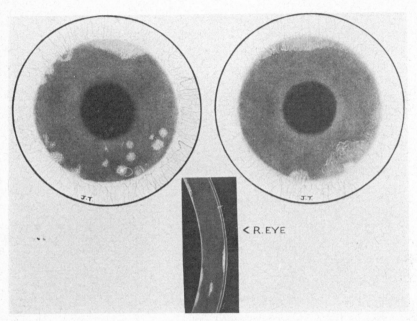

Figure 4.43. Nummular corneal opacities which preceded a diffuse anterior scleritis in a young woman of 24. The superficial corneal opacities resolved leaving permanent changes.

In the absence of syphilis, this type of 'keratitis profunda' has been described as being related to infirmity and chronic sepsis, although Nantz inculpated an allergic response to tuberculin, pyogenic cocci or coliform organisms (Spicer, 1924; Nantz, 1952).

The corneal lesions and mild uveitis are very similar to those described by Cogan (1945) and Norton and Cogan (1959) when reporting and reviewing cases of non-syphilitic interstitial keratitis associated with auditory and vestibular symptoms (Cogan's syndrome). The corneal infiltrates are patchy and deep and fluctuate in intensity and distribution; they are associated with deep vascularisation if they persist long enough. The underlying endothelium shows nonspecific guttate changes.

These patients with scleritis were young but not deaf nor did they have any connective tissue disease. We have seen one case of Cogan's syndrome (Figure 7.37) in a 27-year-old female which was associated with a marked episcleritis, a positive antinuclear factor, and the recent development of joint disease. This patient was very similar to a case described by Bennett (1963).

Limbal guttering. Limbal guttering is occasionally seen, especially in association with diffuse scleritis; the thinned area is not quite adjacent to the sclera, does not extend more than 2 mm into the cornea, and may progress to an area of ectasia rather than guttering. The guttering seen in these types of scleritis is slow to occur, never dramatic and rarely causes complications (Figures 4.44 and 4.45). The gutters usually start between the 9 and 11

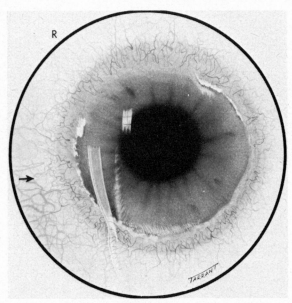

Figure 4.44.   An almost circumferential limbal gutter associated with recurrent diffuse anterior scleritis. Lipid has become deposited at the edge of the gutter.

o'clock positions on the cornea or between 2 and 3 o'clock. Either they extend from the edges to join up above and below, or new areas of peripheral thinning occur in the previously normal sclera. The gutters are not necessarily directly associated with areas of scleral disease although this can happen. Brown and Grayson (1968) described nine cases of marginal furrows of the cornea, of similar type, affecting patients suffering from rheumatoid arthritis of more than five years' duration. The furrows were seen most commonly at the inferior aspect of the limbus and were bilateral in four of the patients. Similar furrows have been described by Collier (1952) and Frasca (1958).

   Patients suffering from long-standing rheumatoid arthritis often display a characteristic corneal lesion (Lyne, 1970). This consists of a partial opacity of the periphery of the cornea involving part or all of its circumference. The cornea in this area is thinned, usually by about one-third of its normal thickness and has a well-demarcated central edge. It is minimally vascularised by superficial vessels crossing the limbus. The appearance is quite striking,

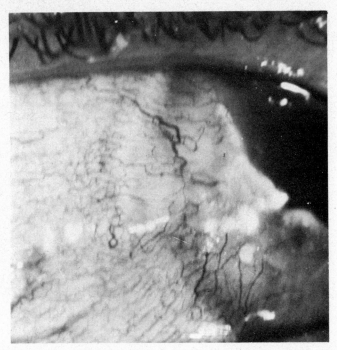

Figure 4.45. Limbal furrowing of gradual onset and of little consequence in a patient who had recurrent attacks of anterior diffuse scleritis.

even upon superficial examination, and resembles that of an eye wearing a microcorneal contact lens, so much so that Lyne calls it 'contact-lens' cornea (see Figure 7.11). Although these changes can occur alone, they are often associated with a diffuse anterior scleritis of long standing and true thinning with increased transparency of the anterior sclera also occurs. When the erosion occurs in the deep layers, the cornea bulges forwards, resembling Terrien's disease. In one patient this has led to an expansion of the eye in the axis of the scleritis to well over 18 dioptres (Figures 4.46 and 4.47). The clinical course of these gutters varies considerably. In some patients they will fill in completely once the scleritis is treated and in others the defect remains. Perforation of these very thin areas is very unusual, so it is unnecessary to do anything about them unless the eye is expanding or vision is affected (Figure 4.48). Even if perforation does occur they are easily treated by annular lamellar grafting or simply by covering the defect with a conjunctival flap.

Lipid deposition. Lipid deposition is always common centrally in a damaged cornea and at the edge of a long-standing corneal gutter, presumably because diffusion of the lipid products of metabolism towards the limbus is impaired. The increased deposition of lipid in the damaged corneal lamellae is not a change peculiar to the corneal involvement in scleral disease but is the same as would occur in any situation where the lamellae of the cornea have been oedematous for a prolonged period.

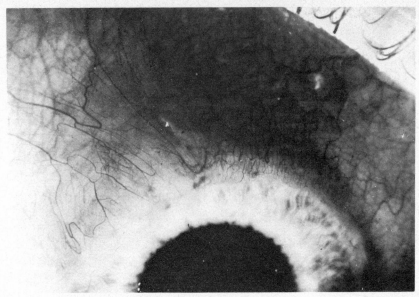

Figure 4.46.   Acute anterior diffuse scleritis adjacent to the limbus in a young man of 30 who had had persistent attacks of similar severity for five years.

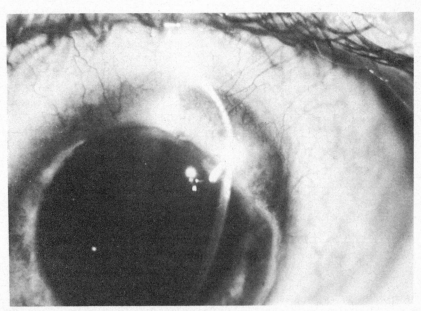

Figure 4.47.   When the scleritis resolved, the deep corneal stroma could be seen to be bowed forwards and thinned as in Terrien's disease. The eyeball expanded and had to be treated by grafting. (See also Figures 9.5 and 9.6.)

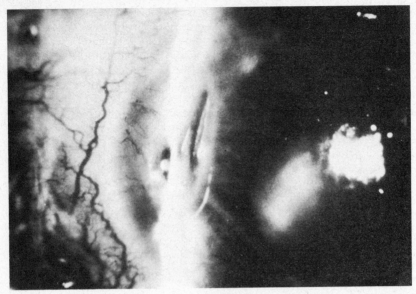

Figure 4.48. Corneal guttering associated with necrotising scleral disease. A deep furrow has formed in soft grey swollen cornea almost to the point of perforation. The gutter has a sharp well-defined margin.

Keratitis associated with necrotising scleritis

The changes seen in necrotising scleritis are similar to but more intense than those seen in diffuse and nodular anterior scleritis. In addition keratolysis of large areas of the cornea can occur.

Acute stromal keratitis. In the severe necrotising scleritis of acute onset the cornea becomes oedematous and dense white infiltrates appear within the stroma (Figure 4.48). They are sometimes central and sometimes peripheral and may coalesce as the disease progresses. If in addition there is anterior chamber activity then keratic precipitates (KP's) adhere to the posterior corneal surface. The opacity is sometimes surrounded by a 'precipitin' ring. The corneal reaction can sometimes be so acute as to reduce the vision temporarily to finger counting only. It may also precede the onset of the scleral inflammation by 24 to 48 hours, although it usually occurs at the same time as, or within 24 hours of, the onset of acute necrotising anterior scleritis.

If the diagnosis is made correctly and treatment is vigorous and instituted at once, the opacities disappear without trace; more usually, however, linear opacities remain within the stroma and, if central, impair vision. In those patients who have not been adequately treated, or have not been treated at all, the corneal changes progress either to a typical sclerosing keratitis with dense corneal opacities or the peripheral or central cornea breaks down with a consequent loss of stromal tissue.

Corneal guttering. The guttering seen in necrotising scleral disease differs from
that seen when the scleritis is less severe. The peripheral corneal gutters,
which start as a grey soft swollen area adjacent to an area of scleritis, rapidly
break down to extend over more than one quadrant of the globe (Figure
4.49). The gutter develops a sharp well-defined border on the corneal side
and the limbal margin may well be undermined. The depth of the ulcer often
contains fine blood vessels but these do not extend beyond the ulcer margins.
The epithelium is almost always intact throughout the course of the disease.
Left untreated these ulcers will extend to include the whole limbus but with
treatment they remain either unaltered or gradually fill in, leaving a small
depression. They do not extend into the corneal stroma and do not of themselves affect vision.

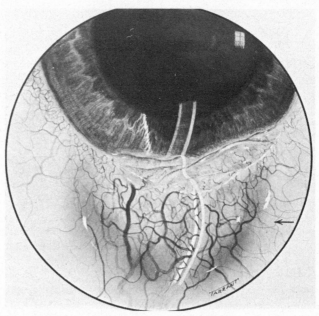

Figure 4.49.   Corneal guttering associated with necrotising scleritis and systemic vasculitis. The
gutter involves both cornea and sclera and consists of multiple deep furrows with everted edges.

This type of limbal guttering can occur with the minimal degree of scleral
involvement and may even precede the scleritis by several months (Ferry
and Leopold, 1970). All the patients we have seen have had gross abnormalities
in the immunoglobulins and almost all have had vasculitis which has been
primary, as in periarteritis nodosa, or secondary, associated with the extra-
articular manifestations of rheumatoid arthritis (Figure 4.49).

The differentiation from Mooren's ulcer is important and difficult. In nearly
20 per cent of cases, Mooren's ulcer was the suspected diagnosis at some
time in eyes with scleritis which eventually came to enucleation, and some
eyes have been removed with Mooren's ulcer as the only diagnosis, the scleritis
being entirely unsuspected. Mooren's ulcer occurs in elderly patients as opposed

to the younger patients with vasculitis. It starts at the periphery in a very similar manner to the guttering found with necrotising scleritis but the corneal margin is undermined and the disease extends towards the centre of the cornea, eventually causing clouding of the cornea and loss of stromal tissue. Both types of ulcers are painful, gradually progressive and neither leads to perforation unless the eye is otherwise damaged. Mooren's ulceration is not associated with any systemic disease, vasculitis or anomalies of immunoglobulins. Any new tissue inserted into a cornea with Mooren's ulceration will be removed in the same way as in the original condition, but, provided the systemic disease is under control, new tissue inserted for any reason into an eye with necrotising scleritis will be retained and remain clear.

Keratolysis. This is the term given to the melting of the cornea sometimes encountered in the severest type of necrotising scleritis and is the most severe of all corneal diseases associated with scleritis and, although rare, happens

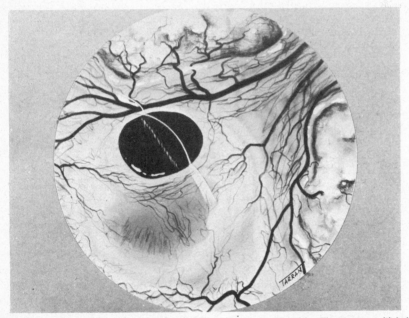

Figure 4.50. Keratolysis in a patient with severe necrotising scleritis. The cornea which had become generally opaque melted away leaving a perfectly clear descemetocoele.

with alarming rapidity. There seem to be two types. In the first is a gradual opacification of the cornea associated with necrotising scleral disease which is increasing in severity. Suddenly, within as short a time as four days, the central stroma of the cornea gives way, the destructive process expands outwards towards the limbus, leaving only Descemet's membrane covered by epithelium, through which the patient can sometimes see extremely clearly (Figure 4.50). If the destructive change is allowed to continue beyond this stage, corneal rupture can occur.

The second type follows a long-standing necrotising scleritis which is circumferential. The cornea, which has been of normal thickness and clarity, thickens, opacifies and begins to lose stromal substance centrally to the extent that a descemetocele occurs. In about half these patients there is also a peripheral corneal gutter (Figure 4.51).

If the destructive process is halted in both these varieties, the area adjacent to the thin cornea which has been oedematous heals, leaving corneal opacities similar to that seen in sclerosing keratitis caused by other forms of scleritis. We have only seen one patient who has had any degree of stromal loss recover any thickness of cornea; all the rest have required corneal grafting to replace the thin atrophic scar or occasionally to repair the ruptured descemetocele.

Uveitis

It has often been suggested that uveitis is a universal accompaniment of scleritis of any severity (Mackenzie, 1830; Duke Elder and Leigh, 1965e). This is not the case (Table 4.4).

Table 4.4. *Percentage anterior uveitis in scleritis*

Type of scleritis		Eyes	Anterior uveitis (%)
Anterior:	Diffuse	119	35
	Nodular	134	17
	Necrotising	29	37
	Scleromalacia		
	perforans	13	100
Posterior		6	66

Only two patients developed a uveitis in the opposite, apparently unaffected eye.
From Watson and Hayreh (1976).

There was some evidence of anterior uveitis in 30 per cent of all those eyes with scleritis which we have studied. It was found universally with those patients with scleromalacia perforans but, surprisingly, did not always occur in patients with necrotising scleritis. This finding is the reverse of what might be expected in that the eyes with relatively little external signs of inflammation always manifested intraocular changes and some patients with very severe necrotising scleritis did not even have any cells in the anterior chamber. The site of the scleral inflammation has some influence on the presence of uveitis: those in whom the inflammation was further back over the ciliary body or involved a great deal of the circumference of the eye had the most severe uveitis (Figure 4.17).

Two-thirds of the patients with posterior scleritis also had some evidence of anterior inflammation in addition to the posterior uveitis universally present, presumably because the choroidal and ciliary vessels are involved in the inflammatory process in the sclera and in the formation of granulomatous tissue.

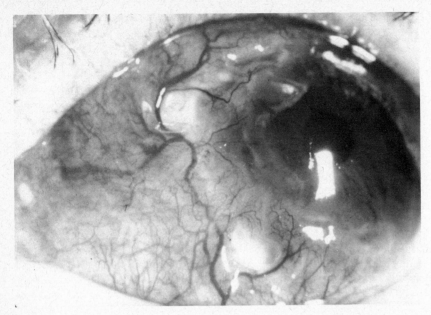

Figure 4.51.   Keratolysis in less acute and long-standing necrotising scleritis. Loss of thickness of the stroma of both cornea and sclera is occurring adjacent to the limbus.

A posterior uveitis is very rare in combination with anterior scleritis. If, therefore, a posterior uveitis is detected in a patient with anterior scleritis, signs of a posterior scleritis must be looked for, even to the extent of using fluorescent angiography to detect any choroidal exudation.

Patients with episcleritis never develop a severe anterior uveitis. Cells in the anterior chamber and a mild aqueous flare were found in four per cent of those patients we have seen and this seemed to be related to the severity of the episcleral inflammation. Synechiae developed in 20 per cent of McGavin et al's patients (1976) with episcleritis and rheumatoid arthritis. This does not accord with our experience and is very surprising in view of the low incidence of a primary uveitis in rheumatoid arthritis which does not exceed that expected in the normal population (Stanworth and Sharp, 1956). It is possible that some of McGavin's patients had otherwise undetected scleral disease or it may be that episcleritis associated with rheumatoid arthritis produces a more violent reaction than when associated with other conditions.

Although uveitis is not a universal accompaniment of scleritis, and there is no particular correlation between the presence of an anterior uveitis with any particular systemic disease, its presence does indicate a more diffuse and severe process, and when also accompanied by glaucoma is a grave and ominous sign. Sixty-eight per cent of all eyes enucleated show signs of having had a severe anterior uveitis (Fraunfelder and Watson, 1976) and the endophthalmitis was so much the predominant feature in two eyes that the presence of scleritis was ignored; a true sclero-uveitis—combination of glaucoma, uveitis and scleritis—should be a strong reason for treating that patient extremely vigorously, particularly if the patient also has a necrotising scleritis. It will be remembered that necrotising scleritis is only associated with anterior uveitis in 37 per cent of patients, but it is this 37 per cent that tend to go downhill quickly unless treated.

When an anterior uveitis did occur it tended to be long-standing and intractable. Mackenzie (1830) described the uveitis which accompanies scleritis thus:

'Dimness of vision uniformly attends this ophthalmia, depending on an accompanying haziness of the cornea and pupil, attended by a slight contraction of the latter, and sluggishness in the movements of the iris. If only one eye is affected, which, at least for some time, is generally the case, the pupil of that eye is seen at once to be less than that of the sound eye. The iris becomes even slightly discoloured; it becomes greenish, for instance, if naturally blue; and the attending iritis may go on to evident effusion of coagulable lymph within the pupil. It must be understood, however, that a severe degree of iritis rarely attends this rheumatic sclerotitis.'

Although flare and cells can occasionally be seen in the anterior chamber of a patient who presents with an anterior scleritis, it is much more common for the cells to appear later in the disease or when the scleritis changes its character to become necrotising. Initially there is little or no exudate, no keratic precipitates and no synechiae. If the condition is allowed to persist (and it will sometimes do this in spite of vigorous treatment) the iris becomes bound down and a plastic exudate fills the anterior chamber and may even extend backwards to involve the vitreous. Scleritis must be considered as a cause of a severe uveitis, particularly if accompanied by a high intraocular pressure.

Glaucoma

As with uveitis, the onset of glaucoma during the course of scleral disease can be an ominous feature and indeed can become so much the predominant feature that in five of 30 eyes examined histologically glaucoma was given as the primary clinical diagnosis, scleritis not being considered as a possible cause. Sevel (1965) also found that 45 per cent of the 43 eyes that he examined had secondary glaucoma. Primary or secondary glaucoma can be expected to be present in 11 per cent of all patients seen in the clinic with scleritis, so that the intraocular pressure must be assessed not only when the patient is first examined but at regular intervals during the course of the disease. Table 4.5 shows distribution of the various types of glaucoma found. Those associated with scleral disease are distinct and their course to an extent is predictable, depending on the severity of scleritis. Of the patients with secondary glaucoma, nine had no abnormality other than scleritis; seven had keratitis and six uveitis. Sclerokeratitis coexisted in some patients. Five patients with episcleritis developed steroid-induced glaucoma (Watson and Hayreh, 1976). It is always important to examine any patient with glaucoma thoroughly, but scleritis adds another dimension because, in most instances, treatment of the scleritis will cure the glaucoma (Watson, 1966; McGavin et al, 1976), thus saving the patient unnecessary medication and possibly surgery.

Table 4.5. *Glaucoma in scleritis*

Type of scleritis	Total eyes	Total with glaucoma	Primary open angle	Primary closed angle	Secon- dary	Steroid- induced
Diffuse anterior	119	12	6	0	6	0
Nodular anterior	134	11	6	0	5	0
Necrotising	29	8	2	0	5	1
Scleromalacia perforans	13	4	0	0	4	0
Posterior	6	0	0	0	0	0
Total	301	35	14	0	20	1

Of the patients with secondary glaucoma, nine had no abnormality other than scleritis, seven had keratitis and six uveitis. Sclerokeratitis coexisted in some patients. Five patients with episcleritis developed steroid-induced glaucoma.
From Watson and Hayreh (1976).

Primary open-angle glaucoma

Five per cent of patients with scleritis have an open-angle glaucoma which can only be classified as primary even though the frequency is more than twice what would be expected in the normal population. A possible explanation of this is that these are patients whose outflow mechanisms would have just been adequate if the eye had not become inflamed, but whose pressure had risen higher than normal and had developed permanent changes in the trabeculae because of slight oedema and infiltration of the outflow channels.

These patients have all the characteristics of idiopathic chronic open-angle glaucoma: gonioscopically normal angles, cupped discs and glaucomatous field defects. They respond to treatment with miotics and acetazolamide, but not to steroids. The intraocular pressure does not return to normal when the scleritis resolves or is treated.

Secondary open-angle glaucoma

Involvement of the drainage mechanism. All the patients in this group differ from those with primary open-angle glaucoma in that until or unless permanent changes occur in the trabecular meshwork, the intraocular pressure falls to normal when the scleritis is adequately treated or quiescent. The underlying mechanism of the glaucoma is uncertain but is apparently due to obstruction of the outflow channels by oedema.

In patients with uveitis the angle can be seen to contain a certain amount of debris and the angle itself appears red and pink.

Recently we have had to operate on a young woman aged 25 who had recurrent scleritis over a period of five to six years which was always most marked within 3 mm of the limbus. With each attack of scleritis the intraocular pressure rose to the mid-40s to 60 mm Hg and returned to normal with each attack. These rises in intraocular pressure were paralleled by a fall in outflow facility which also returned to normal. This satisfactory situation persisted for three to four years. Following this the intraocular pressure and the outflow facilities remained abnormal, the disc began to cup and early field changes appeared. Trabeculectomy was therefore performed on the eye. It had to be done during the active phase of the scleritis and, because the scleritis was circumferential, it also had to be done through an area of intense inflammation. The area adjacent to the scleral spur which contained the trabecular meshwork was red, oedematous and boggy (Figures 4.52 and 4.53). Histologically the specimen showed the trabecular meshwork to be infiltrated with inflammatory cells and was extremely oedematous.

It appears that before any rise occurs in the intraocular pressure the sclera itself must be involved and not just the episcleral outflow channels because we have not seen any glaucomatous changes in all those cases with episcleritis, some of whom had very intense inflammation and oedema.

Neovascular glaucoma

Although we have not observed this clinically, examination of histological sections of patients with both anterior and posterior scleritis reveal the presence of central retinal vein occlusions or branch arterial occlusions, cupped discs and the new vessels on the iris or in the angle.

Steroid-induced glaucoma

Topical corticosteroids are commonly used to increase the comfort in the treatment of patients with episcleritis and scleritis. Topical application of local steroid can induce a rise of 5 to 15 mm Hg in susceptible individuals. This susceptibility is probably genetically determined (Armaly, 1963). The rise in pressure is even greater in older patients or if they have had incipient or manifest open-angle glaucoma. It may be so large as to cause permanent damage which may be irreversible when the drug is stopped. Although very unusual, steroid glaucoma can follow the prolonged use of systemic steroids. A large number of patients are therefore potentially at risk of developing this condition. McGavin et al (1976) found this complication in 16 per cent of the eyes he treated with scleritis and rheumatoid arthritis.

Primary closed-angle glaucoma

Acute closed-angle glaucoma attacks can be induced by an attack of scleritis or episcleritis in a patient with narrow angles and a small eye. The attack is presumably induced by the combination of the slight dilatation of the pupil which often accompanies an attack and the slight congestion and swelling of the ocular tissues in the region of the angle.

The treatment of this type of glaucoma is the same as if the angle closure attack had occurred de novo, that is, systemic treatment with ocular hypotensive agents with or without miotics, to be followed as soon as the eye has become quiet with bilateral peripheral iridectomies.

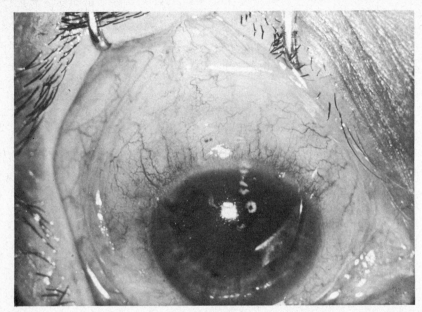

Figure 4.52. Multiple scleral nodules at the limbus in a young woman of 25. The intraocular pressure on intensive local and systemic medication was 40 mm Hg.

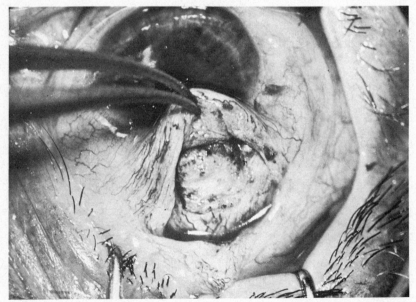

Figure 4.53. Trabeculectomy through one of the nodules. The superficial flap is held forwards revealing the marked oedema of the sclera in the region of the scleral space and trabecular meshwork.

Secondary closed-angle glaucoma

Peripheral anterior synechiae

Following multiple attacks of scleritis and uveitis, particularly if there is a plastic uveitis, peripheral anterior synechiae can be formed and in severe cases a completely occluded false angle can be produced. Fortunately this complication is rare and although it can occur following recurrent circumferential perilimbal scleritis, it occurs mainly in eyes which are severely damaged by necrotising scleral disease in which case the glaucoma may be the terminal event. Vigorous treatment, which may include surgery, is needed to prevent staphyloma formation and loss of vision (Figure 4.54).

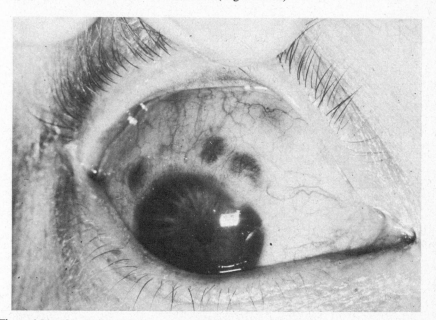

Figure 4.54.   Staphyloma formation in a patient with severe secondary closed-angle glaucoma following scleritis complicated by anterior uveitis.

Surgical treatment, on conventional lines, using a trabeculectomy from behind the scleral spur (Watson, 1966) is surprisingly effective. This particular method of approach has considerable advantages (page 429) because it is possible to dissect away the synechiae under direct vision not only from the area of the trabeculectomy but also from those adjacent to it. The presence of a retained superficial flap of sclera particularly if the operation is performed in an area of relatively normal sclera, prevents the dehiscences of ciliary tissue into the wound which can happen with other glaucoma techniques in which the whole of the sclera is transected.

Angle closure due to ciliary oedema in posterior scleritis

We have recently seen two patients who presented with typical acute closed-angle glaucoma attacks but in whom the opposite anterior chamber was deep and the angle wide open (see Figure 10.21). Examination revealed a posterior scleritis and when the cornea was cleared there was an obvious annular ciliochoroidal detachment which was so large as to displace the lens iris diaphragm forward and close the angle. Treatment with acetazolamide and systemic Tanderil was sufficient to bring the inflammation and the glaucoma under control without the necessity for surgery.

Cataract

Senile cataracts which are present in one eye when the scleritis starts advance more rapidly than in the unaffected eye, but only if the scleritis is severe. Cataract formation which is caused by the sclero-uveitis only seems to occur in those patients who have severe necrotising scleritis or when the disease has been unremitting over several years and has progressed in an annular fashion around the globe. In these patients no change can be observed in the lens whilst there is an arc of 5° of normal sclera, but once the scleritis has involved the sclera through 360° the lens rapidly becomes opaque. The lens changes are very similar to those seen following the anterior segment necrosis produced by encircling operations for retinal detachment. In this situation, the whole lens opacifies at the same time, presumably because the nutrition of the anterior segment is diminished and lens capsule damaged (Figure 4.55).

Posterior subcortical cataracts can be expected to occur in about 15 per cent of patients receiving long-term systemic or local corticosteroid preparations

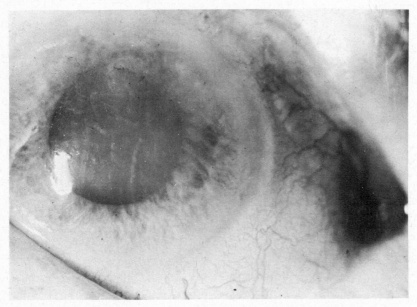

Figure 4.55.   Dense cataract and corneal oedema resulting from a necrotising circumferential scleritis. The clinical picture is very similar to anterior segment necrosis of other causes.

for any reason (Black et al, 1960) and it appears that the combination of anterior scleritis and corticosteroid therapy increases the risk of developing this type of cataract to around 36 per cent (McGavin et al, 1976). Whilst it is advisable to refrain from the use of steroids for the treatment of scleritis in favour of a non-steroid anti-inflammatory agent because of the danger of developing cataracts, it is not justifiable to let the scleritis progress because the treatment is not effective. The cataracts can always be removed, and when dealing with severe disease, it is always worth accepting the small risk involved in the use of steroids.

Cataract extraction has always been uncomplicated. Even in the presence of active scleral disease, the corneoscleral wound has healed normally even though the limbal wound has been adjacent to a dehiscence in the sclera. This implies that the processes involved in wound healing are unaffected by those which cause the scleral inflammation and necrosis. On the other hand, we have seen five patients who had developed scleritis following cataract extraction and scleritis at the site of the corneoscleral wound. Whether this is because the antibody is precipitating at the site of the previous trauma or whether it is related to the use of α-chymotrypsin (a known sensitiser; Watson, 1963) which was used for all the extractions, is at present uncertain.

Oculomotor Pareses

Quite apart from the limitation of movement caused by infiltration of the muscles by granulomata, true oculomotor pareses can occur, presumably due to direct involvement of the nerve supply in the orbit (Davies and Karseras, 1971).

REFERENCES

Alt, A. (1903) Episcleritis and scleritis. *American Journal of Ophthalmology*, **20**, 101–111.

Anderson, D. & Margolis, C. (1952) Scleromalacia: clinical and pathologic study of a case, with consideration of differential diagnosis, relationship of collagen disease and effect of ACTH and cortisone therapy. *American Journal of Ophthalmology*, **35**, 917–931.

Armaly, M. F. (1963) Effect of corticosteroids on intraocular pressure and fluid dynamics. I: The effect of dexamethasone in the normal eye. *Archives of Ophthalmology*, **70**, 482–491.

Barraquer, M. J. (1965) La discontinuité localisée du film lacrymale précornéen: cause des excavations marginales de la cornée de Fuchs, de la progression du pterygion et de certaines necroses de la cornée au voisinage des keratoprosthèses et keratoplasties. *Ophthalmologica*, **150**, 111–122.

Benedict, W. L. (1924) Aetiology and treatment of scleritis and episcleritis. *Transactions of the American Academy of Ophthalmology and Otolaryngology*, **29**, 211–221.

Bennett, F. M. (1963) Bilateral recurrent episcleritis associated with posterior corneal changes, vestibuloauditory symptoms and rheumatoid arthritis. *American Journal of Ophthalmology*, **55**, 815–818.

Bertelsen, T. I. (1960) Acute sclerotenonitis and ocular myositis complicated by papillitis, retinal detachment and glaucoma. *Acta Ophthalmologica*, **38**, 136–152.

Birsch-Hirschfeld, A. (1910) Zur Pathologie und Therapie der Orbitalphlegmonie hochgradige Verbiegung und lakunäre Faserdegeneration im Optikus. *Albrecht v. Graefes Archiv für Ophthalmologie*, **71**, 333–349.

Black, R. L., Oglesby, R. B., von Sallmann, L. et al (1960) Posterior subcapsular cataracts induced by corticosteroids in patients with rheumatoid arthritis. *Journal of the American Medical Association*, **174**, 166–171.

Böck, J. (1929) Uber einen Fall von Periarteritis nodosa mit histologische nachgewiesenen Veränderungen von Muskel und Ziliargefässen des Auges. *Zeitschrift für Augenheilkunde*, **69**, 225–230.

Boylan, C. E. (1964) Case of misdiagnosed scleromalacia perforans. *Survey of Ophthalmology*, **9**, 252–256.

Brenner, E. H. & Shock, J. P. (1974) Proptosis secondary to systemic lupus erythematosus. *Archives of Ophthalmology*, **91**, 81–82.

Brown, S. I. & Grayson, M. (1968) Marginal furrows: a characteristic corneal lesion of rheumatoid arthritis. *Archives of Ophthalmology*, **79**, 563–567.

Campbell, D. M. (1903) Episcleritis. *Ophthalmic Record*, **12**, 517–522.

Clearly, P. E., Watson, P. G., McGill, J. I. et al (1975) Visual loss due to posterior segment disease in scleritis. *Transactions of the Ophthalmological Societies of the United Kingdom*, **95**, 297–300.

Coats, G. (1907) Posterior scleritis and infarction of the posterior ciliary arteries. *Transactions of the Ophthalmological Societies of the United Kingdom*, **27**, 135–149.

Cogan, D. G. (1945) Syndrome of non-syphilitic interstitial keratitis and vestibuloauditory symptoms. *Archives of Ophthalmology*, **33**, 144–149.

Collier, M. (1952) Dystrophie marginale bilaterale de la cornée, ectatique à droite et kerato-conjonctivité sêche. *Bulletin de la Société d'Ophtalmologie de France*, **52**, 380–384.

Critchett, G. (1854) Lectures on disease of the eye. *Lancet*, **ii**, 205–207.

Dalrymple, J. (1852) *Pathology of the Human Eye*. London: Longman.

Davenport, R. (1958) discussion on Graham, P. A.: Unusual evolution of retinal detachments. *Transactions of the Ophthalmological Societies of the United Kingdom*, **78**, 370.

Davies, M. S. & Karseras, A. G. (1971) Oculomotor nerve paresis in a case of scleritis. *British Journal of Ophthalmology*, **55**, 196–198.

Dellaporta, A. (1950) Transitory myopia in scleritis. *Klinische Wochenschrift*, **62**, 308.

Derby, G. S. & Verhoeff, F. H. (1916) Massive granuloma of sclera (brawny scleritis) with a report of an unusual case. *Archives of Ophthalmology*, **45**, 20–32.

Donaldson, D. (1964) Sarcoid nodules of iris and paralimbal sclera. *Archives of Ophthalmology*, **71**, 246.

Drouet, P. & Thomas, C. (1952) Episclérité periodique et système endinocrino-vegatif. *Bulletin de la Société d'Ophtalmologie de France*, **7**, 682–685.

Duke Elder, S. & Leigh, A. G. (1965) *System of Ophthalmology*, Vol 8. (a) p. 1008; (b) p. 1009; (c) p. 1008; (d) p. 1083; (e) p. 1013. London: Kimpton.

Eden, K. C. & Trotter, W. R. (1942) Lid retraction in toxic diffuse goitre. *Lancet*, **ii**, 385–387.

Ferry, A. P. & Leopold, I. H. (1970) Marginal (ring) corneal ulcer as a presenting manifestation of Wegener's granuloma. *Transactions of the American Academy of Ophthalmology and Otolaryngology*, **74**, 1276–1282.

Franceschetti, A. & Bischler, V. (1950) La sclérité nodulaire necrosante et ses rapports avec la scléromalacie. *Annales d'Oculistique*, **183**, 737–744.

Frasca, G. (1958) La degenerazione marginale della cornea nel quadro delle cosidette malattie del collageno. *Rassegna Italiana d'Ottalmologia*, **27**, 255–273.

Fraunfelder, F. T. & Watson, P. G. (1976) Evaluation of eyes enucleated for scleritis. *British Journal of Ophthalmology*, **60**, 227–230.

Fuchs, E. (1895) Ueber episkleritis periodica fugax. *Albrecht v. Graefes Archiv für Ophthalmologie*, **41**, 229–273.

Fuchs, E. (1902) Skleritis posterior. *Sitzungsberichte der Ophthalmologischen Gesellschaft in Wien*, **1903**, 71–77.

Gass, J. D. (1974) *Differential Diagnosis of Ocular Tumours.* 198 pp. St. Louis: Mosby.

Goder, G. (1969) Posterior pseudotumorous scleritis. *Klinische Monatsblätter für Augenheilkunde,* **155,** 200–214.

Graham, P. A. (1958) Unusual evolution of retinal detachments. *Transactions of the Ophthalmological Societies of the United Kingdom,* **78,** 359–371.

Heinonen, O. (1923) Über Episcleritis periodica fugax und Erblichkeit. *Acta Ophthalmologica,* **1,** 166–177.

Heinonen, O. (1927) Nachtrag zu meiner Arbeit 'Über episcleritis periodica fugax und Erblichkeit'. *Acta Ophthalmologica,* **4,** 278–280.

Holt-Wilson, A. D. & Watson, P. G. (1974) Non-syphilitic deep interstitial keratitis associated with scleritis. *Transactions of the Ophthalmological Societies of the United Kingdom,* **94,** 52–57.

Holthouse, F. H. (1893) Unusual case of ulceration of the conjunctiva and sclera. *Royal London Hospital Report,* **13,** 415–418.

Hurd, E. R., Snyder, W. B. & Ziff, M. (1970) Choroidal nodules and retinal detachments in rheumatoid arthritis. *American Journal of Medicine,* **48,** 273–278.

Inman, W. S. (1955) Nine monthly scleritis in a childless woman. *British Journal of Medical Psychology,* **28,** 177–182.

Kamocki, V. (1892) Selbsthielung einer Lederhäutentzündung und Netzhautablösung. *Zentralblatt für praktische Augenheilkunde,* **16,** 15–17.

Kennedy, A. C. & McGavin, D. D. M. (1975) Rheumatoid scleritis producing exophthalmos. *British Journal of Clinical Practice,* **29,** 73–76.

Kiehle, F. A. (1946) Scleromalacia. *American Journal of Ophthalmology,* **29,** 862–863.

Kimura, S. J. & Hogan, M. J. (1964) Chronic cyclitis. *Archives of Ophthalmology,* **71,** 193–201.

Klein, M., Calvert, R. J., Joseph, W. E. et al (1955) Rarities in ocular sarcoidosis. *British Journal of Ophthalmology,* **39,** 416–421.

Lasco, F. & Nicolesco, M. (1960) The ophthalmological manifestations of collagen disease. *Archives d'Ophtalmologie,* **20,** 602–615.

Leira, H. (1975) Sclerotenonitis and orbital myositis. Occurrence in collagenous disease. In *Modern Problems in Ophthalmology.* Vol. 14, *Orbital Disorders,* pp. 669–674. *Proceedings of the 2nd International Symposium on Orbital Disorders, Amsterdam, 1973.* Basel: Karger.

Lyne, A. J. (1970) 'Contact lens' cornea in rheumatoid arthritis. *British Journal of Ophthalmology,* **54,** 410–415.

Mackenzie, W. (1830) *A Practical Treatise on Diseases of the Eye.* London: Longman.

Marquard, H. A. (1956) Two sisters with scleromalacia perforans. *Acta Ophthalmologica,* **34,** 245–249.

Maumenee, A. E. (1956) Ocular manifestations of collagen disease. *Archives of Ophthalmology,* **56,** 557–562.

McGavin, D. D., Williamson, J., Forrester, J. V. et al (1976) Episcleritis and scleritis: a study of their clinical manifestations and association with rheumatoid arthritis. *British Journal of Ophthalmology,* **60,** 192–226.

Moench, L. M. (1927) Gynaecologic foci in relation to scleritis and episcleritis and other ocular infections. *American Journal of the Medical Sciences,* **174,** 439–448.

Nantz, F. A. (1952) Keratitis profunda due to bacterial hypersensitivity: identified by tissue culture and treated by specific desensitization. *IV Congreso Pan-Americano de Oftalmologia.* **2,** 1241–1250.

Norton, E. W. & Cogen, D. G. (1959) Syndrome of nonsyphilitic interstitial keratitis and vestibuloauditory symptoms. *Archives of Ophthalmology,* **61,** 695–697.

Pal, D. (1953) An interesting case of transient and periodic episcleritis. *Advances in Medicine.* **5,** 361.

Parsons, J. H. (1902) Annular scleritis. *Ophthalmic Review,* **21,** 181–186.

Paufique, L. & Etienne, R. (1949) L'étiologie génitale de quelques affections oculaires chez la femme. *Archives d'Ophtalmologie,* **9,** 157–175.

Purtscher, O. (1891) Drusen-bildung in Schnervenkopfe. *Zentralblatt für Praktische Augenheilkunde*, **15**, 292–294.

Roca, P. D. (1974) Necrotising (rheumatoid) disease of the sclera. *New York State Journal of Medicine*, **74**, 1982–1988.

Rosen, E. S. & Lyne, A. J. (1968) Uveal effusions. *American Journal of Ophthalmology*, **65**, 509–518.

Rucker, C. W. & Ferguson, R. H. (1964) Ocular manifestations in relapsing polychondritis. *Transactions of the American Ophthalmological Society*, **62**, 167–172.

Rundle, R. (1941) A study of the pathogenesis of thyrotoxicosis. *Lancet*, **ii**, 149–152.

Sampson, R. (1945) Periarteritis nodosa affecting the eye. *British Journal of Ophthalmology*, **29**, 282–288.

Schepens, C. L. & Brockhurst, R. J. (1960) Uveitis. II: Peripheral uveitis, clinical description, complications and differential diagnosis. *American Journal of Ophthalmology*, **49**, 1257–1266.

Schlodtmann, W. (1897) Über sulzige infiltration der conjunktiva und sklera. *Albrecht v. Graefes Archiv für Ophthalmologie*, **43**, 56–82.

Sevel, D. (1965) Rheumatoid nodule of the sclera. *Transactions of the Ophthalmological Societies of the United Kingdom*, **85**, 357–367.

Sevel, D. (1967) Necrogranulomatous scleritis. *American Journal of Ophthalmology*, **64**, 1125–1134.

Spicer, W. T. (1924) Parenchymatous keratitis; interstitial keratitis, uveitis anterior. *British Journal of Ophthalmology*, Monograph Supplement, **1**.

Stallard, H. B. (1954) Annular peripheral retinal detachment. *British Journal of Ophthalmology*, **38**, 115–118.

Stanworth, A. & Sharp, J. (1956) Uveitis and rheumatic diseases. *Annals of the Rheumatic Diseases*, **15**, 140–150.

Suganuma, S. (1939) Über die klinischen und histologischen Befunde eines Falles von primärer hinterer skleral-tuberkulose. *Klinische Monatsblätter für Augenheilkunde*, **103**, 208–211.

Sym, W. G. (1896) Scleritis. *American Journal of the Medical Sciences*, **112**, 62–67.

Uhthoff, W. (1900) Weiterer Beiträg zur pathologischen Anatomie der Skleritis. *Albrecht v. Graefes Archiv für Ophthalmologie*, **49**, 539–560.

van der Hoeve, J. (1931) Scleromalacia perforans. *Nederlandsch Tijdschrift voor Geneeskunde*, **75**, 4733–4735.

van der Hoeve, J. (1934) Scleromalacia perforans. *Archives of Ophthalmology*, **11**, 111–118.

Villard, E. (1930) Episclérite cataméniale. *Archives d'ophtalmologie*, **47**, 534–538.

von Graefe, A. quoted by Duke Elder S. in *System of Ophthalmology*, Vol. 8, p. 1009. London: Kimpton.

von Szily, A. (1913) Uber die Bedeutung der Anaphylaxie in der Augenheilkunde. *Klinische Monatsblätter für Augenheilkunde*, **15**, 164–180.

Wagenmann, A. (1903) Zur Kenntnis der Skleritis posterior. *Zeitschrift für Augenheilkunde*, **10**, 343–346.

Wagenmann, A. (1906) Weitere Mitteilungen über Skleritis posterior. *Albrecht v. Graefes Archiv für Ophthalmologie*, **64**, 380–390.

Wardrop, J. (1818) Account of the rheumatic inflammation of the eye with observation on the treatment of the disease. *Medico-Chirurgical Transactions*, **10**, 1–5.

Watson, P. G. (1963) Anaphylactic reaction caused by intramuscular injection of lyophilized alpha-chymotrypsin. *British Journal of Ophthalmology*, **48**, 35–38.

Watson, P. G. (1966) Management of scleral disease. *Transactions of the Ophthalmological Societies of the United Kingdom*, **86**, 151–167.

Watson, P. G. & Hayreh, S. S. (1976) Scleritis and episcleritis. *British Journal of Ophthalmology*, **60**, 163–191.

Watson, P. G. & Lobascher, D. (1965) The diagnosis and management of episcleritis and scleritis. *Transactions of the Ophthalmological Societies of the United Kingdom*, **85**, 369–378.

Watson, P. G., McKay, D. A., Clemett, R. S. et al (1973) Treatment of episcleritis. A double blind trial comparing betamethasone 0.1%, oxyphenbutazone 10% and placebo eye ointments. *British Journal of Ophthalmology*, **57**, 866–870.

Williamson, J. (1974) Incidence of eye disease in cases of connective tissue disease. *Transactions of the Ophthalmological Societies of the United Kingdom*, **94**, 742–752.

Wolfe, E. (1882) *On Diseases and Injuries of the Eye*. London: Churchill.

CHAPTER FIVE

Morphological Changes in Inflammatory Scleral Disease

'Pathology is the accomplished tragedy; physiology the basis on which our treatment rests.' (Edward Martin, 1859–1938).

The value of histopathological studies in the determination of the pathogenesis of both joint and scleral disease has been diminished because sections of affected tissue have necessarily been from patients with the severest types of disease in organs which have also been damaged by secondary changes. Biopsy of synovial tissue in the early stages of disease has recently become possible and has contributed a great deal to the understanding of the underlying pathological processes. Unfortunately, biopsy of scleral tissue can be hazardous.

Because of the difficulty of diagnosing the underlying disease, a surgeon was persuaded by his medical colleagues to undertake a biopsy of a scleral nodule in the patient shown in Figure 10.9. The episcleral tissue was normal but slightly congested and the nodule looked large and firm. As soon as the surface of the nodule was scraped it ruptured, releasing a large amount of pultaceous material, the histology of which showed degenerate collagen infiltrated with lymphocytes and a few polymorphs. The sclera failed to heal and the patient has been left with an unsightly scleral defect; no aetiological diagnosis has been made.

We have heard of two similar cases in which biopsy has led to near disaster. Verhoeff and King (1938) also had an exactly similar experience when attempting to biopsy the lesion from the eye that they eventually obtained for histology. The purulent material they obtained contained pus cells and a few plasma cells and the adjacent biopsy tissue many eosinophils.

In the few episcleral biopsies which we have performed we have noted hyperaemia, oedema and lymphocytic infiltrates which have not materially assisted in the diagnosis. In view of these experiences and because biopsy always leaves a conjunctival scar which would not otherwise be present, we have been most reluctant to undertake biopsies in scleral disease.

Friedman and Henkind (1974) have been more fortunate: they report five cases in which biopsy performed because of failure of treatment to help the condition, contributed to a definitive diagnosis. The first patient had a scleritis; the second was due to a foreign body granuloma; the third was the presenting feature of an orbital granuloma, pseudotumour; the fourth was of a patient with sarcoidosis who presented with erythema nodosum; the fifth was a patient with Weber–Christian disease. Hogan and Zimmerman (1962) reported biopsies of scleral nodule in polyarteritis nodosa and cranial arteritis which they found to contain mononuclear cells, some giant cells and areas of lymphocytic and plasma cell infiltration. McCarthy (1961) biopsied an episcleral nodule in erythema nodosum and found masses of lymphocytes, fibrocytes and nuclear debris.

Mundy et al in 1951 studied three biopsies in patients with rheumatoid arthritis which showed the typical changes of pallisading inflammatory cells around areas of fibrinoid necrosis identical to that found in rheumatoid nodules. Feinberg and Colpoys (1951), Ferry (1969) and Edström and Österlind (1948) found exactly similar changes and went one step further by obtaining nodules before and after steroid therapy. They were able to compare these nodules with systemic nodules taken at the same time and were finally able to compare these findings with the changes found after a postmortem examination.

The findings of these authors are clearcut and because of our own experiences we would not regard it as justified, in fact it should be regarded as positively meddlesome, to perform a biopsy on a patient who is known to have rheumatoid arthritis or any other connective tissue disease. This is not to say that they should never be done, for as Freidman and Henkind (1974) have shown, they can be very helpful, but they should only be undertaken with the greatest circumspection after full discussion and with a knowledge of the hazards involved.

In view of the embargo that we have imposed on biopsy, most of our personal knowledge of pathology has come from excised eyes of patients with scleral disease. In a surprising number of these, the diagnosis of scleritis had never been made in life. Wolter and Bentley (1961) had noted this and we have recently surveyed all the eyes which were received by Professor Norman Ashton at the Institute of Ophthalmology in London, in which the principal histological diagnosis was scleritis (Fraunfelder and Watson, 1976). Of the 28 eyes examined over a ten-year period, 43 per cent had not had the diagnosis of scleritis made in life, most of the patients having been diagnosed as having secondary glaucoma from a primary anterior uveitis. In five patients, the clinical diagnosis was a Mooren's ulcer and in five more the diagnosis was of a retinal detachment. There is no doubt that the diagnosis can be difficult because the oedema caused by the inflammation hides the underlying necrotising process, and, as we have seen, the pathological process is not necessarily confined to the anterior segment. Because the surface of the sclera rarely ulcerates, the disease can nibble away inexorably, and often unsuspected, until it is too late to treat it.

The major difficulty in agreeing a standard classification of scleral disease has been the difficulty in correlating the clinical with the pathological appearances. Clinically, only a very few patients with scleral disease progress to the stage that the eye needs to be removed, so that inevitably those eyes which are available for histological evaluation show evidence of a necrotising reaction, not necessarily present in the average case of anterior scleritis. Those biopsies which are available from anterior or nodular scleritis not associated with rheumatoid arthritis or connective tissue disease show a nonspecific inflammatory reaction and contain lymphocytes, plasma cells and polymorphs. They have not shown any specific staining with fluorescent antibody techniques, nor have they shown any fibrinoid necrosis.

Histologically the inflammatory connective tissue diseases all show fibrinoid necrosis, abnormal cellular reactions and fibrin deposition which give rise to granulomas. The amount and extent of the three components of these reactions differ in the different diseases but they are all present in some form or other.

FIBRINOID NECROSIS

Fibrinoid necrosis was first described by Neumann in 1880. This term is applied to eosinophil fibrillar and amorphous material seen in haematoxylin and eosin stained sections. This material undoubtedly contains fibrin as has been shown by the use of immunologically specific reagents labelled with fluorescein (Gitlin, Craig and Janeway, 1957). It contains other proteins and immunoglobulin is present in some cases, e.g. in rheumatoid nodules (Vasquez and Dixon, 1958). Two varieties of collagen are present in fibrinoid areas: the first is normal collagen, present in coarse bundles; the second consists of fine fibrils which can be seen among the bundles of normal collagen, giving the impression that they have been derived by fibrillation of the coarse collagen bundles.

With the discovery of mammalian collagenase active at a pH of about 7 it was felt that enzymatic digestion was the reason for the collagen breakdown. Unfortunately the enzyme is strongly inhibited in the presence of serum (Evanson, Jeffrey and Krane, 1968). It is therefore likely that other factors may be at least as important as collagenase in the breakdown of collagen in fibrinoid areas.

The resistance of native collagen to proteolysis is the result of the tertiary structure of its molecules, a structure largely maintained by hydrogen bonds within and between the individual peptide chains which make up the tropocollagen molecule (see Chapter 2). It is now thought that inflammatory exudates rich in fibrin, immunoglobulins and other plasma components can disrupt hydrogen bonds and so lead to enzymatic removal of collagen. If this is the case, why is this not a more frequent and conspicuous feature of acute inflammatory processes? Dumonde and Glynn (1965) demonstrated that the fate of implanted fragments of fibrin is affected by the presence of humoral antibodies to fibrin itself. They concluded that the presence of an antigen–antibody reaction seriously impairs the normal mechanism for the organisation and removal of fibrinous exudate. The presence of immunoglobulin in one form of fibrinoid (Vasquez and Dixon, 1958) suggests a similar mechanism may be responsible for the persistence of the exudate and thus provides time for the redistribution of the collagen fibrils.

It is now realised that the eosinophilic material described at the base of peptic ulcers, in aneurysms and around placental villi, which is common to connective tissue diseases, is not a single, chemical homogeneous entity but a variety of substances (Gitlin and Craig, 1957) derived from blood plasma and varying in composition in different diseases, whilst retaining identical staining characteristics with dyes of low chemical specificity (Gardner, 1965). The suggestion that the presence of 'fibrinoid' might imply identity of origin was suggested by Klinge (1934) on the basis of his work with rheumatic fever and with arthritis in rabbits provoked by injection of horse serum. This hypothesis was rejected by Klemperer, Pollack and Baehr (1942) even before the heterogeneity of fibrinoid was established. It is also obvious that although fibrinoid is present in, it is not pathognomonic of the connective tissue group of diseases.

Histochemical differences exist between fibrinoid present in different collagen diseases. Fibrinoid in disseminated lupus erythematosus and scleroderma appears to be the result of metabolic disturbances in DNA and in protein chemistry, while that seen in rheumatic fever and polyarteritis is related to the hypersensitivity reaction to a variety of agents. In rheumatoid arthritis and disseminated lupus erythematosus there is an increased concentration of gammaglobulin similar to that found in the Arthus reaction and in thrombocytopenic purpura there is a concentration of fibrinogen and fibrin characteristic of a Shwartzman reaction. Thus similar morphological changes do not imply common pathogenesis.

CELLULAR RESPONSE

Associated with fibrinoid necrosis and occurring at the same time there is a cellular reaction. Lymphocytes, plasma cells, macrophages and multinucleated giant cells aggregate around the site of the inflammation. The presence of these cells in the tissues also suggests that the lesion is caused by a hypersensitivity reaction.

FIBRIN DEPOSITION

Fibrin can always be found in the tissues from the individuals with chronic inflammation in necrotising scleral disease and in connective tissue disease. Whether this is part of the inflammatory reaction, or whether it is a result of haemorrhage, vascular permeability or attempts at repair is uncertain. Gitlin, Craig and Janeway (1957) have shown, using fluorescent antibody techniques that fibrin is deposited in and around the arterioles in these conditions. Morphologically identifiable fibrin can be recognised within rheumatoid synovial cells and rheumatoid synovial fluid polymorphs (Riddle, Bluhm and Barnhart, 1965). The presence of fibrin of altered antigenicity may account for the chronicity of rheumatoid inflammatory reaction (Glynn, 1968) and this change in fibrin structure may also perhaps contribute to an unusual resistance to physiological fibrinolytic mechanisms.

VASCULITIS

Depending on the type of the disease, vascular changes also occur consisting of vasculitis, endothelial proliferation and fibrinoid degeneration of the vessel wall which may lead to thrombosis and infarction of the tissues supplied by the vessel (Figure 5.1). The vasculitis not only involves the vessels normally present at that site but also the new vessels produced as a result of the disease. The pattern in the sclera and the joints follows that found elsewhere in the body, for instance patients with polyarteritis nodosa or Wegener's granulomatosis will show histological features in which the vasculitis is very obvious and prominent, whereas those with no other known systemic disease, or patients with rheumatoid arthritis will show a much more granulomatous reaction.

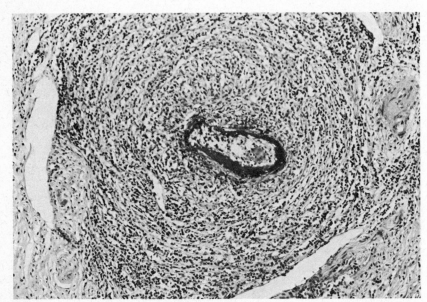

Figure 5.1. Vasculitis of a small artery. There is fibrinoid necrosis in the media and it is surrounded by a cuff of inflammatory cells. Picro Mallory, × 105.
Courtesy of D. Wight, Cambridge.

Jayson and Jones (1971) and Williamson (1974) found that compared with age and sex-matched patients there was a very high mortality in those patients where rheumatoid arthritis was complicated by scleritis and there was also a high proportion of severe invasive seropositive erosive arthritis and an extensive systemic vasculitis. This implies that there can be a change in the histological manifestations of the disease during its course and tends to confirm the view that the histological changes simply reflect the virulence of the connective tissue disorder.

PATHOLOGICAL CHANGES FOUND IN THE SCLERA

Rarely are the histopathological changes in the sclera characteristic of a particular disease. Usually the changes are less specific, being seen most commonly anterior to the equator of the eye (56 per cent), but often extending into the posterior segment (43 per cent). Histologically the posterior segment is rarely, if ever, involved alone, even though clinically this almost certainly happens (Figures 5.2, 5.3 and 5.4). The inflammatory processes can be seen to involve the episclera over the areas of affected sclera (Figure 5.5). Where the posterior segment is involved the underlying choroid is also affected and this gives rise to retinal detachments (21 per cent), choroidoretinitis, macular oedema, intraocular or subretinal haemorrhages (21 per cent) and central retinal vision occlusion (10 per cent), all of which have been noted to occur clinically (Figures 5.3 and 5.4). When the anterior segment is severely affected the cornea becomes involved with central or peripheral ulceration or descemetocele formation (21 per cent) and many of these patients have a severe and obvious anterior uveitis and glaucoma (68 per cent). When glaucoma and uveitis complicate scleritis, then staphyloma formation may occur, but it is very rare to see this complication in the absence of glaucoma.

The histological appearances were well described in the late nineteenth century and early this century by Kostenitsch (1894), Fuchs (1895), Parsons (1904) and others. Their observations concerning the cellular infiltrations, the increased vascularity and the breakdown of tissue in fibrinoid necrosis have stood the test of time. Recently, the use of histochemical and fluorescent antibody techniques has helped to elucidate the changes which can be seen with the light microscope. When viewed with the polarising microscope, the scleral collagen is birefringent and appears luminous and glistening. Loss of birefringence is said to be due to disorganisation of the helical arrangement of the collagen molecules and loss of the mucopolysaccharide coat. This has been

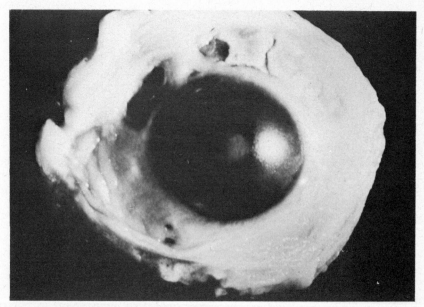

Figure 5.2. Necrotising scleritis which clinically appeared to be entirely anterior. The lens was opaque. The eye was removed for intractable pain and loss of vision, the patient being unable to tolerate steroids. Courtesy of Professor Norman Ashton, London.

confirmed by electron microscopy, as has the type of cells found in the infiltrate but this method of investigation has not yet contributed anything to our understanding of the underlying pathogenesis.

On superficial inspection the affected sclera appears to be sharply demarcated

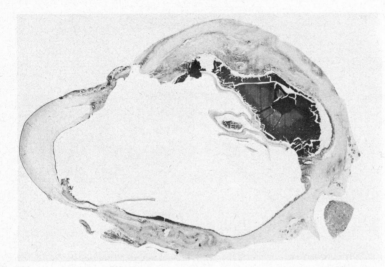

Figure 5.3.   Section of the same eye as Figure 5.3 shows a massive involvement of the posterior segment with an exudative retinal detachment. The very thin area close to the equator still has a fine film of collagen over it. It is most unusual to find true spontaneous perforations in histological specimens. × 5. Courtesy of Dr Smith, Boston.

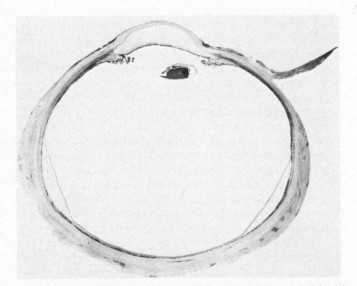

Figure 5.4.   An eye of a patient with posterior scleritis in which there is minimal involvement of the anterior segment. × 5. Courtesy of Dr D. G. Cogan, Boston.

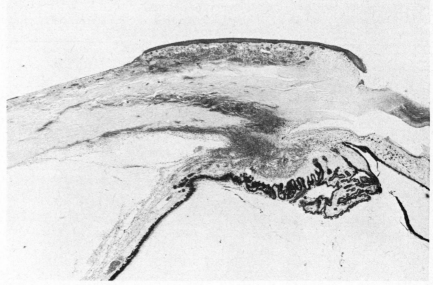

Figure 5.5.   Necrotising anterior scleritis. Intense congestion of all the vessels of the episclera and the perforating anterior ciliary vessels which are surrounded by inflammatory cells. The granuloma also involves the root of the iris and the region of the trabecular meshwork. × 15.

from the rest of the sclera which seems completely healthy (Figure 5.6). However colloidal iron staining reveals a generalised change in mucopolysaccharides of the sclera (Francois, 1970) in these areas. Adjacent to the region which contains the obvious granuloma is a zone of mucoid oedema in which, although the fibres themselves appear to be quite normal, the lamellae of the collagen bundles are forced apart (Figure 5.8). The mucoid oedema, which stained strongly with mucopolysaccharide stains, exists in small 20-μm patches in areas remote from the granuloma, but these become more obvious and larger closer to the lesion. There is no cellular reaction in this region except for the apparent increase in sclerocytes first noted by Kostenitsch (1894).

As the granuloma is approached, plasma cells and lymphocytes infiltrate into the intercellular space until an area is reached adjacent to the central necrotic area which shows a marked cellular reaction consisting of plasma cells, lymphocytes, giant cells and macrophages. Fibroblasts are often present in large numbers but eosinophils and polymorphonuclear leucocytes are few. The collagen fibrils lose their birefringence in polarised light and fibrils themselves become unravelled so that they appear 'as if the scleral lamellae were ending in the form of brushes, the bristles of which have been splayed apart' (Francois, 1970) (Figures 5.7, 5.8, 5.9 and 5.10). Similar changes have been found in the cornea in those cases in which the cornea is involved. Close to the necrotic area a large number of abnormal capillary vascular tufts can be found, some of which can be traced back to their origin from the vessels of the episclera and choroid (Figures 5.11, 5.12 and 5.13). Both the newly formed vessels and their parent vessels, particularly the choroidal ones, are dilated, cuffed with lymphocytes and show medial necrosis with mucopolysaccharide deposition in their walls. In some instances they are thrombosed. Fibrin deposition may be absent from the sclera but present around the vessels.

In the necrotic centre the collagen fibres are indistinguishable, there is very little mucopolysaccharide and the cells are barely recognisable, degenerate and pyknotic. Fibrinoid necrosis is the prominent feature.

Clinically, these granulomas tend to progress circumferentially round the globe and, following natural resolution or treatment, the necrotic area becomes transparent or thin but very rarely sequestrates (Figures 5.3 and 5.4). Histologically the changes which correspond to the clinical appearances can be studied in areas which were known to have been affected and have since healed. The collagen in these areas appears to be diminished in amount but is again birefringent and of the same type as normal scleral collagen. The linear orientation of the fibres is lost at least in relatively recently affected areas, even though it may possibly be restored later. This tissue has most of the characteristics found in scleral wounds which have healed normally.

This scleral healing normally takes place by an ingrowth of vessels. When injured, bleeding occurs, a clot forms and in an exactly similar way to other tissues, ingrowth of new vessels occurs from the neighbouring major vessels, in this case the episcleral and uveal vessels which bring with them the haematogenous fibroblasts (Renard, Lelièvre and Naniex, 1952). This leads to the formation of a fibrous scar which is laid down in an irregular fashion initially

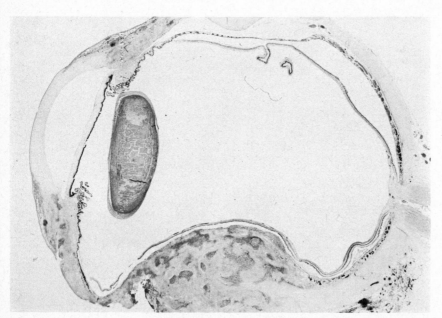

Figure 5.6. The eye of a patient with severe anterior necrotising scleritis in whom the vision ocular movements were restricted, presumably due to the granuloma which involved the sclera behind the equator. The sclera between the granulomas appears to be normal. × 5. Courtesy of Dr W. Lee, Glasgow.

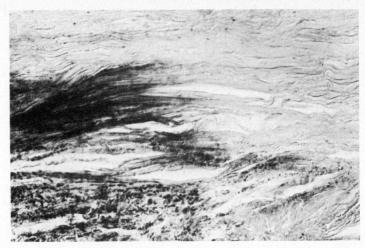

Figure 5.7. An area adjacent to the granuloma in an eye removed with anterior necrotising scleritis viewed in polarised light. As the granuloma is approached, the fibres become forced apart by oedema and the fibrils lose their normal birefringence and appear dark. × 135.

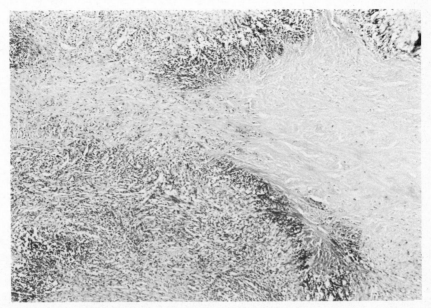

Figure 5.8. The scleral fibres being separated and eaten away by the inflammatory cells to such an extent that the normal architecture is indistinguishable. × 56.

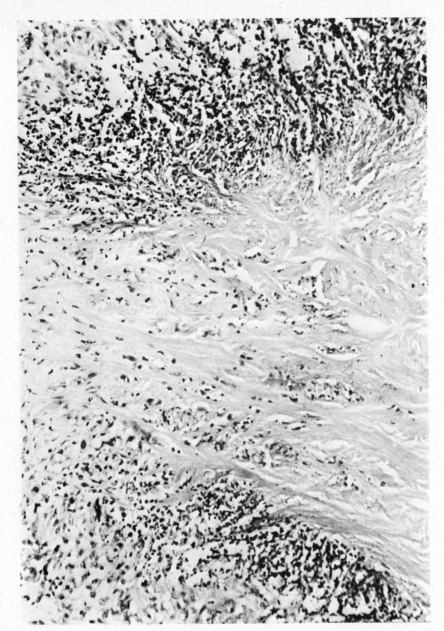

Figure 5.9. The same eye as Figure 5.8, × 200, showing that the inflammatory cells have penetrated the relatively normal scleral tissue a long way from the advancing edge of the granuloma.

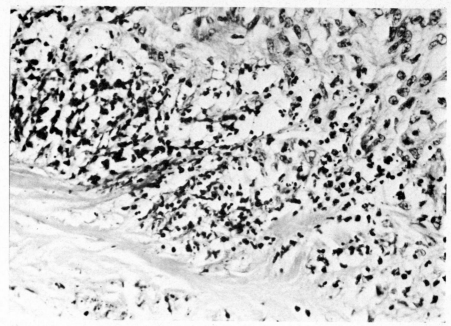

Figure 5.10. The same eye as Figures 5.8 and 5.9, × 405, to show that the cells attacking the scleral fibres are lymphocytes. There are a few plasma cells and further from the edge macrophages and fibroblasts which are removing and remodelling the tissue.

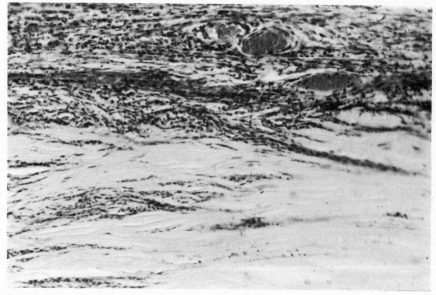

Figure 5.11. Intense congestion of the episcleral and deep vessels adjacent to the granuloma.
× 60.

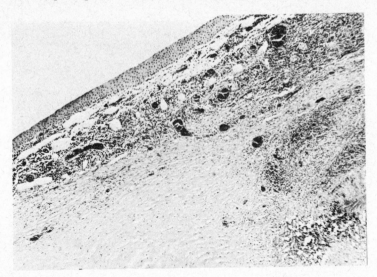

Figure 5.12.   Episcleral congestion with extension of the inflammation between the scleral lamellae. × 135.

but may be reorientated later. There is little, if any, active participation of scleral cells in this process. In the presence of inflammation, the new vessels are already present and the fibroblasts are present within the inflammatory exudate, so that when the inflammatory reaction is suppressed for any reason, repair can take place immediately. It is the experience of retinal detachment surgeons that when the sclera has healed by first intention where the vascular supply is limited, these wounds are weak and can easily be opened years afterwards. The scar is firm if there is an organised clot and often less firm if there is no clot present at the time of injury or surgery. When the eye has been inflamed, however, the scars seem extremely strong, being able to withstand relatively high intraocular pressure over a prolonged period and even quite severe direct injury. Presumably this must be due to the presence of an abnormally large blood supply at the time of healing.

The increased transparency of the sclera seen clinically following scleral inflammation seems to be caused partly by physicochemical changes in the mucopolysaccharide coat and partly by the abnormal reorientation of the collagen in which the lamellae of the collagen fibres are present but disorganised so that the original interlacing has disappeared.

Sequestration of the scleral tissue seems to occur only in severe long-standing rheumatoid arthritis in which there is very little surrounding inflammatory reaction (scleromalacia perforans). Where there is a marked inflammatory reaction with multiple new vessels, the destroyed collagenous tissue is reabsorbed, sometimes almost completely, the subsequent defect being filled by a fine film of collagen, apparently derived from the remaining episclera or conjunctiva.

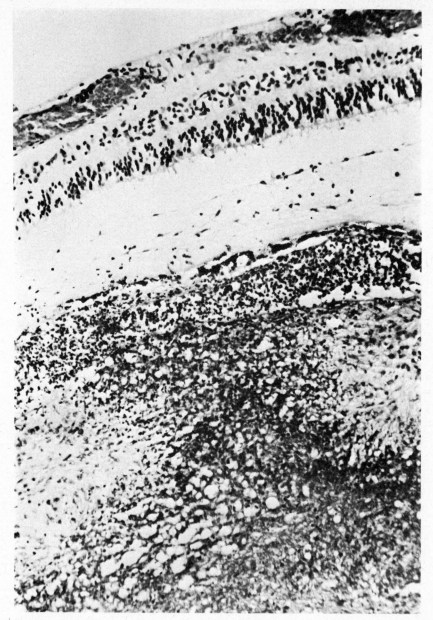

Figure 5.13.   Inflammatory cells in and around the vessels of the choriocapillaris in the region of the granuloma. × 200.

REFERENCES

Dumonde, D. C. & Glynn, L. E. (1965) The reaction of guinea pigs to autologous and heterologous fibrin implants. *Journal of Pathology and Bacteriology*, **90**, 649–657.

Edström, G. & Osterlind, G. (1948). Case of nodular rheumatic episcleritis. *Acta Ophthalmologica*, **26**, 1–6.

Evanson, J. M., Jeffrey, J. J. & Krane, S. M. (1968) Studies on collagenase from rheumatoid synovium in tissue culture. *Journal of Clinical Investigation*, **47**, 2639–2651.

Ferry, A. P. (1969) Histopathology of rheumatoid episcleral nodules, an extra-articular manifestation of rheumatoid arthritis. *Archives of Ophthalmology*, **82**, 77–78.

Fienberg, R. & Colpoys, F. L. (1951) Involution of rheumatoid nodules treated with cortisone and of non-treated rheumatoid nodules. *American Journal of Pathology*, **27**, 925–949.

François, J. (1970) Ocular manifestations in collagenases. *Advances in Ophthalmology*, **23**, 1–54.

Fraunfelder, F. T. & Watson, P. G. (1976) Evaluation of eyes enucleated for scleritis. *British Journal of Ophthalmology*, **60**, 227–230.

Friedman, A. H. & Henkind, P. (1974) Unusual cases of episcleritis. *Transactions of the American Academy of Ophthalmology and Otolaryngology*, **78**, 890–895.

Fuchs, E. (1895) Uber episkleritis periodica fugax. *Albrecht v. Graefes Archiv für Ophthalmologie*, **41**, 229–273.

Gardner, D. L. (1965) *Pathology of the Connective Tissue Diseases*. London: Arnold.

Gitlin, D. & Craig, J. M. (1957) Variations in the staining characteristics of human fibrin. *American Journal of Pathology*, **33**, 267–283.

Gitlin, D., Craig, J. M. & Janeway, C. A. (1957) Studies on the nature of fibrinoid and the collagen diseases. *American Journal of Pathology*, **33**, 55–77.

Glynn, L. E. (1968) The chronicity of inflammation and its significance in rheumatoid arthritis. *Annals of the Rheumatic Diseases*, **27**, 105–121.

Hogan, M. J. & Zimmerman, L. F. (1962) *Ophthalmic Pathology*. 2nd edition, p. 337. Philadelphia: W. B. Saunders.

Janeway, C. A., Gitlin, D., Craig, J. M. et al (1956) Collagen disease in patients with congenital agammaglobulinemia. *Transactions of the Association of American Physicians*, **69**, 93–97.

Jayson, M. I. & Jones, D. E. (1971) Scleritis and rheumatoid arthritis. *Annals of the Rheumatic Diseases*, **30**, 343–347.

Klemperer, P., Pollock, A. D. & Baehr, G. (1942) Diffuse collagen disease, acute disseminated lupus erythematosus and diffuse scleroderma. *Journal of the American Medical Association*, **119**, 331–332.

Klinge, F. (1934) Die rheumatischen Erkrankungen der Knochen und Gelenke und der Rheumatismus. In *Handbüch der Speziellen Pathologischen Anatomie und Histologie* (Ed.) Lubarsch, O. & Henke, F. Vol. 9, part 3, pp. 107–251. Berlin: Springer.

Kostenitsch, J. (1894) Über einen Fall von Skleritis; pathologische-anatomische Untersuchung. *Archiv für Augenheilkunde*, **28**, 27–35.

McCarthy, J. L. (1961) Episcleral nodules and erythema nodosum. *American Journal of Ophthalmology*, **51**, 60–70.

Mundy, W. L., Howard, R. M., Stillman, P.M. & Bevans, M. (1951) Cortisone therapy in the case of rheumatoid nodules of the eye in rheumatoid arthritis. *Archives of Ophthalmology*, **45**, 531–538.

Neumann, E. (1880) Die Picrocarminforbung und ihre Anwendung auf die Entzundungslehre. *Archiv für mikroscopische Anatomie, und Entwicklungsmechanik,* **18**, 130–150.

Parsons, J. H. (1904) *Pathology of the Eye.* Vol. 1, p. 271. London: Hodder and Stoughton.

Renard, G., Lelièvre, A. & Naniex, G. (1952) The healing of wounds of the sclera. *Archives d'Ophtalmologie*, **12**, 5–18.

Riddle, J. M., Bluhm, G. B. & Barnhart, M. I. (1965) Interrelationship between fibrin, neutrophils and rheumatoid synovitis. *Journal of the Reticuloendothelial Society*, **2**, 420–436.

Vasquez, J. J. & Dixon, F. J. (1958) Immunohistochemical analysis of lesions associated with fibrinoid change. *Archives of Pathology*, **66**, 504–517.

Verhoeff, F. H. & King, M. J. (1938) Scleromalacia perforans: report of a case in which the eye was examined microscopically. *Archives of Ophthalmology*, **20**, 1013–1035.

Williamson, J. (1974) Incidence of eye disease in cases of connective tissue disease. *Transactions of the Ophthalmological Societies of the United Kingdom*, **94**, 742–752.

Wolter, J. R. & Bentley, M. D. (1961) Scleromalacia perforans and massive granuloma of the sclera. *American Journal of Ophthalmology*, **51**, 71–80.

CHAPTER SIX

Pathogenesis

'The physician who is attending the patient . . . . . . has to know the cause of the ailment before he can treat it.' Ethical and Political Works (Motzu, 5th–4th century BC).

Our knowledge of the pathological changes within the inflamed sclera is limited, but the cellular reaction in which lymphocytes and plasma cells predominate is very similar to that found in the synovial tissue of joints in rheumatoid arthritis. The latter has been studied in detail. The similar pathological changes seen in infectious diseases such as tuberculosis and syphilis and in the other connective tissue diseases can also be interpreted in the light of modern cell biology.

The changes found in scleral disease and in the joints in rheumatoid arthritis are consistent with a continuing antigen-provoked immune response, but how does it all begin? Two fundamental questions common to both scleritis and rheumatoid arthritis have yet to be answered. What is the nature of the stimulus which initiates inflammation of the sclera and joints, and what are the factors which lead to chronicity and give rise to two types of immune injury which coexist in both tissues? In the joint there is a humoral response which is limited to the synovial fluid and involves polymorphonuclear cells; in the synovium itself there is a cellular immune response.

It is currently fashionable to consider that both conditions arise because a person develops a pathological immune response to his own tissue antigens; one of the more perplexing problems in medicine and immunology concerns the immunological differentiation of 'self' from 'non-self'. Why does not everyone react to their own antigens? Ideally, in order to be considered an autoimmune phenomenon, a pathological process should meet a series of criteria, similar to Koch's postulates for tuberculosis. The criteria for autoimmunity as defined by Milgrom and Witebsky (1962) are:

1. The presence of either a circulating antibody or a cell-mediated immune reaction which is directed at antigens of the target organs.
2. Identification of a specific antigen within the involved organ which is the target of the immune response.

171

3. Immunisation of experimental animals with this specific antigen must elicit an immune response.
4. The disease must be produced in an experimental animal.
5. The disease can be transferred from an immunised animal to a normal recipient by serum and/or immunologically competent lymphocytes.

Many clinical disorders, presumed to be of an autoimmune aetiology, can fulfil one or more of these postulates, but none meets all five. No single explanation can account for the genesis of all autoimmune diseases and in all probability these diseases are the end result of an interaction involving several factors. Four theories have been proposed to explain the development of immune responses directed at self-antigens in a genetically susceptible individual.

1. Sequestered antigen theory.
2. Structural similarity between tissue constituents and exogenous antigens.
3. Breakdown of tolerance by alteration of self-antigens.
4. Alterations in cells capable of controlling the immune response.

Endophthalmitis phaco-anaphylactica is believed to be an example of the sequestered antigen theory (Silverstein, 1968). Normally the lens of the eye is considered a hidden antigen; however, release of antigen either through trauma or cataract can expose lens antigens. As a result lymphocytes reactive to the individual's own lens antigen develop, and these autoreactive cells can cause a uveitis in the opposite eye. However, apart from this condition it appears that this theory has limited application, as antigens are not usually 'hidden' from the immune system.

The second theory of autoimmunity suggests that antigenic similarities exist between self-antigens and those of an exogenous agent. Thus, the immune response directed at foreign antigens elicits an antibody response which can cross-react with the host's own tissues. Rheumatic heart disease may be due to cross-reacting antibodies elicited by certain strains of beta-haemolytic streptococci (Zabriskie, 1967). The pathogenesis of acute rheumatic fever is believed to be as follows. A beta-haemolytic streptococcal infection elicits an immune response with antibodies which, in susceptible individuals, are capable of cross-reacting with myocardial tissue. Another example of cross-reacting antibodies is that produced by *Mycoplasma pneumoniae*, which also react with the I-antigen of human red cells (Thomas, 1964). These antibodies can cause a transient haemolytic anaemia of the cold agglutinin type.

The first three theories of autoimmunity suggest a breakdown in tolerance; the fourth theory is based on alterations in the immune apparatus rather than in the antigenic environment. This theory represents a modification of Burnett's original 'forbidden clones' theory.

The eye is only rarely affected in rheumatic fever, and in tuberculous and syphilitic scleritis there is no evidence to implicate these organisms as participating directly, although they may induce an immune response against 'self'-antigens. Organisms have been constantly sought for as a cause of arthritis and much of this work is relevant to the study of scleral disease, even though it may not be possible to draw any direct conclusions.

INFECTIOUS AGENTS

Recently there has been a revival of interest in the possible role of micro-organisms in rheumatoid arthritis, and indeed, in many of the other forms of chronic inflammatory disease accompanied by intense immunological activity. This revival is due to two main developments. First, we now know that many forms of virus infection may not give rise to obvious signs. Second, many apparently autoimmune phenomena are found in chronic inflammatory diseases known to be provoked by microorganisms.

As with anterior uveitis the search for aetiological agents is unrewarding. Certainly recurrences of scleritis can be induced by systemic infections and psychological upsets, but only in herpes zoster does there seem to be a clearcut association between a known aetiological agent and subsequent recurrent disease. We have isolated herpes simplex from one episcleral lesion which occurred many times at the same site, but after the first occasion no virus could be detected.

It is possible that scleritis can be induced by a viral infection as in herpes zoster or by a bacterial infection. One of our patients had a chronic stitch granuloma from an infected silicone plomb used for replacing his retinal detachment. Pieces of suture were removed on two separate occasions, but the eye remained inflamed. Six weeks later he developed a typical anterior necrotising scleritis underlying the line of the conjunctival incision. Arkin (1951) has reported a similar sequence of events following squint and detachment surgery.

An unequivocal demonstration of a transition from microbial polyarthritis to a sterile arthritis of rheumatoid type has not been made in man, but is commonplace in some animals, especially the pig. A systemic infection with *Erysipelothrix insidiosa* is frequently observed, polyarthritis being one of its characteristic features. Although there is usually recovery from the systemic illness, the arthritis persists. In many instances the affected joints prove sterile (Ajmal, 1971).

There are several viral infections, such as rubella, which produce transient arthritis, and viruses have been implicated in a number of animal diseases such as Aleutian mink disease. However, there has been complete failure to recover such agents from joint tissues or to observe viral particles with the electron microscope.

Grayzel and Beck (1972) have found that fibroblasts derived from rheumatoid synovial membranes are more resistant to infection with rubella virus than are cell lines from normal synovium, suggesting that resistance may be due to the presence of some form of intracellular organism.

Recently great interest has been directed towards the possible implication of Mycoplasma (Williams, 1968; Williams, Brostoff and Roitt, 1970). These organisms lack a cell wall, but are able to grow on artificial media and are associated with arthritis in cattle. Although reports of isolation of Mycoplasma from joint fluid have appeared, it is possible that accidental contamination has occurred since the chances of contaminating cultures with mycoplasma from the laboratory environment are high (Sabin, 1967). The organisms may, however, simply act as immunological adjuvants, perpetuating an inflammation already established. Williams, Brostoff and Roitt (1970) showed that 67 per cent of 43 patients with rheumatoid arthritis had delayed hypersensitivity to

Mycoplasma fermentans, a form of immunological reactivity not shown by control subjects.

Although there have been many claims for an aetiological role for many types of organism isolated from the joints of rheumatoid arthritis patients, none has generally been agreed to play an active role. A number of factors suggest that an infectious agent is present:

1. Acute onset in some patients.
2. Failure to demonstrate genetic pattern of disease.
3. Presence in animals of arthritis of infective origin.
4. Induction of rheumatoid factor in certain known infections.
5. Failure to grow rubella virus on rheumatoid synovia.

Before the pathogenesis of any disease can be said to be due to an infection it must fulfil criteria laid down by Koch in 1882.

1. That the organism must always be found in a given disease.
2. That the organism must not be found in other diseases or in health.
3. That the organisms must be cultivated artificially and reproduce the given disease after inoculation of a pure culture into a susceptible animal.
4. That the organism must be recoverable from the animal so inoculated.

Duthie et al (1967) have been able to isolate organisms from the synovial cells of about 30 per cent of synovial membranes which are classified as 'diphtheroid' bacilli or corynebacteria. Their presence does not, however, fulfil Koch's postulates. Bacteria have been isolated, but it has not been shown that reinjection into an animal can cause the disease, nor is there immunological evidence of the formation of antibodies against these organisms. Their presence inside synovial cells seems to be almost coincidental; they appear to be present as passengers, inert and evoking no response.

In general antibodies to diphtheroids or Mycoplasma have not been detected more frequently or in higher titre in patients with rheumatoid arthritis than in other conditions or in controls (Stewart, Alexander and Duthie, 1969; Williams, Brostoff and Roitt, 1970). Furthermore, the finding that a joint is infected by a particular microorganism does not prove that this has a primary aetiological role. The vascular synovial membrane with its rich content of macrophages is an obvious nidus for secondary infection, and septic arthritis is a recognised complication of the disease (Kellgren et al, 1958).

Much interest centres around the possibility that systemic lupus erythematosus may arise from an interaction of genetic factors and viral infection. This arose because myxovirus-like particles were found in renal biopsies of patients with SLE (Pineus et al, 1970). While not specific for SLE they are found with high frequency in this disease. Whether or not these particles represent actual viruses or alterations in endoplasmic reticulum brought about by viruses is uncertain.

Animal models have provided much information concerning pathogenetic mechanisms of this disease. In the most intensively studied animal, the New Zealand hybrid (black/white) mouse, antinuclear antibodies appear at about three months of age and include those against double-stranded DNA. These animals show a basic defect in their capacity to generate certain immune responses. This defect is present prior to the onset of autoimmunity (Dauphinee et al, 1974). It has been suggested that, as one manifestation of this defect, these animals are unable to recognise and suppress the activity of autoreactive lymphocytes, which proliferate and initiate immune injuries. The animals go on to develop many features of SLE and ultimately die of nephritis. Complexes containing DNA, DNA nucleoprotein and 'Gross-like' viral antigen have been demonstrated in the kidney. However, these virus particles are not themselves the cause of the disease, because Lewis and his colleagues (1973) who raised a colony of dogs which developed serological abnormalities such as antinuclear antibody found that when cell-free filtrates prepared from the spleens of these animals were injected into various species of newborn animals, only the canine recipients developed positive ANF and LE cell tests.

HOST RESPONSES

The suspicion that patients with rheumatoid arthritis suffer from some form of peculiar tissue response to an antigen in microbial agents has led to an intensive study of the factors which influence host responses in chronic inflammation. Population studies have shown only minor differences in the incidence of rheumatoid arthritis in various regions and have not produced any clues to its aetiology. Although there may be familial aggregation in rheumatoid arthritis (Lawrence, 1970), no single genetic mechanism can explain its incidence and distribution. Our own observations indicate that scleral disease has a similar incidence in different races and populations and we have no evidence that genetic factors play a significant role (pages 95 and 103).

Epidemiological studies in Western Nigeria suggest that the incidence and expression of polyarthritis may be modified by immunological factors. The incidence of rheumatoid arthritis there was low (Greenwood, 1968) while its clinical and serological features differed from those in Caucasians (Greenwood and Herrick, 1970), possibly reflecting the effects of chronic parasitic infection in the Nigerian patients (Greenwood, Herrick and Voller, 1970).

Rheumatoid arthritis is a chronic inflammatory disease which predominantly affects the joints, but probably no tissue of the body is entirely exempt. The most commonly affected tissues after the joints are other synovial-lined spaces such as tendon sheaths, the subcutaneous tissues at sites of pressure, the lungs and heart and blood vessels. This diversity is perhaps less interesting than the observation that collagenous connective tissues outside synovial joints, with the exception of the sclera, the tendons, ligaments and subcutaneous tissue, are for the most part spared. The joint pathology of rheumatoid disease is essentially a synovitis with effusion in which the inflamed synovial membrane develops increasing cellularity, with increasing disease activity. All evidence suggests that the pathological changes begin in the synovium or extra-articular tissues, not the cartilage, the cartilage being 'attacked' by enzymes from the invasive mesenchymal tissue at its periphery and by enzymes from the synovial fluid continually bathing it. (The latter may be of less importance as there are inhibitors, e.g. α-macroglobulin, present in the synovial fluid.) It is believed that after an early synovitis synovial cells adhere to the surface of the articular cartilage. Here and at the deeper margin adjoining the cartilage, the synovial cells and phagocytes progressively destroy the cartilage, not in the same manner as an invasive malignant tumour but rather by a kind of replacement fibrosis in which the ground substance of articular cartilage is lysed and replaced by young inflammatory connective tissue. As there are no known pathogens that produce toxins responsible for local inflammation and tissue injury, it must be considered that joints finally destroy themselves, and that mediators released during inflammation become diverted to an attack upon the host.

This is analogous to the situation in the sclera when the avascular scleral tissue appears to be attacked by cells whose origin is from the adjacent vascular episcleral and choroidal tissue and which usually, but not exclusively, takes the form of replacement fibrosis, little of the original tissue remaining. If the intensity of the inflammation is very severe, then the necrotic, destructive phase, rather than the reparative phase becomes the most prominent feature of the condition.

Electron microscopy of rheumatoid synovial/cartilage interface at the periphery of a metacarpophalangeal joint removed during insertion of a prosthesis demonstrated a narrow band several microns wide separating cartilage from invasive cells (Harris, DiBona and Krane, 1970). In this zone were found amorphous material, a few presumably partially degraded collagen fibrils and then processes of macrophage-like cells containing numerous mitochondria and granules. Very similar changes have been noted in the areas adjacent to the granuloma in necrotising scleritis (François, 1970). The interpretation of these findings was that cartilage and sclera were being destroyed in a defined limited zone where substrate was in intimate contact with cells capable of releasing enzymes.

Rheumatoid synovium does appear to have invasive properties. When cultured in vitro in highly enriched culture medium on everted intestinal segments, the synovium proliferated and invaded through the collagenous serosa of the gut segments (Harris et al, 1970). Similarly fragments of rheumatoid synovium cultured on autologous joint capsules were shown to proliferate and invade the collagenous capsule (Harris, DiBona and Krane, 1970). Obviously no similar experiments can be undertaken with scleral and episcleral tissue but the invasiveness of episcleral tissue has been suspected in limbal guttering and has led Brown (1975) to suggest removal of episcleral tissue adjacent to a scleral gutter.

Detection of collagenase in synovium obtained by closed needle biopsy (Harris, DiBona and Krane, 1970) from various conditions, such as Reiter's syndrome, pseudogout and degenerative arthritis suggests that collagenase production is related more to the degree of proliferative and inflammatory change in the synovium than to a specific pathological entity. It is our belief that the collagenase released in scleral necrosis is also the result rather than the cause of the lesion. It remains to be determined whether individual cells in the sclera and rheumatoid synovium produce more collagenase than normal cells, or whether the increased collagenase production reflects primarily the summation of collagenase production by an increased population of cells found in the proliferative lesion. However, the ability of rheumatoid synovial collagenase to degrade polymeric collagen is debated (Leibovich and Weiss, 1971) and the position is equally uncertain with respect to the sclera.

Like the early lesions of inflammatory scleritis, the early synovial changes in rheumatoid arthritis are dominated by vascular changes, suggesting the walls of small vessels as a target tissue with permeability of the small vessels.

The surface is covered by a fibrinous inflammatory exudate, the fibrin having been exuded through synovial capillaries, the permeability of which has changed as part of the inflammatory response. Fibrin present in scleral lesions probably has a similar origin. Glynn (1968) considers that the persistence of fibrin in the joint space plays a part in the persistence of the arthritis, and might account for the chronic unremitting course of some patients with marked scleritis. The exudate in synovial fluid and the early scleritis contains predominantly polymorphs. Synoviocyte proliferation is also early, there being a relative increase in the number of Type B synthetic cells, hyperactivity of the 'phagocytic' type A cells and giant cells appear (Muirden, 1970; Bhan and Roy, 1971). Similar cell types may exist in scleral disease but have not been identified. On the synovial surface of the joint, the Type A cells show characteristic changes (Ghadially and Roy, 1969). The main changes are the presence of large vacuoles and of electron-dense lysosomal bodies. We know that these bodies contain proteolytic enzymes. Giant cells are similar in both scleral and joint disease as in the infiltration of both the sclera and synovial membrane with lymphocytes, plasma cells and macrophages after the end of the acute stage of the disease in both joint and sclera.

These cells form perivascular collections, which in their early stages under the electron microscope appear to be composed mainly of small lymphocytes with neighbouring perivascular collections made up of lymphocytes, lymphoblasts, plasmablasts, plasma cells and macrophages (Kobayashi and Ziff, 1973). Cellular transformation occurs around the vessels and as the lesions mature they become composed mainly of plasma cells (Figure 6.1).

Even when the synovial lesions have become pronounced, scleral or joint destruction does not take place if the disease remits. Neither acute nor chronic inflammation can account for destructive lesions, which are due to scleral

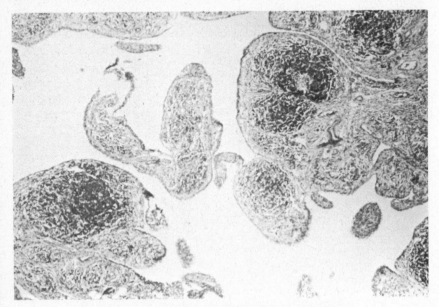

Figure 6.1. Rheumatoid synovium showing lymphoid follicles.

or cartilage collagen digestion. In the joint the destruction is greatest in those areas directly in contact with 'pannus'. 'Pannus' is granulation tissue (fibroblasts and mononuclear cells) which extends marginally on to the surface of the cartilage where enzymes are released from polymorphs and macrophages. A similar granuloma can be found at the site of scleral destruction. A synovial collagenase is activated (Evansson, Jeffrey and Krane, 1967). The earliest changes occur at the margin of the synovial joint. At the articular margins, pannus replaces bone, and in this position the loss of bone gives rise to the radiologically visible erosions which are characteristic of the disease. Pannus may also extend

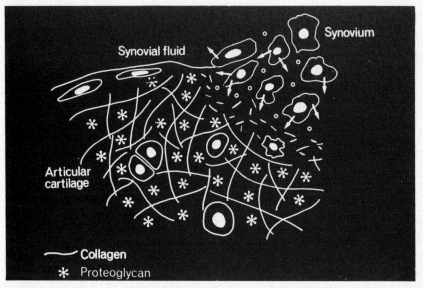

Figure 6.2.   Diagram of the destruction of articular cartilage by enzymes released from the pannus cells of the rheumatoid synovium.
Courtesy of Dr J. Dingle, Cambridge.

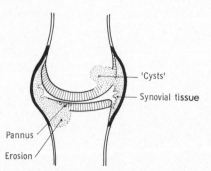

Figure 6.3.   Joint changes in rheumatoid arthritis. The synovial tissues are inflamed. Pannus causes erosions by extending into marginal bone producing 'cysts', eventually leading to destruction of articular cartilage.

through the subchondral bony plate to occupy spaces within the subchondral bone, and in this position gives rise to radiologically visible cysts (these are pseudocysts since they contain solid material).

When the cartilage is involved there is diffuse loss of metachromasia (leaching out of the glycoaminoglycans or mucopolysaccharides), focal dissolution of matrix around chondrocytes, and later cartilage erosion with the death of chondrocytes (Figure 6.2). Cartilage can survive the loss of proteoglycans (split from their protein by acid and neutral cathepsins) and recover its resilience. Articular cartilage in arthritis remote from granulomas is frequently depleted of proteoglycans (Hamerman, 1969). Cartilage in this state has a decreased capacity to resist deformation (Harris et al, 1972). However, once collagen, which forms the structural skeleton of the tissue is lost, cartilage degradation becomes irreversible (Figure 6.3). Similarly reparative processes can restore the scleral collagenous architecture almost to normal whilst there is no actual destruction of tissue, but once collagen destruction has occurred, only a thin layer of fibrous tissue will remain after treatment.

IMMUNOLOGICAL MECHANISMS

Immunological mechanisms appear to play a major part in the pathogenesis of both rheumatoid arthritis and scleritis. The immune mechanisms activated in scleritis associated with rheumatoid arthritis and other connective tissue diseases are similar to those found in common viral or bacterial disease, but there is a major difference and that is the persistence and perpetuation of the response. The factors that regulate and influence remission in these connective tissue diseases are not understood. Occasionally, cases of scleritis and rheumatoid arthritis remit permanently; pregnancy and jaundice also have beneficial effects. Sometimes the histological features that indicate active arthritis may be found in the absence of many of the clinical features of active rheumatoid synovitis, namely anaemia and a raised erythrocyte sedimentation rate.

It is still much too soon to suggest that scleritis and rheumatoid arthritis are due to the presence of an exogenous antigen within the affected tissue, which when replaced by an autoantigen causes the disease to pursue its typically relentless progress; however, there is evidence to suggest that not only do immunological reactions play a major role in the pathogenesis but also in the perpetuation of rheumatoid inflammation. The significance of the immunological findings is difficult to assess because some may be epiphenomena while others are probably concerned with actual pathogenesis. The mechanisms by which these various immunological factors give rise to the granuloma are becoming clear. Although interrelated, these are perhaps best considered in terms of humoral and cellular mechanisms.

Evidence for Immune Mechanisms in Rheumatoid Arthritis

1. Lymphocytic infiltration of synovium with follicle formation complete with germinal centres (Glynn, 1972).

2. Local synthesis of IgG and rheumatoid factor.
3. Depression of complement components in synovial fluid (Hedberg, 1967).
4. Occasionally decreased serum complement.
5. Presence of antigen—antibody complexes (predominantly) IgG—IgG rheumatoid factor) in synovia (Bonomo et al, 1970).
6. Presence of IgG—IgG complexes, IgM and complement components in leucocytes and synovia (Agnello, Winchester and Kunkel, 1970).
7. Presence of lymphokines (macrophage migration inhibition factor) in synovial fluid.

In considering immunological mechanisms to account for tissue damage, one has to look for reactions which lead to activation of tissue enzymes and other mediators of inflammation. There is increasing circumstantial evidence that immune complexes, i.e. the complexes of specific antibody with antigen, the interaction of which leads to fixation and activation of the complement cascade, play a significant role both in rheumatoid synovitis and in the extra-articular lesions such as vasculitis which are characteristic features of rheumatoid disease.

Humoral reactions

The early synovial lesion is nonspecific and heterogenous. Giant cells, lymphocytes and plasma cells, fibroblasts and endothelial cells all exist together. The synovial lining cells may proliferate to more than 20 times their original number. Type B cells and cells 'intermediate' between Types A and B predominate and both have prominent rough endoplasmic reticulum. As the rheumatoid synovial lesion progresses, many foci of lymphocytes and plasma cells develop amidst the proliferating synovial cells and sometimes the synovium takes on the appearance of a lymphoid tissue. Similar cell types are found in the earliest scleral lesions.

Immunofluorescent studies have shown that most of these cells contain IgG and rheumatoid factor. Immune globulins are synthesised in small amounts by normal synovial membrane (Jasin and Ziff, 1969). In rheumatoid synovitis deposits of IgG, IgM and β1C are present (Brandt, Cathcart and Cohen, 1968) in interstitial tissue, the cytoplasm of infiltrating inflammatory cells and in and near blood vessels. Synovial cells have been shown to carry on an active synthesis of immunoglobulin; indeed this local synthesis may result in higher immunoglobulin concentration in synovial fluid than in serum and synthesis is at approximately the same rate as lymphoid tissue (Smiley, Sachs and Ziff, 1968). It has also been demonstrated that synovial lymphocytes do not respond as do circulatory cells by producing antibody to specific antigens such as tetanus toxoid and it has been suggested that this is because synovial lymphocytes and plasma cells may be pre-committed to synthesis of antibody to other, as yet unknown antigens (Herman et al, 1971). Some of the immunoglobulins have antiglobulin activity of the same sort and specificity as the rheumatoid factors present in the serum. These antibodies are autoantibodies, able to interact with the patient's own IgG molecules (whether as antibody in specific combination with any antigen, or as free IgG in tissue fluids or serum). Although there is as yet no proof, similar changes may be occurring in scleral lesions. The scleral nodule in rheumatoid arthritis is identical to that found elsewhere in the body (Ashton and Hobbs, 1952) and the cellular patterns of the nodules found in other patients with scleritis are histologically almost indistinguishable from those found in RA. It is not unreasonable therefore to draw comparisons here between the changes found in the rheumatoid synovium and the changes in scleritis.

Immunoglobulins

Five major structural types or classes of immunoglobulin are described: IgG, IgM, IgA, IgE and IgD. Antigenic analysis has shown that IgG can be grouped into four subclasses. Two subclasses of IgA and of IgM have also been found. Fractionation using gel filtration reveals two sizes of peptide chain termed light and heavy chains. All the differences in the IgG classes lie in the heavy chains. These heavy chains have certain structures in common with each other—the ones which react with specific anti-IgG antisera—but each has structural differences in primary amino acid composition and in disulphide bridging. These give rise to differences in biological behaviour.

Porter proposed a symmetrical four-peptide model for antibody consisting of two heavy and two light chains linked together by interchain disulphide bonds (Figure 6.4). Each chain has a variable portion, in which amino acid

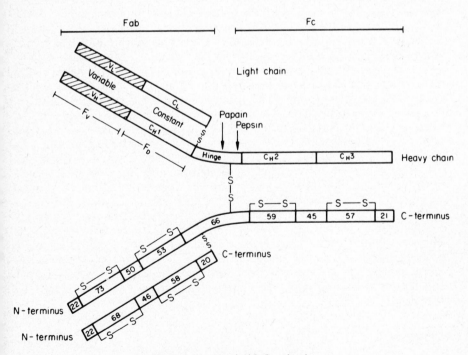

Figure 6.4. A typical IgG molecule.

sequences can differ, and a constant portion in which they remain the same. The enzyme papain can cleave the molecule producing three pieces. The single piece of two COOH ends of heavy chain held together by an SS bond is called the Fc fragment. The other two pieces are identical and consist of the N-terminal end of the heavy chain (the Fd fragment) and the whole of the light chain. Together these are known as the Fab or antigen-binding fragment. IgG is a monomer of this structure but IgM is a pentamer, the individual bonds themselves being held together by SS bonds. Each class of immunoglobulin has its own specific type of heavy chain, γ for IgG, α for IgA, etc., whereas there are only two light chain types, κ and λ common to all classes. In each case about 60 per cent of the light chains are κ and 30 per cent are λ. Immunoglobulin G comprises 80 per cent of the total immunoglobulin and during the secondary response IgG is probably the major immunoglobulin to be synthesised. IgG diffuses more readily than the other immunoglobulins into the extravascular body spaces where, as the predominant species, it carries the major burden of neutralising bacterial toxins and of binding the microorganisms to enhance their phagocytosis.

Immunoglobulin M is produced early in the immune response and is largely confined to the bloodstream. It is a very effective agglutinator and first line defence and is of particular importance in cases of bacteraemia.

Immunoglobulin A is the major immunoglobulin in seromucous secretions where it defends external body surfaces. Immunoglobulin E is raised in parasitic infections and is responsible for symptoms of atopic allergy.

Immunofluorescence studies of rheumatoid synovial membrane have shown that plasma cells produce both IgM antiglobulin and IgG antiglobulin (Winchester, Agnello and Kunkel, 1969) and recent work has shown that so-called 'seronegative' patients may be producers of IgG antiglobulin in 'hidden forms' which require special techniques to reveal their presence (Munthe and Natvig, 1972). This is important as IgG–anti-IgG rheumatoid factor complexes have been demonstrated in synovial fluid (Agnello, Winchester and Kunkel, 1970). These complexes have complement fixing and activating properties and complement bound in association with IgG has been demonstrated both in synovial membrane and within the phagocytic cells in rheumatoid synovial effusions (Ziff, 1973). Complement levels are reduced in synovial effusions and it is thought that these antiglobulin reactions in the rheumatoid joint may themselves well be enough to initiate and continue the inflammatory processes we recognise in the joint. The presence of soluble immune complexes (Ziff, 1973) in the synovial fluid has provided an excellent opportunity to identify the nature of the antigenic moiety. Dissociates of the complexes and their separation on appropriate columns has, however, so far revealed only denatured IgG as antigen. Although disturbances of the normal ratio of these substances in the circulation and an increase in circulating immunoglobulins can be found in scleral disease, the presence of these substances in excess in scleral lesions has yet to be demonstrated. The normal levels have been investigated by Allansmith et al (1973).

Complement

The existence of complement was recognised at the end of the nineteenth century when serum was found to contain a heat-labile factor necessary for lysis of red cells by antibody (Bordet, 1895).

The complement system comprises a series of nine serum proteins known as 'components', symbolised by the letter C and a number, e.g. C1, C2, C3, etc. (C3 is present in greatest concentration). C1 consists of three subunits. The term 'haemolytic complement' describes the end-result of the interaction of all the proteins in the complement system. In the process active enzymes are developed from serum protein precursors; these cleave other serum proteins and lead to the release of substances with important biological effects (Figure 6.5). The following inflammatory products are liberated:

C-kinin: Increases capillary permeability.

C3a | Liberates histamine from mast cells.
C5a | Chemotactic for leucocytes.

C36: Enhances phagocytosis of immune complexes.

C567: Sensitises innocent bystander cells for lysis.
Chemotactic factor.

C5 C9: Membrane damage, osmotic lysis and cell death.

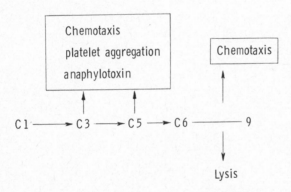

Figure 6.5. Products of complement activation.

Like so many mediators of immune response, the complement system is an indispensible part of the host's defence against infections. Nevertheless it may also contribute to tissue damage in allergic reactions. Complement is essential for the lysis and phagocytosis of bacteria and viruses coated with antibody; as a result patients with various forms of complement deficiency are vulnerable to infections (Alper et al, 1972). In contrast complement damages tissues both by its direct action on cell membranes and by the secondary action of other immunopathological processes resulting from complement activation. Thus disease may be caused either by the persistent activation of complement by immunological stimuli (and in particular antigen—antibody complexes) or as a result of intrinsic defects of the complement system which allow its spontaneous activation.

Complement activation in human disease can be detected by three principal methods. Firstly, concentrations of complement components may be shown to be reduced in the serum and inflammatory fluids but it is essential to correlate the concentration in effusions with those of other serum proteins in order to prove that the depletion of complement is specific. For clinical purposes it is usually enough to find a general indication of complement consumption in the form of a reduced concentration of C3 or of total haemolytic activity, which measures the integrity of the whole system. The second method is the detection of complement components by immunofluorescence in diseased tissues or in phagocytic cells in inflammatory exudates. Thirdly, activated complement components may be identified in the serum and tissues. In scleral disease the volume of involved tissue is so small that these methods are generally too insensitive to be of value.

Complement system activation begins with the union of the first component, C1, with an altered immunoglobulin. Antibodies which have combined with their specific antigen to form immune complexes have this property. This leads to cleavage of C4 and C2, and then to C3 cleavage (the classical complement pathway). Another system involving three or more factors, P, B and D, is able to induce C3 cleavage bypassing the early components (C1, C4 and C2) of the classical pathway (Figure 6.6). Properdin activation

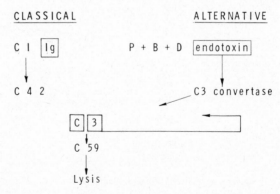

Figure 6.6. Complement activation showing classical and alternative pathways. The generation of the classical C3 convertase has the characteristics of an enzyme cascade.

of C3 and the terminal complement components seems to be triggered by certain polysaccharides (including endotoxin) or by IgA immunoglobulins. Although the biological properties of the properdin protein are not yet fully understood, their effects on C3 and C5 C9 are identical to the results of the classic pathway. Precisely the same release of chemotactic factors, histamine liberators and the final membrane damaging complexes occur. It has recently been shown that a breakdown product of C3 itself, C3b, is a necessary component of the alternative pathway, and that its involvement constitutes a feedback pathway of complement activation. These steps in complement activation may be reversed by a series of inhibitors and they play a critical regulatory function in the complement sequence.

Though serum levels of total complement activity or the individual components are usually normal or elevated in rheumatoid arthritis, synovial fluid levels are often much lower than would be expected on the molecular weight of these proteins (Ruddy and Austin, 1973). This implies that the complement components are being used up in complement-fixing immune reactions within the joints. Studies support the concept that complement components are activated and breakdown products of the third component have been found in the fluid. Studies (Weinstein et al, 1972) have shown an increased functional catabolic rate and a decreased half-life of C3 in rheumatoid vasculitis. Although complement activation must occur in destructive scleral disease, changes in serum complement levels have not been detected in patients with scleritis in whom no other systemic cause can be found. No attempt has been made to assess its activation in diseased scleral tissue.

Immune complexes

Immune complexes can be detected in both serum and synovial fluid but the changes of the complement system are more intense in the joint spaces. Breakdown products of some complement components (C3, C4, properdin factor B) can be quantified and are demonstrated in high amounts in synovial fluid from patients with rheumatoid arthritis. Immune complexes are also present in rheumatoid cartilage (Cooke et al, 1972), in which they collect either as a result of diffusion or local precipitation. In the cartilage the immune complexes may serve as a reservoir for unidentified antigens involved in the rheumatoid process, and they also serve as a stimulus for pannus formation. The activation of complement by synovial fluid complexes leads to the formation of C5, C6, C7 chemotactic factor complex and a C5a complex that attracts polymorphonuclear cells into the fluid; this explains the high concentration of these cells in most rheumatoid fluids.

It is the formation of IgG–anti-IgG rheumatoid factor complexes that appears to be mainly responsible for the reduced levels of complement in rheumatoid effusions leading to fixation and activation of the complement cascade. The contribution of IgM rheumatoid factor to complement utilisation in the rheumatoid effusion is not clear, although depression of synovial fluid complement levels has been observed more frequently in patients with positive tests for IgM rheumatoid factor in the serum. Ruddy and Austin (1973) have attributed this greater diminution in seropositive disease to the further interaction of the IgG–anti-IgG factor complex with IgM rheumatoid factor. IgM rheumatoid factor can convert soluble immune complexes to complement-fixing aggregates. Therefore rheumatoid factors may exaggerate the inflammatory properties of altered gammaglobulin, either by augmenting complement fixation, or by changing the size or solubility of the complexes, thereby enhancing their phagocytosis by leucocytes. Immune complexes have been looked for in two patients with scleral disease but could not be found.

Rheumatoid factor (RhF)

RhF is predominantly an antibody of the IgM class and reacts specifically to various determinants present in immunoglobulin of the IgG class. It is probable that the antigenic determinants are actually present in the individual patient's own IgG molecules even if some of these require some alteration in configuration from the native state before their reactivity with the appropriate rheumatoid factors becomes detectable. This forms the basis of the sheep cell agglutination test and the latex fixation test for rheumatoid arthritis.

Whilst RhF is present in most patients with rheumatoid arthritis (60 to 70 per cent), this is not in itself the cause of the disease and can be found in patients with other connective tissue diseases and in some normal individuals in low titre. RhF may, however, be implicated in the production of some of the more serious manifestations of the condition in that patients with rheumatoid arthritis with a high titre rheumatoid factor frequently have a more serious type of disease—subcutaneous nodules, arteritis, scleritis and peripheral neuropathy (Cathcart and O'Sullivan, 1969). The titre should therefore be assessed in all patients with scleral disease.

The role of RhF is therefore still controversial; we have no idea whether it plays a prime part in the disease process, and in any case the role it plays may vary quantitatively. There is conflicting evidence whether RhF is damaging or protective.

Since rheumatoid factors can occur in non-rheumatoid individuals with various chronic infective conditions, the probable stimulus to their production is the presence of IgG whose configuration has been changed by combination with antigen. In chronic infective states, the rheumatoid factors virtually disappear when the infection is overcome. The characteristic persistence of RhF in rheumatoid arthritis may therefore be taken either as evidence of a persistent infective agent or alternatively of the persistence of some other antigen whose combination with IgG constitutes an adequate stimulus for its production.

McCormick et al (1969) showed that if an experimental renal injury is

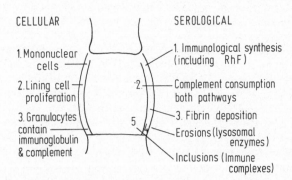

Figure 6.7.   Summary of the possible immunopathological events involved in joint destruction in rheumatoid arthritis.

produced by a sensitisation technique and RhF is added to the nephrotoxic serum, the injury produced is more severe than if the RhF is not present. This suggests that RhF may be able to injure tissue. There is converse evidence which suggests a protective effect. For example, we know that plasma complement has a capacity for attracting white cells to sites where antigen–antibody reactions are taking place. RhF can interfere with this property of complement. In addition RhF can regulate antibody production (Brown and Epstein, 1969), help in the clearance of antigen–antibody complexes from the blood (Lightfoot, Drusin and Christian, 1969) and neutralise infectious virus–antibody complexes in the presence of complement (Ashe et al, 1971). Thus much work remains to be done before its detection in the serum of patients with scleral disease can be regarded as significant (Figure 6.7).

Summary

The presence of complexes of IgG and β1C and of IgM and IgG in the synovial tissues of rheumatoid joints suggests that most if not all of the inflammation at this site is mediated by these immune complexes. The role and the mechanism of action of such complexes in a variety of inflammatory states are now established, but so far their role in scleral disease has not been determined. The activation of complement by immune complexes leads to many of the vascular changes of inflammation and to the release of chemotactic factors responsible for the accumulation of the polymorphonuclear cells and macrophages that are found in both the sclera and in joints. The phagocytosis of complexes leads to a release of lysosomal enzymes which have the potential for initiating further tissue injury. Lysosomal enzyme release (Hembry, 1976, personal communication) has been demonstrated in experimentally induced scleral and corneal disease, but whether this is due to the phagocytosis of immune complexes has yet to be determined.

Evidence for Cell-Mediated Mechanisms in Rheumatoid Arthritis

This discussion of the pathogenesis of scleritis and rheumatoid arthritis has so far emphasised the humoral immune mechanisms involving antigen–antibody complexes and complement in the production of joint inflammation. However, several lines of evidence suggest a role for cell-mediated immune reactions in the production of rheumatoid arthritis. What importance this has in the development of scleral lesions is obscure, but because lymphocytes are prominent in the histological specimens and biopsy specimens taken in the acute inflammatory stage, they may be of great significance. The cell-mediated mechanisms will be discussed in detail because it is possible that future methods of diagnosis and treatment will be based on an understanding of their function.

Lymphocyte subpopulations

During the past few years it has become apparent that peripheral blood lymphocytes are comprised of heterogenous populations of cells. Those processed by the thymus (T-type or thymus-dependent lymphocytes) play a major role in cell-mediated immune responses or type IV delayed hypersensitivity. T-lymphocytes are most heavily concentrated in the paracortical regions of lymph nodes and in the periarteriolar areas of the white pulp of the spleen. The B (bursa-equivalent) cells are not processed by the thymus and come to lie at, or near the germinal centres of lymph nodes and spleen. They play a major role in humoral antibody responses and mature to form antibody-producing plasma cells. Some small lymphocytes survive and ultimately carry on an immunological memory so that if stimulated again they can produce an accelerated response to an antigen (Figure 6.8).

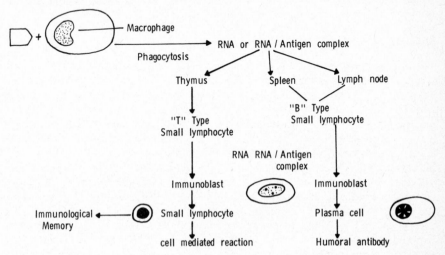

Figure 6.8. Derivation of T- and B-lymphocytes which give rise to the cell-mediated and humoral antibody reactions.

In normal human peripheral blood T-cells comprise some 40 to 70 per cent of lymphocytes and B-cells 15 to 30 per cent. About ten per cent of circulating lymphocytes appear to be neither T- nor B-cells and among these are the so-called K or killer cells which are not themselves specifically sensitised but which can gain specific cytotoxic properties in the presence of antibody or antigen–antibody complexes on the surface of target cells.

Neither light nor electron microscopy can distinguish between T- and B-cells. A variety of methods has been developed in recent years allowing quantitative and qualitative characterisation of T- and B-lymphocytes (Rowlands and Daniele, 1975). These methods depend on the different cell-surface characteristics of T- and B-lymphocytes.

B-lymphocytes synthesise and excrete specific antibodies and a variety of techniques, including fluorescent antisera, can be used to detect immunoglobulin on their surface. B-cells also possess a surface receptor for the Fc component of immunoglobulin; this receptor is not possessed by the T-cell but is found on macrophages. B-cells also possess surface receptors which interact specifically with certain complement components; these receptors can be detected using sheep red cells coated with anti-sheep cell antibody plus complement.

T-cells possess the unique property of forming rosettes with unsensitised washed sheep red blood cells which can be readily coated and examined by light microscopy. Although the precise nature of the receptors involved has not been clearly defined, this reaction has been widely exploited as a means of identifying and quantifying T-lymphocytes.

These techniques are subject to a number of technical and other difficulties. For example, the mere presence of immunoglobulin (Ig) at the surface of a cell does not necessarily mean that Ig was produced by that cell. Moreover surface Ig is lost as B-lymphocytes mature into plasma cells.

Some of the antisera used are of uncertain specificity and some of the reagents are themselves immunoglobulins and may bind nonspecifically to receptors for immunoglobulin molecules. The differences between these sub-populations are not as rigid as was once imagined, and some lymphocytes have been shown to combine the surface features of both the T- or B-cell populations (Chiao, Pantic and Good, 1974). Furthermore, classifications of this sort are too rigid; for instance many substances—and not just the thymic hormone thymosin—modulate the surface of B-lymphocytes and induce some of the antigens regarded as characteristic of T-lymphocytes.

B-cells are often able to respond to antigenic stimuli only in collaboration with T-cells (*Transplantation Review*, 1974); they then form plasma cells and produce circulatory antibodies against antigen. Antigens are first 'neutralised' by phagocytic macrophages—a nonspecific response—and then T-lympho-cytes, either by direct transfer of surface receptors to macrophages help orient or focus antigen for presentation to B-cells, or by release of soluble mediators called 'lymphokines' ensure maximal and sustained response of B-lymphocytes.

The concept of T–B-lymphocyte cooperation is essential to an understanding of the development of certain autoimmune diseases. The exact mechanisms involved in T–B cooperation are not known, but it appears that in the case of complex antigens, the T-cell reacts with one portion of the immunogenic molecule whereas the B-cell reacts with another region (Katz and Benacerraf, 1972).

Lymphokines may have far-reaching biological functions. One or more of them has the effect of arresting the migratory activity of neighbouring macro-phages. As has been shown, macrophages may well be a necessary intermediary in the cooperation of T- and B-cells to respond to antigen.

Studies in animal models have shown that an immune synovitis can be transferred to normal recipients by cells (Pearson and Wood, 1964). A disorder similar to rheumatoid arthritis may occur in patients with agamma-globulinaemia (Good and Rotstein, 1960) and these children have abundant T-cells in their synovial tissue. It has also been shown that the removal of primary T-lympho-cytes by thoracic duct drainage results in marked clinical improvement in patients with severe rheumatoid arthritis (Pearson, Paulus and Machlede, 1975).

Recently attention has been given to the mononuclear cells infiltrating the synovial tissue; some of these cells contain immunoglobulins or can synthesise immunoglobulin. It has also been shown that the majority of these cells are T (thymus-dependent) lymphocytes (van Boxel and Paget, 1975). The absence of such cells in the mature areas of the synovial membrane, which consist mainly of plasma cells, suggests that recirculating T-lymphocytes leave the synovial membrane and enter the synovial fluid as the immunological process becomes more differentiated.

Stastny et al (1973) have shown that lymphokine-inhibiting factors are detectable in rheumatoid synovial fluid and are indeed synthesised in the rheumatoid synovial membrane providing further evidence for the blastic transformation of T-lymphocytes.

Sheldon, Papamichail and Holborow (1975) have shown that while the ratio of T-lymphocytes to B-lymphocytes is somewhat greater in the synovial fluid than in the blood of rheumatoid patients, the T-cells in synovial fluid have to a great extent lost their ability to respond to the mitogen phytohaemagglutinin. They therefore behave like cells which have undergone antigen stimulation and this suggests that they may have already encountered antigen in the joint. We are, of course, ignorant of the nature of the antigenic stimulus, but there are a number of hypotheses as to its nature (virus, altered self-antigen or a fetal antigen expressed by synovial cells whose differentiation is deranged). The increase may not be antigenically induced but may be due to a defect in the normal regulation of these cells. Another feature of cells from inflammatory joint effusions is cytotoxicity. This was first described by Hedberg (1967) who showed that joint fluid cells from arthritic patients were cytotoxic to monolayers of human fetal fibroblasts. MacLennan and Loewi (1970) confirmed this using Chang cells (liver tumour cells) and demonstrated the nonspecific nature of this type of cytotoxicity. No explanation can at present be offered for the increased cytotoxicity of joint effusion lymphocytes.

Another parameter of lymphocyte reactivity is furnished by the mixed lymphocyte reaction. Hedberg et al (1971) have examined this in rheumatoid arthritis. A significantly low response was found when lymphocytes from pairs of patients with rheumatoid arthritis were cultivated together in a mixed reaction. It is likely that this impaired response is due to a chronic disease state rather than a fundamental immune abnormality.

The description of the immunopathological process fails to explain why rheumatoid arthritis is a chronic disease. No characteristic pattern of response or immunological aberration has been shown consistently in patients with rheumatoid arthritis, whether in the form of increased or reduced responsiveness to antigenic challenge. It is attractive to postulate that rheumatoid arthritis is initiated by delayed hypersensitivity to microorganisms duplicating within macrophages in the synovial membrane. If these widely distributed micro-organisms do initiate this chronic destructive process, host factors must also play a major part in determining why only a small percentage of the population develops the disease. Similarly only a minority of people exposed to group A streptococci develop rheumatic fever. Though the belief that rheumatoid arthritis is primarily an autoimmune disease has lost ground in recent years, many would agree that patients with this disorder may have an immunological defect as a result of which a short-lived infection induces a persisting response either to microbial antigens or cross-reacting tissue antigens.

AMYLOIDOSIS

Amyloidosis, which is found as a later complication of rheumatoid arthritis, has been cited as evidence of the immune basis for the disease. The reported incidence varies widely, but some studies suggest that amyloid is present in 10 to 15 per cent of postmortems. It is known that amyloid deposition in horses results from prolonged immunisation with commercial products of antisera, and it has long been suggested that the amyloidosis of rheumatoid arthritis is a sign of prolonged excess response to antigenic stimulation. Amyloid has not been detected in the lesions of scleritis even though in many cases the eye examined has been inflamed for many years.

In the pre-antibiotic era, by far the highest incidence of amyloidosis was seen in association with chronic infection such as osteomyelitis and pulmonary tuberculosis. The metabolic steps between immune stimulation and amyloid deposition are far from clear. Immunoglobulin constitutes only a minor component of amyloid.

ANIMAL MODELS

Animal experiments support the immunological nature of the synovial lesion. There are innumerable ways of producing experimental arthritis; the only ones producing anything resembling the rheumatoid lesions are those in which an allergic reaction is involved. Two methods are commonly used: adjuvant arthritis in rats and allergic arthritis in rabbits. In both these methods tubercle bacilli play a major role. In the Glynn model, rabbits immunised with a protein antigen, e.g. ovalbumin in Freund's complete adjuvant, will develop an arthritis similar to rheumatoid arthritis if the same antigen is injected into one knee joint. The inflammation may persist for many years (Glynn, 1972), possibly due to retention of the injected antigen in the form of immune complexes in avascular tissue (Hollister and Mannik, 1974), but this appears unlikely (Dumonde and Glynn, 1965). A more probable explanation is that one or more new antigens appear to be derived from the joint itself or from the inflammatory exudate. Attempts to induce a persisting scleral reaction from antigen injected into the sclera of these animals has so far failed, although perforation of the sclera has occurred (see Figure 6.12). In these animals perforation of the sclera occurred at a site remote from the antigen injection site about ten days after the local stimulus. The period of inflammation, however, was not prolonged. The eye became red in the region of the perilimbal plexus of vessels, necrosis occurred, the eye perforated, and after a few days the inflammation disappeared. Histologically the inflamed sclera was similar to that found in the human disease but the scleral changes rapidly returned to normal after perforation had occurred. It would seem that the lesion produced was a necrotising vasculitis rather than a chronic granuloma.

VASCULITIS

Vasculitis is a feature of pathological specimens of eyes with scleritis whatever the underlying cause, and involves not only the vessels already present but also the newly formed vessels. Acute necrotising lesions as in polyarteritis are indeed uncommon, but a less acute form of vasculitis involving small veins as well as arteries may be widespread and probably plays a part in the typical nodule formation in the subcutaneous tissues and, more rarely, in the lungs of patients with rheumatoid arthritis.

Rheumatoid vasculitis is closely associated with IgM rheumatoid factor seropositivety and the other extra-articular features of rheumatoid arthritis, and immunofluorescent studies show the presence of IgG and complement in the vessel wall (Bonomo et al, 1970). It has been suggested that rheumatoid factors of the IgG variety may participate in the formation of immune complexes involved in the development of vasculitis (Theofilopoulos et al, 1974). IgG rheumatoid factors have been demonstrated in the serum of patients with rheumatoid arthritis (Torrigiani et al, 1970) and Theofilopoulos et al (1974) found a correlation between IgG RhF and vasculitis and also between low molecular weight IgM RhF and vasculitis. In addition they found a correlation between IgG RhF, low molecular weight IgM RhF and vasculitis. These results suggests that IgG–IgG–RhF complexes may be involved in the pathogenesis of rheumatoid vasculitis.

Vasculitis is the prominent feature of polyarteritis nodosa and complexes of Australia antigen and antibody and complement have been demonstrated on vessel walls. Hypersensitivity angiitis also seems to have an immunological basis; a disease can be produced in animals which is very similar to drug-induced hypersensitivity angiitis in man (Tucker and Wyatt, 1967).

OTHER MEDIATORS OF INFLAMMATION

There are a number of mediators of inflammation in the rheumatoid joint and in uveitis. How these relate to the sclera is at present unclear. The theoretical possibilities are great since practically every active substance extracted from blood or tissues has at one time or another been incriminated as a mediator of inflammation. Histamine and serotonin, polypeptide kinins (Eisen, 1970) and prostaglandins are present in acute inflammation during the early reversible changes of tissue injury. They all possess potent vasoactive, chemotactic and pain-producing properties. The role of kinins as mediators of joint inflammation is unclear (Phelps, Prockop and McCarthy, 1966). The prostaglandins have recently stimulated much interest, and it has been suggested that defective reactivity of lymphocytes to prostaglandin could offer the basis for chronicity in rheumatoid arthritis (Morley, 1974) and presumably for scleritis.

Prostaglandins

These are naturally occurring substances which have been detected in a wide variety of human and animal tissues. Their chemical structure is related to unsaturated fatty acids such as arachidonic acid which is one of their precursors. They have a wide spectrum of biological activity and were initially identified through their vasodepressor actions and effects on smooth muscles. Synthesised in many tissues, they appear to act as local mediators or hormones which modulate cellular activity. As with classical hormones, this modulation goes through the second messenger system of cyclic nucleotides: cAMP (cyclic adenosine monophosphate) which tends to stabilise membranes, and cGMP (cyclic guanosine-3′,5′-monophosphate) which tends to destabilise membranes. Several classes of prostaglandins have been described according to their chemical structure and prostaglandin E (PGE) and prostaglandin F (PGF) are probably the most important. It seems that macrophages are the primary source of PGE in inflammation (Bray et al, 1974) and PGE also inhibits lymphocyte formation. Table 6.1 shows some of their biological properties.

Table 6.1. *Biological properties of the prostaglandins*

Respiratory system: bronchodilation.

Gastrointestinal: contraction of isolated smooth muscles;
　　　　　　　　inhibition of basal gastric secretion.

Inflammation: increased amount in inflammatory tissue.

Stimulation of epidermal proliferation.

Potentiation of pain induced by various mediators (histamine, bradykinin).

Pyretic properties.

Prostaglandins are present in inflammatory exudates and can mediate various inflammatory reactions. An increase in prostaglandins is found in the skin after exposure to the sun and it has been shown that indomethacin and aspirin inhibit prostaglandin synthesis in lung homogenates (Vane, 1971). Recently the newer non-steroidal anti-inflammatory agents have been found to have similar properties (Ferreira and Vane, 1973).

There is no doubt that prostaglandins are involved in inflammation because:
1. Prostaglandin production can be suppressed by anti-inflammatory drugs.
2. Prostaglandin can mimic features of inflammation.
3. There is prostaglandin in synovial effusions.
4. Prostaglandin is produced by culture of inflammatory cell populations.

CHANGES IN THE CONNECTIVE TISSUE

The changes in collagen seen in granulomatous scleral disease correspond exactly with what is known about the degradation and regeneration of this substance and other collagenous structures elsewhere. Under normal circumstances the proteoglycan filler and the collagen fibres themselves are in dynamic balance between synthesis and destruction of both cellular and extracellular macromolecules. The rate of turnover of the various molecules varies from hours to perhaps hundreds of days. Nevertheless this catabolic activity of cells in organised tissues is as characteristic of life as is cell division. It seems reasonable as a working hypothesis to view both the increased breakdown seen during physiological remodelling and that associated with pathological damage as a local exaggeration of a normal process. The process itself is thought to involve the combination of extracellular enzyme action and concurrent or perhaps subsequent endocytic activity and intracellular digestion.

Proteoglycans create a swelling pressure between the collagen fibrils, keeping them in their proper anatomical relationship, and also by steric exclusion of other solutes prevent the underlying collagen from attack (Stockwell, 1974).

Proteoglycans can be attacked by numerous enzymes but the protein core has to be broken for the enzymes to come into contact with the underlying collagen fibril. These enzymes are normally intracellular, in the lysosomes. A variety of agents are known to be able to cause tissues to secrete lysosomal enzymes, including vitamin A, complement sufficient antisera, antibodies and sensitised lymphocytes. The molecule is broken down in a systemic synergistic fashion. Cathepsin D has been shown to be localised within the lysosomes, and immunocytochemical techniques, involving tissue culture in the presence of specific anti-D immunoglobulin G followed by fixation and staining with a fluorescein-labelled antibody to this immunoglobulin G, have indicated release of cathepsin D into the matrix immediately round the cells (Figure 2.17).

It seems likely that some or all of these enzymes (cathepsin B1, cathepsin D, cathepsin E, cathepsin F, collagenase, neutral proteinase, elastase) may act synergistically. Their relative importance may vary with the tissue, the stimulus for activity, and the precise pericellular or extracellular site of action. Dingle (1973) has suggested a 'two-step' hypothesis for the degradation of extracellular macromolecules including proteoglycans and collagen; the initial extracellular attack is followed by phagocytosis of portions of the aggregates whose digestion could be completed within the vacuoles, or secondary lysosomes of cells such as fibroblasts where the pH conditions are optimal.

One enzyme which could be involved in the extracellular stage of digestion of both macromolecules in acute inflammatory conditions in which there is infiltration of polymorphonuclear leucocytes is elastase. This degrades proteoglycans and elastin. Once the collagen fibril has been exposed, it can be attacked by collagenase, there being a considerable time lag between the breakdown of the proteoglycans and the collagen (Dingle at al, 1975). The protein core of collagen is unusually resistant to proteolytic degradation, and whilst collagenases have been known to be present in bacteria such as *Clostridium histolyticum* for a considerable time, animal collagenases were only identified from the tails of metamorphosing tadpoles in 1962 (Gross and Lapiere, 1962). Fibroblast-like cells in tissue culture can be made to secrete collagenases and their characteristics determined. They cleave collagen across all three chains of the triple helix at a point three-quarters of the way from the amino end (Dingle, 1973). It is likely that cathepsin B1 can also attack the cyclical region of collagen. Cathepsin B1 probably acts on pieces of collagen fibres in the intracellular phase of digestion whilst collagenase is mainly responsible for the extracellular attack. The collagenases and their possible involvement in disease have been the subject of a detailed review by Harris and Krane (1974).

The different types of collagen vary in their resistance to destruction by proteolytic enzymes: Type 1 is five times less resistant to collagenase than Type II and Type II ten times less resistant than cathepsin B1. Corneal collagenase which acts on Type I and Type III collagens appears to be adherent to the surface of the collagen fibril in the cornea rather than being tightly bound in the glycoprotein shell, as in joint collagen and in the sclera (Hembry, unpublished results, 1976), so it is possible that corneal collagenase can be more readily activated in the cornea than in the sclera, and in part accounts for the higher resistance of the sclera to destruction in patients with corneal necrotising disease, Mooren's ulcers, etc.

In one patient with scleritis and progressive corneal guttering the collagenase, normally present on the surface of the fibrils, had practically disappeared, indicating that it had been activated to take part in collagen breakdown in a similar manner to that which occurs in the uterus at parturition (Harkness and Moralee, 1956).

Irreversible injury to tissue results from enzymatic breakdown and the enzymes contained within lysosomes seem to be responsible for much of the tissue injury seen in rheumatic diseases (Weissmann, 1972). These enzymes have many actions, including: degradation of collagen (collagenase), degradation of elastin (elastase), breakdown of cartilage proteoglycans (acid and neutral proteases), digestion of nucleic acids (RNAase and DNAase), and depolymerisation of hyaluronate (hyaluronidase).

Tissue depleted of proteoglycan is stimulated to synthesise this component more rapidly, suggesting that the degradation of proteoglycan in connective tissue may normally be reversible and that disease results when the process of synthesis and degradation move out of phase. Excessive depletion, aided in cartilage for example by mechanical wear, may lead to loss of collagen, which may be irreversible in the sense that newly synthesised collagen is seldom laid down with the same organisation of the fibres as that in undisturbed tissue.

In rheumatoid arthritis it is assumed that weakness of cartilage by pannus is due to degradation of proteoglycans by acid and neutral cathepsins and that its final erosion is mediated by collagenases (Harris, DiBona and Krane, 1969, 1970).

The major catabolic enzymes responsible for the degradation of cartilage matrix have now been identified. These are cathepsins D, B1 and F and a group of neutral proteinases of varying specificities, including elastase, collagenase and a metal-dependent neutral proteinase.

Inflammatory synovial fluid contains many enzymes, including cathepsin D and collagenases. Cathepsin D appears to be mainly responsible for the breakdown of protein polysaccharide (Dingle, Barrett and Weston, 1971), allowing access to cartilage and possibly collagen fibres. The entry and persistence of antigen–antibody complexes together with complement in the superficial layer has been demonstrated in experimental arthritis (Cooke et al, 1972). Fell and Barratt (1973) have shown that articular cartilage can lose its proteoglycans in the presence of connective tissue, this effect being markedly exaggerated when complement-fixing complexes are present. This work, done in explanted tissues, shows destruction which is not dependent on invading cells and that antibodies and complement can reach tissues by diffusion rather than via blood vessels. Gammaglobulin could penetrate into the matrix where prior loss of metachromasia was produced by the connective tissue. Depletion of the matrix, which seems to be the initial process, is not dependent on loss of chondrocytes.

Werb and Reynolds (1975) have shown that fibroblasts from synovium can be made to secrete 12 to 15 times their normal secretion of collagenase and neutral proteinases if made to digest foreign matter, suggesting that if the digestion of the secondary lysosome system is disturbed, extralysosomal enzyme production is increased.

Proteolytic enzymes are inhibited by tissue and serum inhibitors, in particular the α2-macroglobulins in the circulation which bind and inhibit the active form of the enzymes (Barrett, 1975). The level of α2-macroglobulin in the synovial fluid of patients with rheumatoid arthritis is often raised considerably. It is therefore likely that cartilage destruction only takes place at the narrow interface between cells in the pannus–cartilage junction. This control system breaks down if there is excessive tissue destruction and insufficient α2-macroglobulin remains in the vicinity of the lesion. The proteolytic enzymes are then present in excess, increasing the rate of destruction of the tissue. α2-macroglobulin will not inhibit the enzyme in the presence of inflammatory cells which in part accounts for the fact that connective tissue can be removed from the site of inflammation but not from adjacent tissues. Once the damaged tissue has been removed, the inflammatory reaction dies down and new fibres are laid down in an irregular fashion.

Synovial lining cell proliferation is accompanied by an altered cell metabolism. Proliferation correlates well with increased utilisation of oxygen and glucose as well as with production of lactate and carbon dioxide (Dingle and Page Thomas, 1956). The increase in blood flow through synovial vessels is not sufficient to meet the increased metabolic demands of the tissue and as a result the extracellular Po_2 of the synovial fluid falls (Falchuk, Goetzl and Kulka, 1970; Goetzl et al, 1971).

Castor (1971) has found a 'connective tissue activating peptide' widely distributed in mammalian cells, including leucocytes and connective tissue cells. When synovial cells are exposed to this polypeptide in vitro there is a prompt increase in metabolic activity and a marked increase in the formation of hyaluronic acid. It is not yet clear whether excess production of this peptide precedes all the changes in synovial metabolism or whether its synthesis is another result of an insult to connective tissue. Antirheumatic drugs inhibit the activation phenomenon in vitro (Castor, 1972).

There is increased collagen production in the subsynovial tissue and joint capsule and the latter becomes less compliant and thicker. The increased permeability of small vessels allows considerable exudate to pass into the synovial membrane and joint space; fibrin accumulates and appears to resist the normal processes of digestion.

INDIVIDUAL SUSCEPTIBILITY

It has been suggested that certain individuals are more likely to develop some connective tissue disorders than others. Credence was given to this suggestion by the discovery that the inherited histocompatibility antigen HLA-B27 is present in a very high proportion of patients with ankylosing spondylitis and other patients with seronegative arthritis (Brewerton et al, 1975).

Patients with scleritis not associated with any known connective tissue disease do not have an excess of any tissue antigen (Joysey et al, unpublished observations, 1976). This is discussed further in Chapter 7.

CONCLUSIONS

It is far too early to consider a unitary concept for the pathogenesis of scleritis, of which the necrotising variety is by far the most important. Leaving aside those granulomatous changes where a specific infectious agent can be isolated from the inflamed tissue, and gout in which the mechanism is also known, the causes of these changes are still in doubt. Partly through direct evidence and partly by analogy with similar conditions, a pattern is emerging.

One problem is to find out why the apparently inert sclera becomes the target of this type of inflammation. Inflammation certainly occurs at the site of the primary inflammation in herpes zoster and in one case we have shown it to follow a herpes simplex infection of the episclera. Reports in the literature suggest that it can occur after tuberculosis. In each case the organism can be found at the time of the initial attack but not thereafter. In herpes zoster the episclera and sometimes the underlying sclera become inflamed at the vesicular stage of the eruption and the inflammation disappears completely as the skin lesions scar up, only to return after a period of two months or sometimes less, with deep scleral inflammation underlying the site of the original lesion. The fact that no aetiological agent has been isolated does not mean that one does not exist because Silverstein (1968) has shown that in anterior uveitis the offending antigen may initiate the inflammation but only be present in the eye for a very short time.

He induced a uveitis by injecting soluble protein into the vitreous. The antigen diffuses very slowly and a spontaneous uveitis then appears about one week after the injection. The aqueous recovered contains lymphocytes, monocytes and plasma cells. The eye returns to a normal state histologically but scattered specifically sensitised lymphocytes remain in the uveal tract; thus, if there is exposure to the original antigen, the uveitis recurs. The uveitis recurs if the antigen is given subcutaneously or even by mouth; no other organs or the opposite eye are affected. This implies that the uveal tract can retain an immunological memory for an antigen within the prior experience of the host but which has not necessarily entered the eye. In this way, at a later date, systemic exposure to the second substance might recall that memory and result in an anterior uveitis. The identification of the initial aetiological agent would not therefore necessarily influence therapy. As these immune competent cells reside in the uveal tract adjacent to the sclera a similar mechanism could be invoked for scleral inflammation provided these cells could reach the source of antigenic stimulus.

To find out whether these cells could arise at such a site, a Shwartzman reaction was induced in the sclera by the injection of *Serratia marcescens* lipopolysaccharide (LPS) B-type into the scleral coat and 24 hours later the animal was challenged systemically with the same antigen. The inflammatory cells, polymorphs and lymphocytes migrated from the choroidal and episcleral circulation to the site of the original scleral injection within as little as half an hour of the systemic challenge, showing that inflammatory cells can readily pass through the scleral stroma in response to an appropriate stimulus (Figures 6.9, 6.10 and 6.11).

Silverstein has also shown, using lymphocytic choriomeningitis virus to induce uveitis, that the virus disappears in the immunologically intact animal after

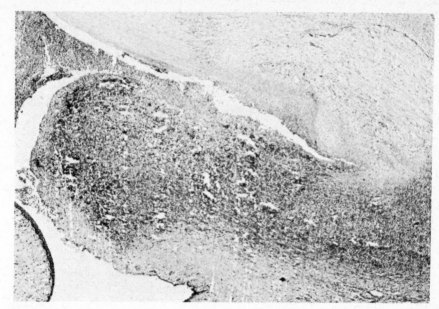

Figure 6.9. Shwartzman reaction in the sclera. Intense polymorphonuclear inflammatory reaction half an hour after systemic challenge with endotoxin of *Serratia marcescens* lipopolysaccharide (LPS) B-type and 24 hours after the local injection of the same antitoxin at this site. The control animals showed very little reaction.

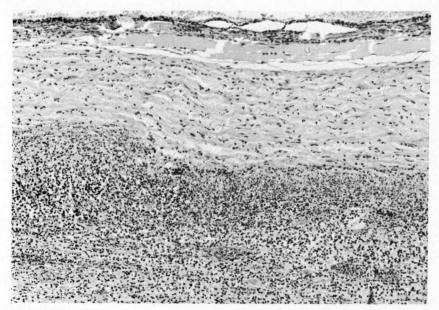

Figure 6.10. The intense polymorphonuclear response remote from the site of infection and related to both episcleral and choroidal vessels. The whole of the sclera is infiltrated with polymorphs half an hour after the systemic challenge.

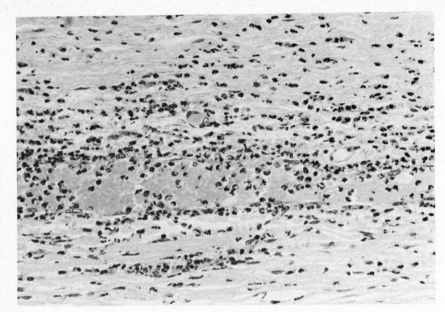

Figure 6.11.   Polymorphs migrating through a vessel in the deep sclera remote from the area of
infection half an hour after systemic challenge.

seven to eight days at the time that the uveitis appears. In scleritis it may
well be that the causative agent is dispersed or is neutralised early, as from
the local site of inflammation, but the tissue becomes marked in situ so that
further exposure to antigenic stimulus gives rise to further inflammation.

In episcleritis and the diffuse anterior and nodular scleritis which comes
and goes without loss of tissue, it is not possible to speculate any further.
Our knowledge of the changes found in the more severe forms of scleritis
and necrotising scleritis is helped by being able to study the histology of
the lesions produced. We are also able to draw some analogies from the
diseases with which these forms of scleritis are known to be associated. The
implications of the observations of the cellular components of the inflammatory
lesion have been discussed in detail. It will be recalled that clinically the
onset of necrotising disease in rheumatoid arthritis, at least, occurs at the
time when other extra-articular manifestations appear and in particular with
the onset of vasculitis. This is sometimes referred to as a change from a benign
to a malignant form of the disease. Necrotising scleritis occurs frequently
in severe vasculitis of other origins.

The inflammatory reaction in rheumatoid arthritis is associated with local
synthesis of antibody and rheumatoid factor. The synovium from morphologic
and functional evidence is seen to act as a lymphoid organ. The antibody
seems to be directed against a locally occurring antigen and to be unrelated
to the overall immune status of the host. In addition lymphokines such as
migration inhibition factor are produced in the rheumatoid synovium (Stastny,
Rosenthal and Andreis, 1973).

Complexes of IgG–IgG rheumatoid factor and IgG–IgM rheumatoid factor fix complement and are present in synovial tissue and fluid (Winchester, Agnello and Kunkel, 1969). The complement pathway is activated and this leads to the formation of chemotactic factors which attract the classic cell of inflammation, the polymorphonuclear leucocyte (Ruddy and Austen, 1973). After phagocytosis of these complexes the neutrophils discharge a variety of hydrolases from their lysosomal granules which are capable of destroying components of joint tissue. Some of these enzymes are capable of activating the complement pathway leading to a self-perpetuating process (Weissmann, 1972). It has been shown that complexes and products of complement activation play a part in the pathogenesis of tissue injury and inflammation in experimental models of arthritis (Cochrane and Koffler, 1973). Although it seems likely that a similar sequence of events occurs in scleral disease, particularly when it is associated with a vasculitis, it has yet to be proved.

The vasculitis leads to vascular occlusion, and indeed clinically areas of apparently avascular episclera are noted in the early stages of necrotising scleritis and what appears to be avascular sequestra occur late in scleromalacia perforans. Thrombosis, occlusion and microaneurysmal changes can all be seen and correlated with the abnormal vascular pattern seen clinically in intense diffuse and necrotising scleritis. The majority of scleral disease is also anterior to the equator which has the best vascular supply. In experimental scleritis induced using the Glynn model, the scleral perforation is related to the limbal vascular plexus, implying that there is indeed a vasculitis at that site (Figure 6.12). Inflammatory changes are necessary to induce necrosis because Sevel (1965) completely deprived the rabbit anterior segment of blood supply without any necrotic change taking place.

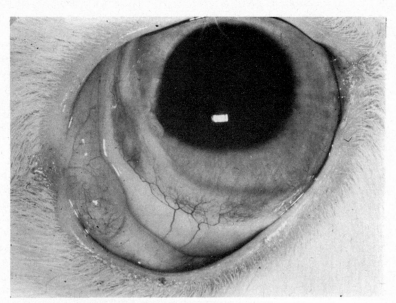

Figure 6.12.   Scleral perforation induced in a rabbit which had been previously sensitised with ovalbumin (Glynn) and then challenged by intrascleral injection. The perforation is at 90° from the site of the scleral injection.

Our present interpretation of these pathological changes is therefore that of a two-phase disease. Phase one results from some systemic infection, by an organism with a tendency to settle in joints or the eye, where it excites an inflammatory response largely as a result of a local immune response. With the elimination of the antigen it eventually subsides. Continuation of the disease activity is the result of the development of autoimmunisation to some antigen or antigens engendered by the initial inflammation itself. The well-known natural disease in pigs, which is due to infection with *Erysipelothrix insidiosa*, seems to follow precisely this pattern (Collins and Goldie, 1940). The products of inflammation lead to release of enzymes, and the degradation of proteoglycan and collagen has been shown to be associated with the extracellular release of proteolytic enzymes, some of which are of lysosomal origin. The process of degradation is thought to involve the combination of extracellular enzyme action and concurrent, or perhaps subsequent, endocytic activity and intracellular digestion.

REFERENCES

Agnello, V., Winchester, R. J. & Kunkel, H. G. (1970) Precipitin reactions of the C1q component of complement with aggregated gammaglobulin and immune complexes in gel diffusion. *Immunology*, **19**, 909–919.

Ajmal, M. (1971) Experimental Erysipelothrix arthritis. I. Observations on specific pathogen free and gnotobiotic pigs. II. Observations on rabbits. *Research in Veterinary Science*, **12**, 403–412.

Allansmith, M., Newman, L. & Whitney, C. (1971) Distribution of immunoglobulin in rabbit eyes. *Archives of Ophthalmology*, **86**, 60–64.

Allansmith, M. R., Whitney, C. R., McClellan, B. H. et al (1973) Immunoglobulins in the human eye. *Archives of Ophthalmology*, **89**, 36.

Alper, C. A., Colten, H. R., Rosen, F. S. et al (1972) Homozygous deficiency of C3 in a patient with repeated infections. *Lancet*, **ii**, 1179–1181.

Arkin, V. (1951) Necrosis sclerae as a post-operative complication. *Klinika Oczna*, **21**, 149–151.

Ashe, W. K., Daniels, C. A. & Scott, G. S. (1971) Interaction of rheumatoid factor with infectious herpes simplex virus antibody complexes. *Science*, **172**, 176–177.

Ashton, N. & Hobbs, H. E. (1952) Effect of cortisone on rheumatoid nodules of the sclera (scleromalacia perforans). *British Journal of Ophthalmology*, **36**, 373–384.

Barrett, A. J. (1975) In *Dynamics of Connective Tissue Macromolecules* (Ed.) Burleigh, P. M. & Poole, A. R. Ch. 10. Amsterdam: North Holland.

Bhan, A. K. & Roy, S. (1971) Synovial giant cells in rheumatoid arthritis and other joint diseases. *Annals of the Rheumatic Diseases*, **30**, 294–298.

Bonomo, L., Tursi, A., Trizio, D. et al (1970) Immune complexes in rheumatoid synovitis: a mixed staining immunofluorescence study. *Immunology*, **18**, 557–563.

Bordet, J. (1895) Les leucocytes et les proprietes actives du serum chez les vaccines. *Annales de l'Institut Pasteur*, **9**, 462–506.

Brandt, K. D., Cathcart, E. S. & Cohen, A. S. (1968) Studies of immune deposits in synovial membranes and corresponding synovial fluids. *Journal of Laboratory and Clinical Medicine*, **72**, 631–647.

Bray, M. A., Gordon, D., Morley, J. et al (1974) Role of prostaglandins in reactions of cellular immunity. *British Journal of Pharmacology*, **52**, 453P.

Brewerton, D. A., Hart, F. D., Nicholls, A. et al (1973) Ankylosing spondylitis and HL-A27. *Lancet*, **i**, 904–907.

Brown, J. C. & Epstein, W. V. (1969) Influence of human rheumatoid factor on numbers of antibody-producing cells. *Arthritis and Rheumatism*, **12**, 1–9.

Brown, S. I. (1975) Mooren's ulcer. *British Journal of Ophthalmology*, **59**, 675–682.

Castor, C. W. (1971) Connective tissue activation. I. The nature, specificity, measurement and distribution of connective tissue activating peptide. *Arthritis and Rheumatism*, **14**, 41–54.

Castor, C. W. (1972) Connective tissue activation. IV. Regulatory effects of anti-rheumatic drugs. *Arthritis and Rheumatism*, **15**, 504–514.

Cathcart, E. S. & O'Sullivan, J. B. (1969) A longitudinal study of rheumatoid factors in a New England town. *Annals of the New York Academy of Sciences*, **168**, 41–51.

Cochrane, C. G. & Koffler, D. (1973) Immune complex disease in experimental animals and man. *Advances in Immunology*, **16**, 185–264.

Collins, D. H. & Goldie, W. (1940) Observations on polyarthritis and on experimental erysipelothrix infection of swine. *Journal of Pathology and Bacteriology*, **50**, 323–353.

Cooke, T. D., Hurd, E. R., Ziff, M. et al (1972) The pathogenesis of chronic inflammation in experimental antigen-induced arthritis. II. Preferential localisation of antigen antibody complexes to collagenous tissues. *Journal of Experimental Medicine*, **135**, 323–338.

Dauphinee, M. J., Talal, N., Goldstein, A. et al (1974) Thymosis corrects the abnormal DNA synthetic response of NZB mouse thymocytes. *Proceedings of the National Academy of Sciences of the U.S.A.*, **71**, 2637–2641.

Dingle, J. T. (1973) The role of lysomal enzymes in skeletal tissues. *Journal of Bone and Joint Surgery*, **55**, 87–95.

Dingle, J. T. & Burleigh, M. C. (1974) Connective tissue and its changes in disease. *Transactions of the Ophthalmological Societies of the United Kingdom*, **94**, 696–711.

Dingle, J. T. & Page Thomas, D. P. (1956) In vitro studies on human synovial membrane. A metabolic comparison of normal and rheumatoid tissue. *British Journal of Experimental Pathology*, **37**, 318–323.

Dingle, J. T., Barrett, A. J. & Weston, P. D. (1971) Characteristics of immunoinhibition and the confirmation of a role in cartilage breakdown. *Biochemical Journal*, **123**, 1–13.

Dingle, J. T., Horsfield, P., Fell, H. et al (1975) Breakdown of proteoglycan and collagen induced in pig articular cartilage in organ culture. *Annals of the Rheumatic Diseases*, **34**, 303–311.

Dumonde, D. C. & Glynn, L. E. (1965) The reaction of guinea pigs to autologous and heterologous fibrin implants. *Journal of Pathology and Bacteriology*, **90**, 649–657.

Duthie, J. J., Stewart, S. M., Alexander, W. R. et al (1967) Isolation of diphtheroid organisms from rheumatoid synovial membrane and fluid. *Lancet*, **i**, 142–143.

Eisen, V. (1970) Plasma kinins in synovial exudates. *British Journal of Experimental Pathology*, **51**, 322–327.

Evanson, J. M., Jeffrey, J. J. & Krane, S. M. (1967) Human collagenase: identification and characterisation of an enzyme from rheumatoid synovium in culture. *Science*, **158**, 499–502.

Falchuk, K. H., Goetzl, E. J. & Kulka, J. P. (1970) Respiratory gases of synovial fluids. An approach to synovial tissue circulatory-metabolic imbalance in rheumatoid arthritis. *American Journal of Medicine*, **49**, 223–231.

Fell, H. B. & Barratt, M. E. (1973) The role of soft connective tissue in the breakdown of pig articular cartilage cultivated in the presence of complement sufficient anti-serum to pig erythrocytes. *International Archives of Allergy and Applied Immunology*, **44**, 441–468.

Ferreira, S. H. & Vane, J. R. (1973) Inhibition of prostaglandin biosynthesis: an explanation of the therapeutic effects of non-steroid anti-inflammatory agents. In *Seminar on Serum Prostaglandins*, pp. 345–357. Paris.

François, J. (1970) Ocular manifestations in collagenoses. *Advances in Ophthalmology*, **23**, 1–54.

Ghadially, F. N. & Roy, S. (1969) Ultrastructural changes in the synovial membrane in lipohaemarthrosis. *Annals of the Rheumatic Diseases*, **28**, 529–536.

Glynn, L. E. (1968) The chronicity of inflammation and its significance in rheumatoid arthritis. *Annals of the Rheumatic Diseases*, **27**, 105–121.

Glynn, L. E. (1972) Pathology, pathogenesis and aetiology of rheumatoid arthritis. *Annals of the Rheumatic Diseases*, **31**, 412–420.

Goetzl, E. J., Falchuk, K. H., Zeiger, L. S. et al (1971) A physiological approach to the assessment of disease activity in rheumatoid arthritis. *Journal of Clinical Investigation*, **50**, 1167–1180.

Good, R. A. & Rotstein, J. (1960) Rheumatoid arthritis and agammaglobulinemia. *Bulletin of the Rheumatic Diseases*, **10**, 203–206.

Grayzel, A. I. & Beck, C. (1972) Rubella infections of synovial cells and the resistance of cells derived from patients with rheumatoid arthritis. *Journal of Experimental Medicine*, **131**, 367–373.

Greenwood, B. M. (1968) Autoimmune disease and parasitic infections in Nigeria. *Lancet*, **ii**, 380–382.

Greenwood, B. M. & Herrick, E. M. (1970) Low incidence of rheumatoid factor and auto-antibodies in Nigerian patients with rheumatoid arthritis. *British Medical Journal*, **i**, 71–73.

Greenwood, B. M., Herrick, E. M. & Voller, A. (1970) Can parasitic infection suppress auto-immune disease? *Proceedings of the Royal Society of Medicine*, **63**, 19–20.

Gross, J. & Lapiere, C. M. (1962) Collagenolytic activity in amphibian tissue: a tissue culture assay. *Proceedings of the National Academy of Sciences of the U.S.A.*, **48**, 1014–1022.

Hamerman, D. (1969) Cartilage changes in the rheumatoid joint. *Clinical Orthopaedics*, **64**, 91–97.

Harkness, R. D. & Moralee, B. E. (1956) The time course and route of loss of collagen from the rat uterus during post-partum involution. *Journal of Physiology*, **132**, 502–508.

Harris, E. D. & Krane, S. M. (1974) Collagenases. *New England Journal of Medicine*, **291**, 557–563, 605–609, 652–661.

Harris, E. D., DiBona, D. R. & Krane, S. M. (1969) Collagenases in human synovial fluid. *Journal of Clinical Investigation*, **48**, 2104–2113.

Harris, E. D., DiBona, D. R. & Krane, S. M. (1970) A mechanism for cartilage destruction in rheumatoid arthritis. *Transactions of the Association of American Physicians*, **83**, 267–276.

Harris, E. D., Evanson, J. M., DiBona, D. R. et al (1970) Collagenase and rheumatoid arthritis. *Arthritis and Rheumatism*, **13**, 83–94.

Harris, E. D., Parker, H. G., Radin, E. L. et al (1972) Effects of proteolytic enzymes on structural and mechanical properties of cartilage. *Arthritis and Rheumatism*, **15**, 497–503.

Hedberg, H. (1967) Studies on synovial fluid in arthritis. *Acta Medica Scandinavica*, Supplement **479**.

Hedberg, H., Kallen, B., Low, B. et al (1971) Impaired mixed leucocyte reaction in some different diseases, notably multiple sclerosis and various arthritides. *Clinical and Experimental Immunology*, **9**, 201–207.

Herman, J. H., Bradley, J., Ziff, M. et al (1971) Response of the rheumatoid synovial membrane to exogenous immunization. *Journal of Clinical Investigation*, **50**, 266–273.

Hollister, J. R. & Mannik, M. (1974) Antigen retention in joint tissues in antigen induced synovitis. *Clinical and Experimental Immunology*, **16**, 615–627.

Jasin, H. E. & Ziff, M. (1969) Immunoglobulin and specific antibody synthesis in a chronic inflammatory focus: antigen induced synovitis. *Journal of Immunology*, **102**, 355–369.

Katz, D. H. & Benacerraf, B. (1972) The regulatory influence of activated T cells on B cell responses to antigen. *Advances in Immunology*, **15**, 1–94.

Kellgren, J. H., Ball, J., Fairbrother, R. W. et al (1958) Suppurative arthritis complicating rheumatoid arthritis. *British Medical Journal*, **i**, 1193–1200.

Kobayashi, I. & Ziff, M. (1973) Electron microscopic studies of lymphoid cells in the rheumatoid synovial membrane. *Arthritis and Rheumatism*, **16**, 471–486.

Koch, E. (1882) Die Aetiologie der Tuberkulose. *Klinische Wochenschrift*, **19**, 221–230.

Lawrence, J. S. (1970) Rheumatoid arthritis: nature or nurture? *Annals of the Rheumatic Diseases*, **29**, 357–379.

Leibovich, S. J. & Weiss, J. B. (1971) Failure of human rheumatoid synovial collagenase to degrade either normal or rheumatoid arthritic polymeric collagen. *Biochimica et Biophysica Acta*, **251**, 109–118.

Lewis, R. M., Andre-Schwartz, J., Harris, G. S. et al (1973) Canine systemic lupus erythematosus. Transmission of serologic abnormalities by cell free filtrates. *Journal of Clinical Investigation*, **52**, 1893–1907.

Lightfoot, R. W., Drusin, R. E., Christian, C. L. et al (1969) The interaction of soluble immune complexes with rheumatoid factors. *Annals of the New York Academy of Science*, **168**, 104–110.

MacLennan, I. C. M. & Loewi, G. (1970) The cytotoxic activity of mononuclear cells from joint fluid. *Clinical and Experimental Immunology*, **6**, 713–720.

McCormick, J. N., Day, J., Morris, C. J. et al (1969) The potentiating effect of rheumatoid arthritis serum in the immediate phase of nephrotoxic nephritis. *Clinical and Experimental Immunology*, **4**, 17–28.

Milgrom, F. & Witebsky, E. (1962) Autoantibodies and autoimmune diseases. *Journal of the American Medical Association*, **181**, 706–716.

Morley, J. (1974) Prostaglandins and lymphokines in arthritis. *Prostaglandins*, **8**, 315–326.

Muirden, K. D. (1970) Giant cells, cartilage and bone fragments within rheumatoid synovial membrane: clinicopathological correlations. *Australasian Annals of Medicine*, **19**, 105–110.

Munthe, E. & Natvig, J. B. (1972) Immunoglobulin classes, subclasses and complexes of IgG rheumatoid factor in rheumatoid plasma cells. *Clinical and Experimental Immunology*, **12**, 55–70.

Pearson, C. M. & Wood, F. D. (1964) Passive transfer of adjuvant arthritis by lymph nodes or spleen cells. *Journal of Experimental Medicine*, **120**, 547–560.

Pearson, C. M., Paulus, H. E. & Machlede, R. (1975) The role of the lymphocyte and its products in the propagation of joint disease. *Annals of the New York Academy of Sciences*, **256**, 150–168.

Phelps, P., Prockop, D. J. & McCarthy, D. J. (1966) Crystal induced inflammation in canine joints. III. Evidence against bradykinin as a mediator of inflammation. *Journal of Laboratory and Clinical Medicine*, **68**, 433–444.

Pineus, T., Blacklow, N. R., Grimley, P. M. et al (1970) Glomerular microtubules of systemic lupus erythematosus. *Lancet*, **ii**, 1058–1061.

Rowlands, D. M. & Daniele, R. P. (1975) Surface receptors in the immune response. *New England Journal of Medicine*, **293**, 26–32.

Ruddy, S. & Austen, K. F. (1973) Activation of the complement system in rheumatoid synovitis. *Federation Proceedings*, **32**, 134–137.

Sabin, A. B. (1967) Nature and source of mycoplasma in various tissue cultures. *Annals of the New York Academy of Sciences*, **143**, 628–634.

Sevel, D. (1966) *Necrogranulomatous Scleritis, a Clinical, Pathological and Experimental Study.* MD Thesis, University of London.

Sheldon, P. J., Papamichail, M. & Holborow, E. J. (1975) Studies on synovial fluid lymphocytes in rheumatoid arthritis. *Annals of the Rheumatic Diseases*, **33**, 509–514.

Silverstein, A. (1968) Allergic reaction of the eye. In *Clinical Aspects of Immunology* (Ed.) Gell, P. G. & Coombs, R. R. pp. 1160–1175. Philadelphia: Davis.

Smiley, J. D., Sacks, C. & Ziff, M. (1968) In vitro synthesis of immunoglobulin by rheumatoid synovial membrane. *Journal of Clinical Investigation*, **47**, 624–632.

Stastny, P., Rosenthal, M. & Andreis, M. (1973) Lymphokinins in the rheumatic joint. *Arthritis and Rheumatism*, **18**, 237–243.

Stewart, S. M., Alexander, W. R. & Duthie, J. J. (1969) Isolation of diphtheroid bacilli from synovial membrane and fluid in rheumatoid arthritis. *Annals of the Rheumatic Diseases*, **28**, 477–487.

Stockwell, R. A. (1974) Fine structure and macromolecular organisation of connective tissue. *Transactions of the Ophthalmological Societies of the United Kingdom*, **94**, 648–662.

Theofilopoulos, A. N., Burtonboy, G., LoSpalluto, J. et al (1974) IgM rheumatoid factor and low molecular weight IgM. An association with vasculitis. *Arthritis and Rheumatism*, **17**, 272–284.

Thomas, L. (1964) Circulating autoantibodies and human disease. *New England Journal of Medicine*, **270**, 1157–1159.

Torrigiani, G., Roitt, M., Lloyd, K. N. et al (1970) Elevated IgG antiglobulins in patients with seronegative rheumatoid arthritis. *Lancet*, **i**, 14–16.

Transplantation Review (1974) T and B cells in humans. *Transplantation Review*, no. **16**.

Tucker, A. D. & Wyatt, J. H. (1967) Possible dietary factors in the aetiology of chronic murine pneumonia, nephrosis and periarteritis. *Nature*, **215**, 976–978.

van Boxel, J. A. & Paget, S. A. (1975) Predominantly T-cell infiltrate in rheumatoid synovial membranes. *New England Journal of Medicine*, **293**, 517–520.

Vane, J. R. (1971) Inhibition of prostaglandin synthesis as a mechanism of action for aspirin-like drugs. *Nature, New Biology*, **231**, 232–235.

Weinsten, A., Peters, K., Brown, D. et al (1972) Metabolism of the third component of complement C3 in patients with rheumatoid arthritis. *Arthritis and Rheumatism*, **15**, 49–56.

Weissmann, G. (1972) Lysosomal mechanisms of tissue injury in arthritis. *New England Journal of Medicine*, **286**, 141–147.

Werb, Z. & Reynolds, J. T. (1975) Stimulation by endocytosis of the secretion of collagenase and neutral proteinase from rabbit synovial fibroblasts. *Journal of Experimental Medicine*, **140**, 1482–1497.

Williams, M. H. (1968) In *Rheumatic Diseases* (Ed.) Duthie, J. J. & Alexander, W. R. 171 pp. Pfizer Medical Monograph, 3, University of Edinburgh.

Williams, M. H., Brostoff, H. J. & Roitt, I. M. (1970) Possible role of Mycoplasma fermentans in pathogenesis of rheumatoid arthritis. *Lancet*, **ii**, 277–280.

Winchester, R. J., Agnello, V. & Kunkel, H. G. (1969) The joint fluid gamma G globular complexes and their relationship to intra-articular complement diminution. *Annals of the New York Academy of Sciences*, **168**, 195–203.

Zabriskie, J. B. (1967) Mimetic relationships between group A streptococci and mammalian tissue. *Advances in Immunology*, **7**, 147–188.

Ziff, M. (1973) Pathophysiology of rheumatoid arthritis. *Federation Proceedings*, **32**, 131–133.

CHAPTER SEVEN

Scleritis in Relation to Connective Tissue Disorders

'*Therefore the moon, the governess of the floods*
Pale in her anger, washes all the air
That rheumatic diseases do abound . . .'
Titania in *A Midsummer Night's Dream* (Shakespeare).

'No matter what form be present, while a certain number of cases are the result of syphilis or tubercle, by far the larger proportion are undoubtedly due to gouty or rheumatic predisposition' (Ramsay, 1909).

Perusal of Table 7.1 rather confirms this nineteenth century view of scleral disease. Although our definitions are somewhat different to theirs it is certainly true that scleritis is most frequently associated with those conditions now known as the connective tissue diseases.

Mackenzie (1830) wrote: 'Were it asked "what is meant by rheumatic ophthalmia?" I should reply that "I mean simply inflammation of the fibrous tissue of the eye (the sclerotica), and of the surrounding parts of similar structure, excited by exposure to cold" '. Whilst this is no longer believed, McGavin et al writing from the same city and institutions in 1976 have looked again in detail at the scleritis occurring in rheumatoid arthritis. One hundred and fifty years of observation in between these two reports confirms the strong and undoubted association between scleritis and the commonest form of connective tissue disease, rheumatoid arthritis. However, scleritis is rather less common in rheumatoid arthritis than in the other connective tissue diseases when the relative incidence of the various conditions is taken into consideration. It has unfortunately become a common habit in clinical practice to equate scleritis with rheumatoid arthritis. Whilst this is far from the truth, there are features of scleral disease which manifest themselves far more commonly in rheumatoid arthritis than in the others so this condition deserves particular attention.

A decade ago it was usual to support the school of 'lumpers' which considered rheumatoid arthritis to be a nonspecific syndrome that could be

206

Table 7.1. *Incidence of associated systemic diseases in episcleritis and scleritis*

Disease	Episcleritis		Scleritis				
	Simple	Nodular	DA[a]	NA[b]	Necrotising[c]	Scleromalacia perforans	Posterior
Rheumatoid arthritis	5	2	8	4	3	6	0
Ankylosing spondylitis	0	0	1	0	0	0	0
Psoriatic arteritis	0	0	0	3	0	0	0
Systemic lupus erythematosus	0	0	0	1	1	0	0
Periarteritis nodosa	0	0	0	0	2	0	0
Systemic vasculitis	0	0	1	0	1	0	0
Wegener's granulomatosis	0	0	0	0	1	0	0
Relapsing polychondritis	0	0	0	0	2	0	0
Rheumatic heart disease	2	1	1	1	0	0	0
Palendromic rheumatism	0	0	0	0	2	0	0
Associated with hypersensitivity disorders							
Erythema nodosum	0	0	0	2	0	0	0
Severe asthma or hay fever	0	0	2	0	0	0	0
Erythema multiforme	1	0	0	0	0	0	0
Schönlein–Henoch purpura	1	0	0	0	0	0	0
Penicillin sensitivity	2	0	0	0	0	0	0
Contact dermatitis following desensitisation vaccination	2	1	0	0	0	0	0
Rosacea	1	2	0	2	0	0	0
Associated with granulomatous conditions							
Tuberculosis: active	1	0	1	0	3	0	0
inactive	1	2	0	0	0	0	0
Syphilis	0	1	1	3	2	0	0
Associated with virus infection							
Herpes zoster	2	1	2	14	0	0	0
Herpes simplex	0	0	0	2	0	0	0
Associated with metabolic disorders							
Gout	6	5	2	3	0	0	0
Other associated conditions							
See footnote	1	0	10	7	1	0	0
Total	27	15	29	42	18	6	0

Footnote: in simple episcleritis one patient had regional ileitis.

[a] In diffuse anterior (DA) scleritis ten patients had other diseases, e.g. orbital granuloma (1), essential hypertension (3) followed irradiation to other eye (1), fragilitas ossium (1), thyrotoxicosis (1), degenerative osteoarthritis (2).

[b] In nodular anterior (NA) scleritis seven patients had other diseases, e.g. Cogan's syndrome (3), thyrotoxicosis (1), ophthalmia nodosa (1), thyrotoxicosis (1), hypertension (1).

[c] One patient with necrotising scleritis had hypertension as the only other systemic disease. There was no other evidence of a generalised systemic vasculitis.

precipitated by widely differing insults such as psoriasis, urethritis or ulcerative colitis. Indeed Reiter's disease, psoriatic arthritis and ankylosing spondylitis were considered atypical forms of rheumatoid arthritis.

Recently the trend has changed in favour of the school of 'splitters' and all so-called variants of classical rheumatoid arthritis in which rheumatoid factor cannot be detected are regarded as discrete entities. Although distinctive features exist for each disorder, considerable evidence has accumulated to support the concept that any of the variant disorders may in time evolve into one of the other syndromes. The discovery that over 90 per cent of patients with ankylosing spondylitis carry HLA-B27 has lent new emphasis to the concept of spondyloarthroses, as have the numerous family studies. These indicate overlap in the arthropathies associated with psoriasis, ulcerative colitis and regional enteritis as well as the close correlation of sacroiliitis with HLA-B27 in these conditions, in Reiter's syndrome and in other reactive arthropathies. The rarer rheumatic disorders which include systemic lupus erythematosus, polymyositis and scleroderma can all be separated from one another, although in practice overlapping features can occur. Finally there is a group of clinical syndromes which is characterised by segmental inflammation of blood vessels. The common property showed by most of the diseases and syndromes is that of involvement of joints and/or para-articular structures.

In the connective tissue diseases listed below there is scleral involvement:

1. Seropositive conditions:
   Rheumatoid arthritis
   Rheumatoid arthritis of juvenile onset
   Systemic lupus erythematosus

2. Seronegative conditions:
   Ankylosing spondylitis — adult, juvenile
   Psoriatic arthritis
   Reiter's disease
   Ulcerative colitis
   Crohn's disease
   Behçet's syndrome

3. Vasculitis:
   Classical polyarteritis nodosa
   Hypersensitivity angiitis
   Allergic granulomatous angiitis including Wegener's granulomatosis
   Giant cell arteritis and polymyalgia rheumatica
   Vasculitis associated with other connective tissue diseases

4. Other connective tissue diseases:
   Erythema nodosum
   Relapsing polychondritis
   Sarcoidosis
   Amyloidosis

Scleral disease has not been described in dermatomyositis, polymyositis and scleroderma (progressive systemic sclerosis) which are commonly grouped with these conditions.

SEROPOSITIVE CONDITIONS

Rheumatoid Arthritis

Rheumatoid arthritis is a generalised or systemic chronic inflammatory condition of unknown aetiology whose distinctive features involve the musculoskeletal system with persistent and symmetrical peripheral inflammatory arthritis. Its diagnosis is made certain by sufficient destructive multisystem features and, equally important, by the absence of the many independent causes of arthritis. Rheumatoid arthritis remains the major entity against which other forms of arthritis are compared because it is the most common (two to three per cent of the population) and the most disabling of the inflammatory arthritides. There is a female predominance of three to one and 70 per cent of cases begin between the ages of 25 and 54. There is an even distribution of the disease in most tropical countries showing that climate has little effect on prevalence; the prevalence of clinical symptoms is, however, higher in cold damp areas.

Clinical features

Characteristically, the onset of rheumatoid arthritis is insidious and many patients complain of ill-defined symptoms which may precede arthritis for weeks. Fatigue, diffuse pains and loss of appetite are the most prominent features, but loss of weight may be noticeable. These symptoms may be followed by the slow onset of polyarticular stiffness, pain and swelling involving the interphalangeal joints of the fingers, the wrists and the metatarsophalangeal joints of the fingers, and subsequently shoulders, knees, ankles, elbows and other joints.

At the other extreme, in about 15 per cent of patients there may be an acute onset of systemic or articular illness. In a few involvement of a single joint may occur, the disease remaining localised to that joint and spreading very slowly. Tendon lesions may be a presenting feature and an episodic or palindromic presentation is well recognised.

Much has been written about predisposing factors occurring at the onset of rheumatoid arthritis: acute infections, emotional loss and hopelessness have all been discussed as potential triggers. Despite this, there is no convincing evidence that any precipitating factor is important in the development of rheumatoid arthritis.

Joint involvement

Patients complain of pain, stiffness and loss of function in the involved joints. In few diseases do patients suffer such unremitting debilitating pain. Morning stiffness is a characteristic feature; the patient feels incapable of moving in the early morning hours. This symptom is the hallmark of inflammatory activity and also a valuable semiquantitative measure of the activity of the inflammatory process. In addition, after periods of relative inactivity the joints often become stiff, a phenomenon known as 'gelling'. These symptoms may be related to fluid retention in the peri-articular tissues.

In the early stages of rheumatoid arthritis, the inflammatory changes may not be localised to the joints. Tender swelling of the entire hands or forearms, or swollen feet and ankles may be the earliest findings. As joint destruction progresses, the anatomical changes themselves produce increasing functional disability.

All joints can be affected—the large (knees, hips, shoulders) and the small (proximal interphalangeal, metacarpal phalangeal, wrists, ankles and feet). The distinctive features of rheumatoid arthritis are the symmetry, the prominent signs of inflammation and, to a lesser degree, the location. The most commonly affected joints (with decreasing frequency) seem to be proximal interphalangeal (see Figure 3.24), metacarpophalangeal (see Figure 3.23), wrists, knees (see Figure 3.19), ankles and metatarsophalangeal joints.

Hands and wrists

The typical patient shows fusiform inflammatory swellings, often with a dusky cyanosis over the inflamed joints. Later there may be marked synovial hypertrophy on the dorsum of the wrist with involvement of the extensor tendon sheath, which may cause rupture of the tendons. In the palmar aspect of the wrist synovial hypertrophy may lead to the carpal tunnel syndrome. The ulnar head may be prominent and extremely tender. Early synovial swelling of the wrist is highly characteristic and is a valuable sign in distinguishing inflammatory from degenerative disease.

Wasting of the dorsal interosseous muscles is often marked and rheumatoid arthritis is the most common cause of wasting of the small muscles of the hand.

Synovial infiltration of flexor tendon sheaths often causes a trigger finger. Palmar erythema is often present. Mild vasomotor disturbances are common in rheumatoid arthritis. Typical Raynaud's phenomenon may occur, but if severe in the presence of mild arthritis then one should reconsider the diagnosis of scleroderma.

Progressive joint destruction by erosive changes leads not only to limitation of movement, but in certain joints to subluxation. This arises from persistent stretching of the joint capsule by effusion and from ligamentous laxity.

Deformity of the hands comprises ulnar deviation of the fingers, the button-hole or boutonnière deformity and the swan-neck deformity (see Figure 3.24). Involvement of the distal interphalangeal joint is rare. Anterior subluxation of the wrist may occur.

Knee joint

Involvement of the knee joint accounts for a great deal of disability. Synovial hypertrophy and effusion are often marked, and the bursae in the popliteal fossa may be swollen and may communicate with the joint cavity. These enlarged bursae are called Baker's cysts. Quadriceps wasting is often marked, even in the early stages of the disease. Flexion contractures may develop and these are especially important because of the obvious disability that they produce. Both the cruciate and lateral ligaments may be destroyed, resulting in gross joint instability and valgus or varus deformity.

Rupture of the joint or of a Baker's cyst, as a consequence of the high intra-articular pressure developed during exercise, causes acute pain in the knee radiating into the calf which becomes swollen and tender on pressure. This often leads to a misdiagnosis of deep venous thrombosis, but an arthrogram will demonstrate the lesion.

Cervical spine

The upper cervical discs are frequently involved, in contrast to lower cervical involvement in osteoarthrosis. The cervical vertebrae may become subluxed and this may cause serious neurological involvement.

The atlantoaxial articulations and their associated ligaments are frequently involved. This is detected by taking lateral radiographs in both flexion and extension, where separation between the odontoid process and the first cervical vertebra exceeds the normal 2 to 3 mm. Patients with this involvement often complain of pain radiating along the distribution of the first and second cervical nerves. Pain commences in the cervical spine and radiates upwards over the occiput and vertex to the forehead. Symptomatic relief may be found with a well fitting cervical collar.

Atlantoaxial dislocation may cause vertebrobasilar insufficiency or may produce neurological signs by direct pressure on the cord. However, neurological sequelae are fortunately less common than might be expected. As this condition is present in 25 per cent of patients requiring reconstructive surgery, it is important that anaesthetists are aware of this potentially fatal lesion.

Involvement of other joints

Pain in the forefoot is commonly due to downward metatarsal head subluxation. The patient complains of a feeling of 'walking on pebbles' and the metatarsal heads are readily palpable on the sole of the foot. The most common deformities are subluxation of the metatarsophalangeal joints with the toes displaced upwards, together with fixed flexion deformities of the interphalangeal joints.

The hip joint is less commonly involved than the knee or metatarsophalangeal joints, but when it occurs it carries with it serious disability. The femoral head may penetrate the acetabulum (protrusio acetabuli) and the femoral head may collapse. This is often referred to as aseptic necrosis and is commoner in corticosteroid-treated patients.

Extra-articular manifestations

Articular symptoms and signs may be sufficiently impressive and disabling to distract one from the realisation that rheumatoid arthritis is a systemic disease. It is important to look for systemic features of rheumatoid arthritis (Table 7.2) for two reasons:

1. Signs of systemic involvement occur in the most active patients and warrant a more aggressive therapeutic approach.
2. Systemic features make the likelihood of early death from rheumatoid arthritis several times that of the patient with non-articular rheumatoid arthritis.

Scleral involvement in rheumatoid arthritis is an extra-articular manifestation of the disease with the same sinister significance and the same necessity for vigorous treatment. The types of scleral change vary with the stage and virulence of the other systemic changes so that a great deal can be learned from careful observation of the scleral signs.

Table 7.2.　*Extra-articular manifestations of rheumatoid arthritis*

Systemic changes	Frequency of complication
Rheumatoid nodules	Common
Systemic vasculitis	Uncommon
Ocular manifestations	
(a) Keratoconjunctivitis sicca	Very common
Keratitis: marginal ulceration marginal thinning	Common
sclerosing keratolysis	Rare
(b) Scleritis: diffuse anterior	Common
nodular anterior	Uncommon
necrotising anterior	In severe systemic disease
scleromalacia perforans	In long-standing disease
posterior	Uncommon
(c) Episcleritis: diffuse	Uncommon
nodular	
(d) Uveitis	Rare
Respiratory changes	Uncommon
Cardiac disease	Uncommon
Lymph nodes and spleen	Uncommon
Amyloidosis	Common

The subcutaneous rheumatoid nodule and the rheumatoid nodule of the eye

The nodule occurs in approximately 25 per cent of patients at some time in the course of their disease. It is the only feature that by itself is pathognomonic of rheumatoid arthritis. It is found characteristically lying in the subcutaneous tissue along the extensor surface of the forearms, but may also be found over other bony protuberances or related to tendons (see Figure 3.20).

Apart from the cosmetic effects and the inconvenience of these firm swellings on pressure areas or on fingers, the two main disabilities produced are ulceration of the overlying skin and pain when the nodules overlie the ischial tuberosities.

There is seldom any difficulty in the diagnosis of rheumatoid nodules, although at the elbow the nodules of rheumatic fever, gouty tophi, granuloma annulare, xanthomas and reticulohistiocytosis may occasionally cause confusion. They sometimes develop before clinical signs of rheumatoid arthritis appear but only in patients who are seropositive. Rarely (Lowney and Simons, 1963) nodules indistinguishable from those of rheumatoid arthritis develop in patients who never develop the disease. Their size varies from time to time in any one patient, and they may completely disappear only to return later. There is no unique significance in subcutaneous nodules as they are the same as nodules found elsewhere. It is their accessibility to physical examination which makes them clinically important. Although they most commonly appear insidiously near body surfaces exposed frequently to pressure or stress, they are not confined to these zones, for example they appear in the lung tissue, pleura, heart and sclera.

The clinical association between inflammatory scleral disease and rheumatoid arthritis is undoubted and the direct histopathological similarities between those changes found in the joint and subcutaneous nodules are remarkable and well documented (van der Hoeve, 1931; Eber, 1934; Kiehle, 1937; Soriano and Riva, 1937; Urrets Zavalia, Maldonado Allende and Obregon Oliva, 1937; Oast, 1938; Verhoeff and King, 1938; Smoleroff, 1943; Franceschetti and Bischler, 1950; Christensen, 1951; Fienberg and Colpoys, 1951; François, 1951; Mundy et al, 1951; Stillermann, 1951; Swan, 1951; Ashton and Hobbs, 1952; Petrohelos and Wolter, 1956; Wolter and Bentley, 1961; Victoria and Fanjul, 1963; Ferry, 1969; François, 1970).

Klinge (1930), Clawson and Wetherby (1932), Dawson (1933) and Collins (1937) studied the subcutaneous rheumatoid nodule in detail and Fienberg and Colpoys (1951) were able to observe the changes which occurred in these nodules as a result of treatment with steroids. The changes which occur in both the rheumatoid nodule and the sclera are of an avascular central necrotic area consisting of a dense network of fibrin, partly digested mature collagen and fragments of cells and nuclear debris surrounded by the cellular proliferation of lymphocytes and plasma cells, dilated capillaries and small blood vessels with swollen endothelia. Multinucleated giant cells can sometimes be found in the histolytic zone or in the surrounding connective tissue.

Characteristically in the rheumatoid nodule are found elongated cells resembling fibroblasts or a palisade layer of histiocytes around the necrotic centre of the nodule (Bennett, Zeller and Bauer, 1940), orientated so that their long axis is perpendicular to the centre of the nodule. Fienberg and Colpoys (1951) felt that the precision of this orientation depended on the activity of the disease process. When the disease is very active the orientation of the cells is very precise, but under the influence of treatment or natural resolution the palisading becomes much less obvious and the cells tend to aggregate to form giant cells. Electron microscopy studies show that the marginal palisade cells of the nodule are at least initially of phagocytic rather than of fibroblastic (secretory) character. As resolution progresses the palisaded cells increase the volume of their cytoplasm and probably begin to lay down fibrous tissue which eventually resolves into a scar.

The necrotic centre of the rheumatoid nodule is interpreted variously as:
1. A result of local ischaemia, due to nearby arterial disease (Sokoloff, 1963).

2. As a reaction to chemical toxins or infectious agents.
3. As a focus in connective tissue of the cytotoxic consequences of an antigen—antibody interaction.

Careful dissection, it is claimed, shows a constant relationship to a diseased artery (Sokoloff, McClusky and Bunim, 1953). Coarse amorphous masses have been seen and are believed, from the evidence of Zucker-Franklin (1968), to be antigen—antibody complexes. This observation suggests that the nodule, like the other lesions of rheumatoid arthritis, may be the result of a direct immunological injury to collagen (Klemperer, Pollack and Baehr, 1942). The possibility that the local accumulation of antigen—antibody complexes can be responsible for granuloma formation is substantiated by recent experimental work (Spector and Heesom, 1969).

A neutral protease and a collagenase similar to the rheumatoid synovial enzymes have been isolated from primary cultures of rheumatoid nodules (Harris, 1972). It was suggested that the collagenolytic enzyme system might contribute to the central necrosis of these nodules by destroying the extracellular matrix to such an extent that cells could not survive.

Attempts have been made to provoke nodule formation in the skin of patients with rheumatoid arthritis and in animals by the injection of insoluble material such as bentonite or fibrin. The reactions are not specific and are not related to rheumatoid arthritis.

Immunofluorescent studies have shown that the exudation and tissue destruction are likely to be the result of interactions between rheumatoid factor as antibody and IgG immunoglobulin as autoantigen (Nowoslawski and Brzosko, 1967). The central necrotic areas contain much IgG in the form of IgG—IgM complex. IgG immunoglobulin occurs as granules and as bumpy deposits filling the distended spaces between collagen fibres.

Studies of the blood vessel walls in or around the nodules have demonstrated fibrin deposition and IgG immunoglobulin. Some blood vessels were occluded by large, bumpy precipitates of globulin and of fibrin or fibrinogen.

The vascular changes, although present, do not form a permanent feature of the clinical picture unless a systemic vasculitis has been present clinically. Similarly there is nothing in the clinical picture to distinguish a rheumatoid nodule of the sclera from scleritis due to other causes. Those patients whose eyes have been examined histologically have all had some necrotising scleritis with or without inflammation (scleromalacia perforans) but these are naturally those patients who have had the most severe disease.

Rheumatoid vasculitis and the effect on the eye

Arteritis occurs in rheumatoid disease. This may conveniently be considered in three categories:

1. Involvement of small end arteries like the anterior ciliary arteries and those in the nail folds, obstruction of which produces characteristic minute ischaemic areas. Whilst these changes are usually of no significance in the nail bed (Figure 7.1), they are of great significance in the eye.

2. Involvement of small and medium-sized arteries such as the vasa nervosum and digital arteries.
3. Involvement of large arterial trunks, e.g. mesenteric or major limb vessels leading to peripheral gangrene, mesenteric occlusion or cerebrovascular accident.

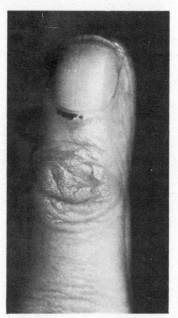

Figure 7.1.   Nail-fold lesions. There is necrosis of the base of the nail which is typical of the endarteritis in rheumatoid arthritis.

The larger the vessel affected, the more severe is the pattern of arteritis. Thus the nail-fold lesions result from bland intimal hyperplasia, but when the medium-sized arteries are involved there is a much more active process with fragmentation of the elastic lamina and cellular infiltration. These destructive changes, which lead to gross necrosis of the arterial wall, can be so severe that they are indistinguishable from polyarteritis nodosa.

Arterial involvement occurs only in the strongly seropositive patient. The eye and nail-fold lesions are often the first warning that the disease is assuming a more sinister character. Occlusion of medium-sized arteries produces necrotic skin lesions and ulceration, usually of the legs, which are not confined to the usual sites for varicose lesions but look like arterial rather than venous lesions, being sharply outlined and punched out (Figure 7.2).

Approximately 25 per cent of patients with rheumatoid arthritis have been found to have vasculitis on postmortem examination (Cruickshank, 1954). However, it is not always the cause of death. The vasculitis found during the normal course of the disease is not confined to joints but involves all veins and arteries and may be widespread, but unlike classical polyarteritis nodosa, it spares the kidneys and only rarely causes hypertension. Williamson (1974) and McGavin et al (1976), comparing 4210 age and sex-matched patients

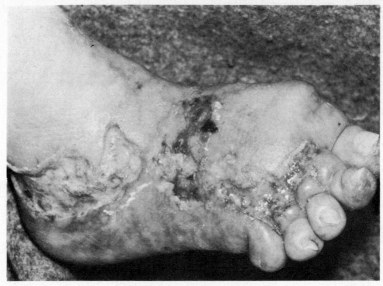

Figure 7.2.   Vasculitis of the skin of the foot in rheumatoid arthritis. This is unlike a varicose
ulcer because of the distribution and the punched-out lesions.

with rheumatoid arthritis found a high proportion of severe erosive seropositive
arthritis, extensive vasculitis and a high mortality in those patients whose
rheumatoid arthritis was complicated by scleritis. This supported the observations of Jayson and Jones (1971) who studied a group of severely ill patients
with arthritis and found that arteritis was present in 10 out of the 16 patients
studied and the mortality in this group of patients was 36 per cent. When
this is compared with the patients seen at Moorfields Eye Hospital, London,
with necrotising scleral disease, it is seen that the 27 per cent mortality rate
is very much the same. Because necrotising scleritis can be the first indication
of a systemic vasculitis, it is of considerable importance to distinguish this
condition as early as possible so that vigorous sytemic treatment can be
undertaken.

Ocular involvement

Keratoconjunctivitis sicca. Keratoconjunctivitis sicca is but one part of a
generalised condition in which there is decreased secretion of the lacrimal,
salivary and mucosal glands of the upper air passages and the vulva. The
lacrimal gland and parotid gland are sometimes enlarged and there may be
an enlargement and associated hypofunction of the thyroid and ovaries,
Hashimoto's thyroiditis, liver and renal disease.

It was von Grosz in 1936 who suggested that the triad of dry eyes, dry
mouth and peripheral arthropathy should be called Sjögren's syndrome, even
though it was described independently by Gougerot in 1926, Mulock-Houwer

in 1927 and Sjögren in 1933. In patients with rheumatoid arthritis between 11 per cent (Williamson, 1974) and 35 per cent (Lackington, Charlin and Gormas, 1951) have been found to have keratoconjunctivitis sicca. The sicca syndrome, which is commonest in middle-aged women, may occur alone or with other connective tissue disorders (Bloch et al, 1965). In Sjögren's syndrome, whether this is accompanied by rheumatoid arthritis or not, the lacrimal gland, salivary and other mucosal glands undergo progressive atrophy and destruction of the secretory epithelium accompanied by a massive infiltration with lymphocytes and plasma cells. The duct epithelium becomes hyperplastic, leading to formation of the characteristic Morgan–Castleman myoepithelial islands (Morgan and Castleman, 1953). These changes result in a reduction of the watery contribution of the tears and the production of an abnormal mucus secretion. Early in the disease lysosome in the tears is reduced and the IgG level in the serum is increased. These findings may be helpful if the diagnosis is in doubt in the very early stages. Later in the disease the gland may become fibrosed with little inflammatory infiltrate remaining.

An antibody to salivary duct cytoplasm has been demonstrated by immuno-fluorescent techniques in 26 per cent of patients with uncomplicated rheumatoid arthritis and in an even higher percentage of patients with Sjögren's syndrome (Feltkamp and van Rossum, 1968). This latter group also has a higher incidence of autoantibodies to gastric parietal cells (Buchanan, Cox and Harden, 1966) and thyroglobulin (Bloch and Bunim, 1963). The evidence supporting an associa-tion between thyroiditis, pernicious anaemia and Sjögren's syndrome is incon-clusive. However, Sjögren's syndrome ranks second only to systemic lupus erythematosus in its abundance of serum autoantibodies, both organ-specific and non-organ-specific. Hypergammaglobulinaemia, usually polyclonal, is almost the rule in this disease. Depending on the method used 75 to 100 per cent of patients can be shown to have rheumatoid factor in their sera, even in the absence of rheumatoid arthritis (Bloch et al, 1965). Antinuclear antibodies are found in roughly two-thirds of patients with Sjögren's syndrome, a speckled or nucleolar pattern being common (Beck et al, 1962).

A patient with keratoconjunctivitis sicca complains of progressive discomfort in the eyes with a sensation of constant pricking and occasionally soreness and she may say that she is unable to cry or that the eyes do not water when she peels onions. As the disease progresses it becomes more and more painful to close the lids so that the rate of blinking is significantly decreased. These symptoms are very much worse in the morning because of the drying of the tears which occurs during the night. The precorneal film when viewed on the slit lamp is obviously abnormal in that it does not cover the corneal surface evenly. If the lids are held open patches of drying can be seen on the cornea because the tears do not flow evenly across its surface. Viscous, thick, tenacious strings of mucus can be seen to pass across the surface of the cornea, and to settle in the lower conjunctival fornix where they remain until they are picked out. These strands of mucus may adhere to the corneal epithelium, stripping it off in a characteristic whirl shape which was first described by Leber in 1882. This accounts for the considerable pain experienced, because each time the patient blinks the lids the epithelium is stripped further from the cornea, giving a feeling that a foreign body is present. Gross examination of the cornea reveals multiple small filaments which can easily be seen because they distort the light reflection of the anterior corneal surface. If there is any doubt the abnormal mucus and damaged epithelium can be easily demonstrated by placing a drop of one per cent Bengal rose in the conjunctival sac. This dye stains epithelium which has become keratinised. Keratinisation of the corneal and conjunctival epithelium only occurs if the tears are abnormal or if the epithelium has been permanently altered by chemical injury or disease. In keratoconjunctivitis sicca, there is a characteristic punctate staining of both the cornea and the bulbar conjunctiva (Figure 7.3). The Bengal rose

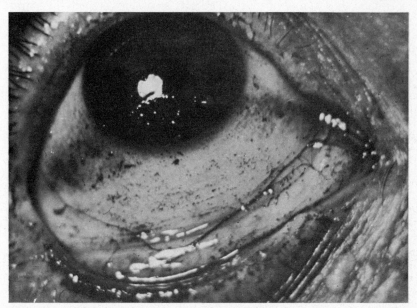

Figure 7.3. Fine punctate staining of both cornea and conjunctiva with Bengal rose found in the earliest stages of keratoconjunctivitis sicca. Note the abnormal mucous adhering to both cornea and conjunctiva.

solution does not cause undue discomfort when it is first applied to the conjunctival sac but after 30 seconds or so produces intense pain which may persist for many minutes—a diagnostic feature of considerable importance. Because of the severe discomfort it causes, once the diagnosis of keratoconjunctivitis sicca has been made, Bengal rose should not be applied again.

Schirmer's test to measure the flow of tears by measuring the rate of absorption of tears into filter papers placed in the conjunctival sac is frequently used as an aid to diagnosis.

SCHIRMER'S TEST

Filter paper strips are made 5 mm wide and about 5 cm long. One end is bent like a stamp hinge and is placed in the conjunctival sac. The strips are left in place for five minutes, after which time the amount of tears absorbed onto the filter paper is measured (minimum value 5 mm; normal value usually between 20 and 15 mm). If the amount in the filter paper is less than 5 mm, then with the strips still in place, a nasal swab is rubbed round the back of the nose. This should increase the flow by at least 10 mm.

However, Sjögren's syndrome may be present even with a normal amount of tears; indeed, in the early stages of keratoconjunctivitis sicca there is often an increase in the amount of watery secretion, so that keratoconjunctivitis sicca may thus still be present in spite of a normal Schirmer's test. We find Bengal rose staining to be a more reliable indicator of the sicca syndrome. If the diagnosis is still in doubt following the use of Bengal rose and Schirmer's test, then it is possible to:

1. Biopsy minor salivary glands to show the characteristic histology and avoid biopsy of the lacrimal gland (Bloch et al, 1965).
2. Measure salivary flow to show impairment of secretion; parotid gland saliva is usually collected (Lenoch et al, 1964).
3. Use radiotechnetium scanning; there is diminished uptake by the salivary glands in Sjögren's syndrome (Stephen et al, 1971).

Fortunately, corneal complications other than filamentary keratitis are uncommon in keratoconjunctivitis sicca because of the protection afforded by the oily secretion of the lids which prevents evaporation of the tears. However, the cornea can ulcerate, the ulcers being central in the interpalpebral region with a slushy necrotic centre. Gradually they become deeper and they may eventually completely destroy the corneal stroma, producing a descemetocele.

Intraocular infections are common in keratoconjunctivitis sicca, particularly with staphylococci, and it is possible that this is partly due to a reduction in tear lysozyme. Thus antibiotic cover for intraocular surgery must always be given in patients with keratoconjunctivitis sicca.

Apart from the eye symptoms, soreness and dryness of the throat are common in patients with Sjögren's syndrome, and dysphagia may occur. Those with severe dysphagia may have postcricoid narrowing similar to that seen in the Paterson–Brown–Kelly syndrome (Doig et al, 1971). Dysphagia in patients with Sjögren's syndrome should be taken seriously because post-cricoid webs may be premalignant, as they are in sideropenic cases. Patients with Sjögren's syndrome also have an unduly high prevalence of lymphoma, pseudo-lymphoma and Waldenström's macroglobulinaemia (Talal and Bunim, 1964).

Many forms of treatment are available for the 'dry eye' and often the simplest succeed. Treatment involves replacement or conservation of tears, control of excess mucus and eradication of secondary bacterial or viral infection. Hypromellose drops are useful as a replacement for tears and may be used as frequently as necessary. The mucolytic N L-acetyl cysteine is painful to use, less satisfactory, but may succeed in controlling excess mucus production if this is the major feature of the condition. If these measures do not produce relief of symptoms, it may be necessary to prevent tear drainage by blocking the lower punctum and canaliculus by cautery. A temporary block should be created first using gelatine rods to ensure that excessive watering will not result from permanent occlusion of the puncta. Treatment of keratoconjunctivitis sicca does not influence the progress of scleritis in the same eye, nor does the presence of one condition seem to have an influence on the other.

Scleral and episcleral changes. Depending on the severity of the illness and the type of hospital in which the survey was undertaken, the estimates of the incidence of scleritis in patients with rheumatoid arthritis vary from 0.15 to 6.3 per cent (Jayson and Jones, 1971). The largest series of 4210 patients by McGavin et al (1976) gives an incidence of 0.67 per cent. Conversely the incidence of rheumatoid arthritis in patients presenting in eye departments with scleritis is about 30 per cent and with episcleritis is five per cent. These figures are similar in all the published series. There is nothing in the clinical features of the episcleritis or scleritis by which the underlying rheumatoid disease can be distinguished and certainly nothing which could justify the phrase 'rheumatoid scleritis' or the rheumatic nodular scleritis described as a separate entity by Duke Elder and Leigh (1965) (Figure 7.4).

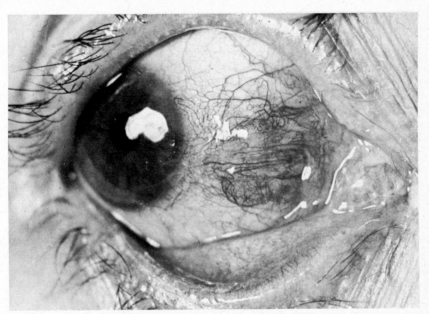

Figure 7.4.   Nodular episcleritis in a patient with rheumatoid arthritis. There is no detectable difference between the episcleral inflammation seen here and that detected in any other cause of nodular episcleritis.

Although McGavin et al's (1976) patients only had simple episcleritis, episcleral nodules certainly occur in rheumatoid arthritis, but they do not differ in any obvious way to the nodular episcleritis occurring in any other condition. Edström and Osterlind (1951) have described the histology of this condition which is typical of the rheumatoid nodule in the episclera. The nodule seen in episcleritis associated with rheumatoid arthritis is usually solitary and tends to recur in the same site. These nodules have been said to extend to involve the sclera. We have only seen this once (Figures 7.4 and 7.5). What happened in another of our patients was that a nodular episcleritis recurred on several occasions but the nodule remained within the episclera throughout the course of the disease and the patient developed a necrotising scleritis in another part of the globe. This we had taken to be an indication

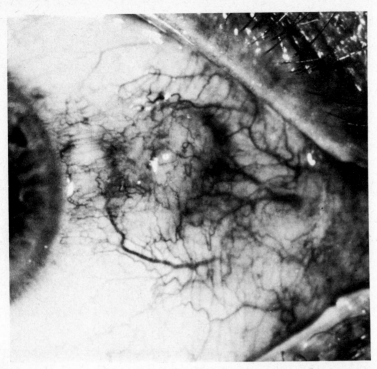

Figure 7.5. The same patient as Figure 7.4 two years later. The nodule on this occasion has involved the sclera. This coincided with a marked deterioration in the rheumatoid arthritis. The transformation from episcleritis to scleritis is an extremely rare occurrence and usually coincides with the onset of vasculitis.

that the inflammation only occurs at the site of antigen–antibody deposition at a previously sensitised site.

The commonest presentation of scleral disease in rheumatoid arthritis is of a patient who has only recently been diagnosed or who has no other overt signs of rheumatoid arthritis. He presents with a diffuse or less often a nodular anterior scleritis which does not differ in any way from that found in other conditions, either in clinical presentation or in its course of recurrences which may or may not need treating over many years. In certain of these patients and in other patients in whom it occurs de novo, a change occurs in the character of the scleritis which indicates that it is moving from a simple, relatively benign anterior scleritis or nodular scleritis to a necrotising disease. This change is usually heralded by an increase in the amount of pain with the attack and observation of the vascular pattern reveals that bypass channels are being formed round certain areas of the scleral tissue which have become relatively avascular. This avascular patch, which will sometimes be obvious during the first attack, is a very important physical sign indicative of an early necrotising scleral disease (Figure 7.6). Once the character of the scleritis has changed, the disease becomes progressive and destructive, involving not only the sclera but also the cornea, uveal tract

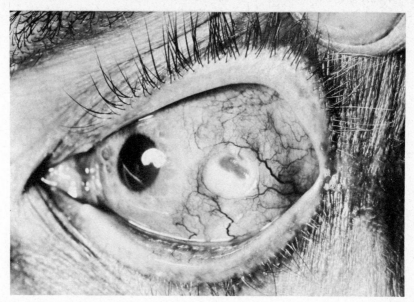

Figure 7.6. Necrotising nodular scleritis in rheumatoid arthritis which again coincided with the onset of vasculitis.

and sometimes the posterior segment. The necrotising lesions of the anterior segment consist of a relatively avascular central area with a markedly inflamed peripheral zone which is also very oedematous, presumably the site of the pannus of new vessels. The episcleral tissue overlying it is also very inflamed. The granulomatous change then begins to reach circumferentially around the globe and, depending on the severity of the inflammation either the collagen disintegrates, leaving a scleral defect, or fibrosis occurs, leaving a thin translucent sclera behind the advancing edge of the inflammation (Figure 7.7).

A systemic vasculitis or other extra-articular manifestation of rheumatoid arthritis can almost always be found in these patients. Treatment is urgent because if uveitis and glaucoma are allowed to develop the chances of saving the eye or eyesight are very slim.

In certain patients, almost all of whom are female and have severe, very long-standing rheumatoid arthritis and destructive joint changes, a series of strange and apparently unique changes occurs in the sclera. Progressively, over a period of many months or even years, the episcleral tissue almost completely disappears (Manschot, 1960). If the conjunctiva and subconjunctival tissue is observed carefully, it will be seen that the vessels seem to peter out, often forming whirls and microaneurysms (see Figures 4.31 and 4.32). This change involves the whole of the anterior segment including the muscle sheaths so that the muscles themselves can be seen beneath the conjunctiva. As the disease progresses, fine, grey chalk-like cracks appear in the superficial sclera, shortly after which the normal smooth outline of the superficial sclera seems to break up inside the area of the crack. Gradually these fibrils seem to agglomerate and a white pultaceous mass forms in the centre, the cracks widen and the centre becomes a sequestrum (Figure 7.8) which will eventually

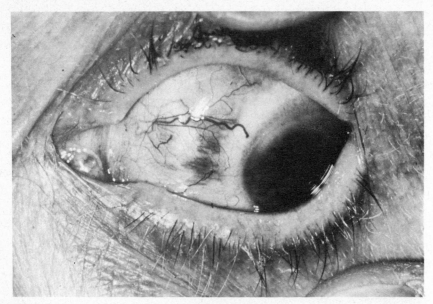

Figure 7.7. Increasing translucency of sclera following a circumferential necrotising scleritis in a patient with rheumatoid arthritis.

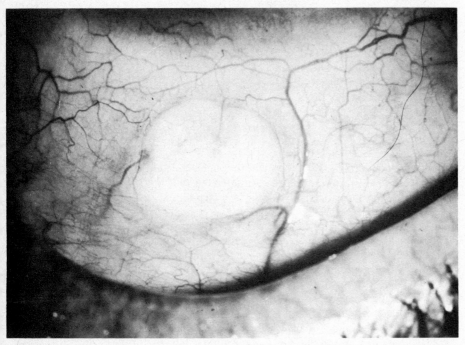

Figure 7.8. Early stage of necrotising scleritis without inflammation in a patient who had had rheumatoid arthritis for 20 years. The episclera is thin and a small well-demarcated white avascular area has appeared.

be thrown off, leaving the underlying choroid completely exposed (Figure 7.9). All of this takes place without any obvious inflammatory change whatever, or at most a very slight flush of the remaining episcleral tissue. This is true scleromalacia perforans, a term which should be reserved for this condition. Histologically these cracks can also be seen filled in by epithelial cells which line the newly formed fistula (Verhoeff and King, 1938). The sequestrum is isolated from the healthier surrounding tissue by a wall of epithelioid cells before the cells in the centre break away. The cell content of the avascular sequestrum

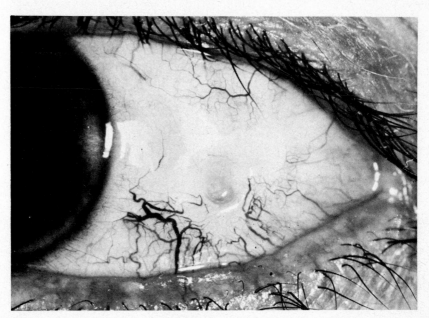

Figure 7.9.   Another quadrant of the same eye as Figure 7.8. The centre of the avascular area has sequestrated.

is sparse, consisting only of polymorphonuclear leucocytes and lymphocytes. This sequestrum formation is so characteristic that it justifies separation clinically from the necrotising scleritis of rheumatoid arthritis and vasculitis, even though the pathological changes, the cellular types, and the collagenous and proteoglycan changes appear to be identical. Provided this necrotising process of either type does not involve the whole of the circumference of the globe, the eye seems to be able to withstand the wholesale destruction of the sclera without any problem (Figure 7.10). If, however, an anterior uveitis develops, or the inflammation becomes totally circumferential or the intraocular pressure rises, then intraocular complications can occur. To prevent staphylomas forming it is important to monitor the intraocular pressure carefully and to treat the glaucoma with surgery if necessary. Glaucoma is the most sinister and blinding of all the complications, but all forms of scleral disease in association with rheumatoid arthritis must be taken seriously because the destructive changes are insidious and take place over such a prolonged period.

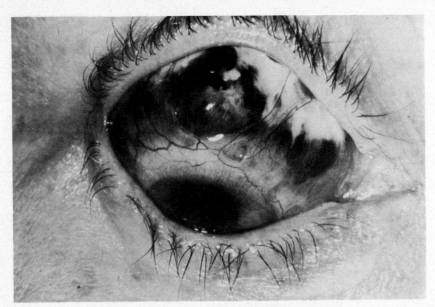

Figure 7.10. Scleromalacia perforans. A wide area of sclera has sequestrated or been absorbed. The underlying choroid is exposed and covered only by thick conjunctiva and a fine film of connective tissue. There is no staphyloma formation.

Corneal changes. Corneal changes associated with scleritis seem independent of those which occur purely as a result of the rheumatoid arthritis and those which occur as a result of keratoconjunctivitis sicca. The changes of keratoconjunctivitis sicca are diffuse and affect the stroma superficially. They may well lead to ulceration and, of course, filament formation. Those associated with rheumatoid arthritis alone are of two sorts: either a marginal guttering in which the cornea becomes very thin peripherally with or without any inflammatory changes and sometimes ulcerates completely, or more commonly, the extreme periphery of the cornea shelves outwards. This process, which eventually progresses through the full circumference of the eye starts between 2 and 3 mm from the limbus, so that whilst the whole cornea is clear, the centre is thicker than the periphery, looking exactly like a contact lens on the surface of the cornea (Lyne, 1970) (Figure 7.11). When the corneal changes are associated with the scleral disease, these are the same as those found from other causes and take the form of infiltrations of the deep corneal stroma with or without peripheral melting of the cornea (Figure 7.12) or corneal guttering adjacent to the site of the scleral inflammation (Figure 7.13). The most severe changes are those which are sometimes seen with necrotising scleritis in which keratolysis occurs in the corneal tissue and the cornea itself can completely disintegrate.

Central corneal changes do not seem to occur in patients with scleromalacia perforans, but peripheral changes are common.

Uveitis. Rheumatic iritis used to be a common diagnosis, but in fact uveitis is an unusual complication of rheumatoid disease, even though rheumatoid

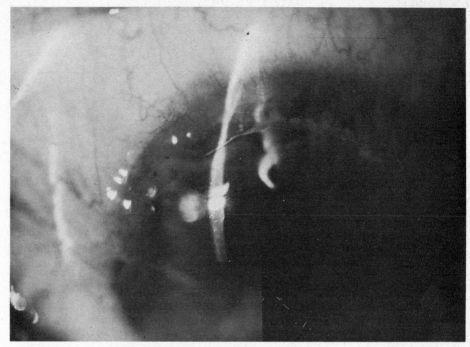

Figure 7.11. 'Contact lens cornea' of long-standing rheumatoid arthritis. The peripheral cornea shelves towards the limbus. The central cornea remains clear and of normal thickness.

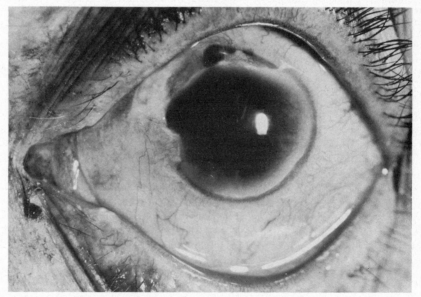

Figure 7.12. Extreme thinning adjacent to the site of necrotising scleritis in rheumatoid arthritis. The peripheral cornea is thin circumferentially and the opacification adjacent to this is due to lipid deposition. The sclera is so thin above that there is a descemetocele.

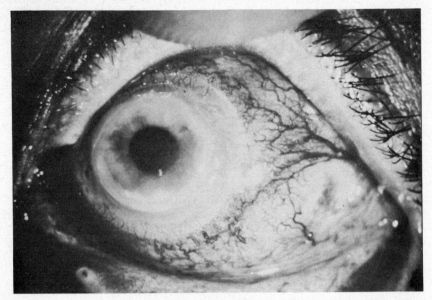

Figure 7.13.   Peripheral corneal guttering associated with necrotising scleritis in RA, involving the whole circumference of the corneal margin. Although the centre is still clear the edge adjacent to the gutter is oedematous. If left untreated this would progress to keratolysis.

factor has been found in 20 per cent of patients with uveitis. It is now generally agreed that adults with classical rheumatoid arthritis do not have a higher incidence of uveitis, except as a complication of scleritis, than other groups of patients. Similarly, there are no specific choroidal, retinal or optic nerve changes which can be related to rheumatoid disease. Posterior scleritis is, however, not uncommon in patients with rheumatoid arthritis (22 per cent) and in McGavin's series gave rise to choroiditis in two patients, a retinal detachment in one and extraocular muscle imbalance in five. If therefore uveitis is discovered in a patient with rheumatoid arthritis, the eye should be diligently examined for signs of other disease, particularly a scleritis in the region of the equator of the globe. The combination of scleritis and uveitis is of sinister significance for the health of the eye: 68 per cent of enucleated eyes have this combination (Fraunfelder and Watson, 1976).

Fundus changes in rheumatoid arthritis.   Fundus changes are the result of inflammatory disease elsewhere in the eye or systemic hypertension. We have found no specific retinal vasculitis which could be attributed to the rheumatoid arthritis, and the only physical sign, even when the rheumatoid vasculitis and cardiac disease is severe, is retinal arterial narrowing. However, Tupikin and Krikunov (1972) felt they could detect retinal vasculitis which became more severe with the degree of arthritis. They observed no change in the physical signs with treatment, even though the patient's symptoms improved. The retina and choroid may be involved if there is a posterior scleritis (Hurd, Snyder and Ziff, 1970) and as a result of the intraocular inflammation which accompanies the final destructive stage of necrotising scleritis. Kolmakova (1965) has described 'interstitial' destructive changes in the retina, optic nerve and chiasma in patients who have died from rheumatoid arthritis but who had obvious eye disease. Mathias (1955) described a case in which there appeared to be an atypical retinitis pigmentosa and there was no family history. Whether this is a chance relationship or is of pathological significance is unclear.

Heart

Although pericarditis is frequently found at postmortem, heart disease is not usually a prominent clinical problem, although both effusion and constriction have been reported in patients with scleritis and rheumatoid arthritis (Smoleroff, 1943; Edström and Osterlind, 1948). McGavin et al (1976) found a marked increase in electrocardiographic abnormalities in those patients who had scleritis and rheumatoid arthritis, as compared with rheumatoid arthritics who did not have scleritis. These included bundle branch block, myocardial infarction and nonspecific S–T wave changes. They also found, as Jayson and Jones had done, that some patients had aortic stenosis and incompetence at postmortem, presumably due to valvular deformity and dysfunction.

Rheumatoid nodules may be found in endocardium, myocardium and pericardium, but seldom cause myocardial dysfunction, unless they happen to occur in strategic positions such as the conduction system.

Cardiac involvement occurs in the following ways.

Pericarditis. At postmortem, 40 per cent of patients with rheumatoid arthritis have evidence of pericarditis, but it is rarely diagnosed clinically. However, Kirk and Cosh (1969) in a careful clinical study of patients admitted to hospital, found evidence of pericarditis in ten per cent. Also Bacon and Gibson (1974) using echocardiography detected effusions in 7 of 22 patients with classical or definite rheumatoid arthritis. Many of the effusions were small and posterior.

Rheumatoid granulomas. These can occur in any layer of the heart valves. They are found in one to three per cent of postmortems. The valve lesions are usually mild and of no haemodynamic significance. This may be due to the fact that the arthritis may restrict activity such that exertion symptoms are not produced. Bacon and Gibson (1974) used echocardiography to measure the diastolic closure rate of the mitral valve. They found very slow closure such as occurs in significant mitral stenosis in 3 out of 22 cases and suggested that this represented rheumatoid granulomas involving the mitral valve cusps.

Myocarditis. Nonspecific interstitial myocarditis and endocarditis occasionally occur presumably secondary to vasculitis. This can be associated with patchy valvular fibrosis.

Coronary arteritis. This is rare and is usually part of a widespread necrotising arteritis clinically indistinguishable from polyarteritis nodosa.

Respiratory complications

McGavin et al (1976) found a striking increase in pulmonary complications, such as pleurisy, pneumonitis, pleural effusion and rheumatoid nodules of the pleura in patients with rheumatoid arthritis and scleritis over those who did not have scleritis. An increased incidence of chest infections occurs in rheumatoid arthritis (Walker, 1967), including pneumonia, chronic bronchitis and bronchiectasis. The following pulmonary manifestations also occur:

1. Pleurisy with or without effusion.
2. Rheumatoid granulomas.
3. Diffuse interstitial pulmonary fibrosis.
4. Rheumatoid pneumoconiosis (Caplan's syndrome).
5. Pulmonary hypertension.
6. Empyema.

Pleurisy with effusion is the commonest pulmonary complication. It occurs most frequently in seropositive patients and is frequently associated with other extra-articular features of the disease. It can, however, occur early, even as a presenting feature. It is usually unilateral and contains lymphocytes and a low glucose content due to reduced diffusion of glucose into the pleural cavity. None of these findings is diagnostic and it is imperative that other causes of effusion are excluded, in particular pulmonary neoplasm and tuberculosis. The pleural reaction is due to rheumatoid granulation tissue of the pleural surface.

Rheumatoid nodules may occur in the lung parenchyma. They are usually single and present radiologically as 'coin' lesions. Differentiation from tuberculosis or carcinoma may prove difficult and biopsy proof may be required. Occasionally cavitation occurs due to central necrosis of the nodule and this may lead to a bronchopleural fistula.

Diffuse interstitial fibrosis is a syndrome that may occur either in isolation or in association with a variety of general disorders, of which rheumatoid arthritis is one. It is associated with seropositive disease. Clinically, there is progressive dyspnoea, and radiographs show diffuse fine reticular shadowing. Respiratory function tests show a restrictive defect and there is a reduction in diffusing capacity (Walker and Wright, 1969).

Pneumoconiosis and rheumatoid disease occurring in the same patient produce distinctive lung changes. Radiographs show a fine reticular pattern, and large opacities, becoming confluent, form in the periphery (Caplan's syndrome) (Caplan, 1953). The nodules represent an exaggerated response to the dust disease and may be related to an altered immune state in these patients.

It seems likely that rheumatoid patients develop chest infections more frequently and patients on long-term corticosteroid therapy may develop pulmonary tuberculosis.

Peripheral neuropathy

Both the peripheral and the central nervous system can be involved in rheumatoid arthritis:

1. Peripheral neuropathy: entrapment, symmetrical, mononeuritis multiplex.
2. Cervical cord and vertebral artery compression: cervical, C1 and C2 subluxation, midcervical subluxation.

In compression or entrapment neuropathy, there is an obvious local cause and the abnormality is confined to one nerve. This usually occurs at one of three sites: compression of the median nerve at the wrist (carpal tunnel syndrome), the ulnar nerve at the elbow, or the posterior tibial nerve behind the medial malleolus (tarsal tunnel syndrome). These are very common problems in rheumatoid arthritis.

Mononeuritis multiplex is the descriptive term given to the clinical picture of ischaemic interruption of peripheral nerve due to occlusive arthritis; for example there may be both motor and sensory features of a median and a lateral popliteal nerve lesion in the same patient. Extraocular muscle pareses are not uncommonly seen in this condition.

A symmetrical peripheral neuropathy also occurs in rheumatoid arthritis and is of two types (Chamberlain and Bruckner, 1970): it may be a purely sensory neuropathy of the fingers and/or toes which carries a relatively good prognosis, or, in the more severe form, sensory and motor signs occur, often in all four limbs. This neuropathy may be difficult to distinguish from mononeuritis multiplex. It carries a grave prognosis and it tends to accompany widespread and florid arteritis.

Lymph nodes and spleen

In early and acute cases of arthritis local lymph node enlargement is present in regional lymph nodes draining affected joints. Occasionally the follicular hyperplasia is of such a degree as to resemble that of giant follicular lymphoma (Butler, 1969).

Splenomegaly occurs in about five per cent of patients with seropositive rheumatoid arthritis. Felty's syndrome is defined as the association of rheumatoid arthritis, splenomegaly and neutropenia, and sometimes leg ulcers. The natural history of Felty's syndrome is variable and unpredictable and sometimes splenectomy is required in the face of critical recurring infections. Splenectomy is sometimes, but not regularly, followed by temporary or even permanent remission (Barnes, Turnbull and Vernon-Roberts, 1971).

A normochromic anaemia is characteristic of active disease. It is most often relieved by controlling the activity of the disease, rather than using iron or other haematin agent. Intramuscular iron is more effective than oral iron (Mowat, 1971).

Amyloidosis

Rheumatoid arthritis is the commonest cause of amyloidosis in the Western world. It is found in 20 to 60 per cent of postmortem examinations. Although it is rarely evident during life it is usually marked by proteinuria due to the deposition of amyloid in the glomerulus.

Prognosis

It is difficult to predict reliably the course that rheumatoid disease will follow since it is characterised by spontaneous exacerbations and remissions. Factors which favour a better prognosis include the absence of rheumatoid factor and a low erythrocyte sedimentation rate, the male sex, absence of erosions, a good initial response to treatment and acute onset.

Of the patients affected severely enough to be admitted to hospital, at the end of ten years only ten per cent will be severely crippled and dependent on others, whilst 60 per cent remain socially and economically independent. However, a few patients pursue a course characterised by gross systemic involvement with evidence of vasculitis, sometimes termed malignant. As a result of either disease or therapy the disease tends to be fatal. It is also in this group that most cases of necrotising scleritis fall and the appearance of this condition in a patient with rheumatoid arthritis has a sinister significance.

Polyarthritis in Children

Should a child who has arthritis develop scleritis, he almost always has detectable rheumatoid factor in his circulation. Most patients who develop arthritis in childhood are seronegative and although they commonly develop an anterior uveitis and keratitis, they virtually never develop scleral disease. As this topic has been a source of considerable confusion, we will discuss it in detail. In order to distinguish juvenile chronic polyarthritis from acute infectious illness, rheumatic fever, Schönlein–Henoch purpura, gout, etc., Bywaters (1967) and Ansell (1974) have suggested the following criteria:

1. Onset before 16 years of age.
2. Inflammatory involvement of four or more joints for a minimum period of three months.
3. If less than four joints are involved, synovial biopsy should show histological changes.

It now seems that the four different types of juvenile chronic polyarthritis can be distinguished by their clinical features (Table 7.3) and their eye signs, should the latter develop (Table 7.4). As there is very little overlap between the types, an indication can be given of the probable general and visual prognosis when the patient is first seen.

An acute febrile onset is associated with systemic manifestations of the type described by Still (1897). A polyarthritis may be present or may develop subsequently. In the polyarticular group arthritis is the dominant feature and affects four or more joints. Systemic manifestations vary. In the monoarticular and oligoarticular groups, one to three joints are involved with minimal systemic disease apart from iridocyclitis.

Table 7.3. *Clinical features of juvenile chronic polyarthritis*

	Still's disease	Juvenile rheumatoid arthritis	Juvenile ankylosing spondylitis	Juvenile antinuclear factor positive polyarthritis
Onset	Acute	Insidious	Acute	Insidious
Age	6–8	9–12	8–12	3–5
Sex	Females predominate	Females predominate	Male	Male and female
Rash	Present	None	None	None
Splenomegaly	Present	None	None	None
Lymph node enlargement	Present	None	None	None
Serum	Negative	Positive	HLA-B27 present Negative to Rose–Waalar test or SCAT	ANF positive in 90 per cent
Joint involvement	Multiple	Multiple	Few	Few

Table 7.4. *Eye changes in juvenile chronic polyarthritis*

Disease	Eye signs
Juvenile chronic polyarthritis (Still's disease)	None
Juvenile rheumatoid arthritis (rheumatoid factor positive)	Scleritis, keratitis
Juvenile ankylosing spondylitis (HLA-B27 positive)	Acute anterior uveitis, usually later in the disease
Juvenile polyarthritis (antinuclear factor positive)	Chronic uveitis throughout the disease, band keratopathy, secondary cataract, glaucoma

Juvenile chronic polyarthritis (Still's disease)

Of the 22 cases of chronic joint disease in children described in 1897 by George Frederick Still whilst he was working at the Hospital for Sick Children, Great Ormond Street, London, 12 were of the type which now classically carry his name.

These children, usually girls of around the age of seven or eight, complain of increasing morning stiffness followed by limitation of movement of many joints, particularly the knees, wrists and perhaps the cervical spine. The condition often starts with an acute febrile illness which is followed by a continuing or remittent low fever, generalised lymphadenopathy, splenomegaly and occasional skin rashes. From the onset of the disease there is a remarkable arrest of physical development but mental development is normal. The joint disease gradually becomes generalised and the child may develop pericarditis and anaemia. The ESR is raised and there is a leucocytosis. Rheumatoid factor or ANF are not present in the sera. Similar cases have been described since

Still's work in 1897, but they add little to his description of the distinctive features of the disease including the disturbance of growth and the absence of valvular heart disease. However, he failed to mention the rash.

Clinical features

Fever and rash. The fever is characteristic; it is present in the majority of children and differs from that of rheumatic fever. The temperature may be normal or subnormal in the morning and the child appears reasonably well, but by late afternoon a temperature of 40°C can be recorded and the child is usually ill. As a rule salicylates control the fever. When high fever precedes arthritis diagnosis can prove difficult, but is often aided by the appearance of the rash. About 40 per cent of the children develop a rash which is evanescent and often appears when the temperature is high. For this reason it may not be seen by the clinician who sees the patient in the morning. The rash is usually macular (Figure 7.14) and pink and does not irritate or spread. The trunk and limbs are usually affected, although it can be widespread and involve face, palms and soles.

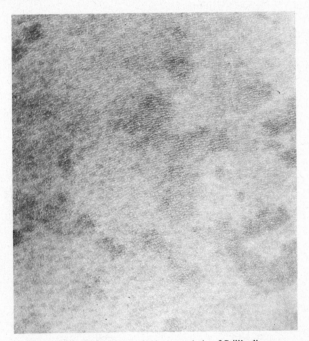

Figure 7.14.   Macular rash characteristic of Still's disease.

Lymph node enlargement and splenomegaly. Generalised lymph node enlargement may be marked and lead to the suspicion of blood dyscrasia or lymphoma. Histology shows reactive hyperplasia and the nodes regress as the disease subsides. Enlargement of the mesenteric glands may cause abdominal pain. Splenomegaly is of moderate degree and if it persists, the complication of amyloidosis should be considered.

Arthritis. Children seem to suffer less discomfort from arthritis than adults, and arthritis is often first suggested by swelling, a limp, or guarding of joints; in any pyrexia of unknown origin a careful examination of the joints should be made. Knees, wrists, hips, ankles and neck are commonly involved at first. Erosion of bone occurs less commonly in juvenile than in adult rheumatoid arthritis. However, local bone growth disturbances, either inhibition or overgrowth, may occur. The bones of the hands may appear small with fusiform swelling (Figure 7.15). The temporomandibular joints are frequently involved and may lead to micrognathia (Figure 7.16). Involvement of the cervical spine is common and leads to pain and limitation of movement. Radiographs show fusion in the later stages of the disease, and subluxation of the upper portions of the cervical spine, particularly the atlantoaxial joint, occurs.

Other clinical features. Subcutaneous nodules can occur but they are not the same as those found in juvenile or adult rheumatoid arthritis, the histological picture resembling that of rheumatic fever.

Pericarditis is detected in seven per cent of patients, but is found in approximately 45 per cent of necropsies. Myocarditis may also occur but endocarditis is not found.

Amyloidosis is a serious complication of the disease and leads to renal failure. It is thought that immunosuppressive therapy may delay progression once diagnosis has been made.

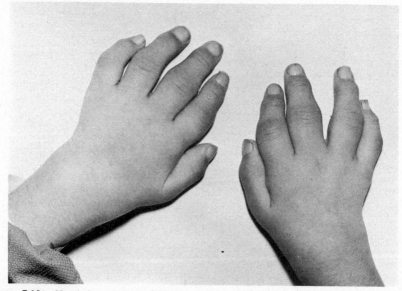

Figure 7.15.   Hands in a patient with Still's disease. The hands are small and there is fusiform swelling of the proximal interphalangeal joints.

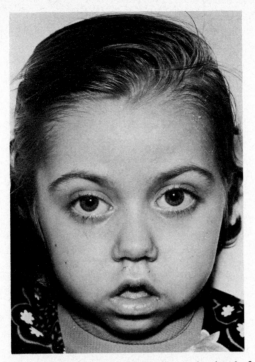

Figure 7.16. Characteristic facial appearance of Still's disease showing the failure of development of the jaw.

Juvenile rheumatoid arthritis

These children account for about ten per cent of those with juvenile polyarthritis. The age of onset is older than those with true Still's disease, being between 9 and 12 years of age, and although they may present with a generalised upset, they more often present with a polyarthritis involving four or more joints. However they do not have the typical rash, nor do they have the splenomegaly and lymph node enlargement. These children, who run a severe course clinically resembling adult rheumatoid arthritis, have rheumatoid factor in the circulation and are best referred to as seropositive juvenile rheumatoid arthritis.

Although eye changes are unusual, they do occur in the form of an anterior, diffuse or nodular scleritis, and very occasionally necrotising scleritis. From these changes stromal corneal opacities may develop (Plate VI). Clinically the scleritis is indistinguishable from that seen from any other cause except that it is somewhat more difficult to see the scleral swelling because of the thickness of the episclera. The scleritis can be the first manifestation of rheumatoid disease and Lyne and Rosen (1968) described a patient with a rheumatoid nodule of the sclera which when treated left an ectatic area near the limbus. We have one seropositive patient who developed an anterior diffuse scleritis at the age of ten, and although his scleritis persisted throughout adolescence, he had no articular symptoms until his mid-twenties, after which he developed severe crippling polyarthritis.

The course of children with juvenile rheumatoid arthritis is progressive and severe, rarely burning itself out; the fatalities in an otherwise relatively benign condition occur in this seropositive group.

Juvenile ankylosing spondylitis

These children, all of whom are boys between eight and twelve, may present with an acute iridocyclitis but more usually present with monoarticular or oligoarticular disease, the lumbodorsal spine and sacroiliac joints being particularly affected. About five years after the start of the arthritis, they develop a severe anterior uveitis, occasionally with hypopyon (Figure 7.17) first in one eye and then in the other. This responds immediately to vigorous treatment with

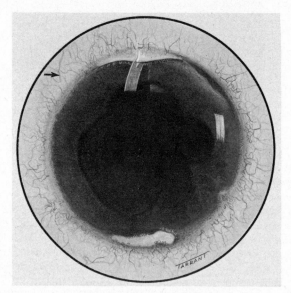

Figure 7.17. Posterior synechiae as a result of recurrent acute anterior uveitis in a child with juvenile ankylosing spondylitis.

mydriatics to keep the pupil from sticking to the lens and local steroids to suppress the inflammatory signs. The steroids can be withdrawn as soon as the cells disappear from the anterior chamber and only need to be given again if the inflammation recurs. We have one patient who requires one drop 0.1 per cent Predsol once every other week. By using this drop when the eye feels slightly uncomfortable he seems to be able to prevent recurrences. Long-term local steroid therapy should be avoided if at all possible because of the complications of glaucoma and cataract formation.

Radiographically the changes typical of ankylosing spondylitis often become apparent many years later and these children have a high incidence of HLA-B27 histocompatibility antigen (see page 247).

Juvenile polyarthritis (antinuclear factor positive)

These children develop their polyarthritis at a very early age (the norm being three to nine years), two-thirds of them being girls. There is no systemic upset, no rash, no fever, no splenomegaly and only a few joints are involved.

The remarkable feature of this group of children is the presence of a chronic iritis, of insidious onset which may precede the joint involvement by as many as 11 years (Smiley, 1974). In one-third the uveitis occurs within a year of the onset of arthritis. The chronic iridocyclitis is often symptomless and in half the cases a diagnosis is only made because it was specifically sought, or because the pupil has become bound down or the vision has deteriorated. The diagnosis was missed in the rheumatic and paediatric clinics in half Smiley's series of 60 patients, the slight inflammation being dismissed as conjunctivitis.

It is essential that patients with chronic polyarthritis who might fit into this group are examined routinely at regular intervals by an ophthalmologist with the slit-lamp microscope. Treatment should be instituted as early as possible to prevent synechiae formation; if treatment is not given, sight will inevitably be lost. Even with treatment the prognosis is poor, 50 per cent being on the partially sighted or blind registers because of the secondary complications of the uveitis, corneal band-shaped opacities, cataract and secondary glaucoma.

The iritis starts insidiously with a few cells in the anterior chamber. Flare is constantly present because of the proteinaceous exudate which eventually coagulates to cover pupil, lens, iris and angle. After a time, the lens gradually becomes opaque, due to poor nutrition, sometimes assisted by the unavoidable use of steroids.

Cataract extraction in young children is usually a very satisfactory procedure and is best achieved by aspiration of the lens, phacoemulsification or the use of the vitreous suction cutter. Surgery should only be attempted when the uveitis is quiescent or adequately suppressed otherwise the eye may react to surgical interference by becoming soft and visionless. This does not mean, however, that lens aspiration should not be attempted and provided every precaution is taken, great success can attend a few.

The secondary glaucoma caused by trabecular damage or rarely by pupil block or seclusio papillae is also resistant to conventional therapy (Smiley, 1974). Long-term therapy with Diamox is usually effective in keeping the pressure at a level where damage to the optic nerve does not occur. Should surgery be essential, trabeculectomy (Cairns, 1968) may control the pressure for a period but the subconjunctival drainage often ceases after about six months because of scarring of the conjunctiva. The operation may be repeated at another site or the original superficial flap raised and the overlying episcleral tissue excised. In these children only the trabecular tissue and Schlemm's canal anterior to the scleral spur should be excised and the posterior edge of the the flap left unsutured. The sclera in these children is very thin and if it is further reduced in thickness by removing the deep flap over the ciliary body, staphylomas could develop. Excising the thick episcleral tissue over the operation site and leaving the posterior flap unsutured has so far led to satisfactory and prolonged control of intraocular pressure in the few patients we have seen who needed surgical treatment. We have not had any success with goniotomy or trabeculotomy.

Another sequel of this type of iritis is the deposition of calcium beneath the corneal epithelium, forming a band keratopathy. Initially the opacity is seen with the slit-lamp microscope at the level of Bowman's membrane at 9 o'clock or 3 o'clock or both, near the corneal limbus. These opacities start as closely grouped grey dots interspersed with clear fenestrations of variable size and spread towards the corneal centre in the exposed intrapalpebral area just below the pupil. Eventually they may form a complete band.

Corneal band opacity commonly occurs in blind, degenerating adult eyes. In children, however, it can develop in a few months in association with chronic iridocyclitis in an eye which is relatively undamaged and retains good vision. The longer the inflammation persists the more likely is the band to spread.

The combination of chronic iridocyclitis, corneal band opacity and complicated cataract has been described as the 'ocular triad' of Still's disease. However, these changes are not specific and not diagnostic and can occur in association with any long-continued iridocyclitis in children.

Eighty-eight per cent of the children reported by Schaller et al (1974) with chronic polyarthritis and chronic iridocyclitis had antinuclear antibodies, which could be detected before the onset of the eye inflammation. This means that young seronegative children without systemic disease, with only a few joints involved and with positive antinuclear factor, are likely to develop chronic iridocyclitis and must be closely supervised by an ophthalmologist.

Systemic Lupus Erythematosus (SLE)

Reports of the incidence of ocular changes in patients with systemic lupus erythematosus vary between 5 and 52 per cent depending on the diligence with which the signs are looked for (Shearn and Pirofsky, 1952—32 patients, 28 per cent; Harvey et al, 1954 and Tumulty, 1954—105 patients, 24 per cent; Larson, 1961—200 patients, 5.5 per cent; Dubois and Tuffanelli, 1964—520 patients, 10.5 per cent; Gold, 1972—46 patients, 52.5 per cent). They may well be the presenting feature in many patients and scleritis is the commonest of these presentations, its intensity being directly related to the severity of the systemic disease.

Systemic lupus erythematosus is an uncommon disease, predominantly affecting young females. The aetiology is unknown, although at present there is much interest in the possibility that the disease may arise from an interaction of genetic factors and viral infection. The diverse clinical features, particularly in skin, kidneys, joints, blood, serous membranes, the nervous system and the eye reflect the multisystem involvement which is characteristic of the disease. Table 7.5 gives the incidence of the other major clinical manifestations of SLE in a series of 150 patients according to Hughes (1974).

Table 7.5. *Major clinical manifestations of SLE*

Manifestations	Percentage incidence
Musculoarticular	95
Cutaneous	81
Fever	77
Neuropsychiatric	59
Renal	53
Pulmonary	48
Cardiac	38

The prevalence of SLE appears to vary from country to country and is about 4 per 100 000 of the population in the U.K. It seems that Negroes are more susceptible than Caucasians. Epidemiological studies have been limited by the comparative infrequency of the disease and have only been possible since the discovery of the LE cell.

There is an increased prevalence of SLE in the families of patients with the disease (Siegel and Lee, 1973) and the incidence of antinuclear antibodies, hypergammaglobulinaemia and false positive serological tests for syphilis is also increased in healthy members of these families. These findings have led to the suggestion that there may be a genetically determined 'lupus diathesis', i.e. a capacity to develop SLE in appropriate environmental circumstances in predisposed individuals.

Clinical features

Musculoskeletal features

The commonest complaint is of joint or muscle pains, and the pain may appear out of proportion to the degree of synovitis. An important clinical point is the rarity of erosions in SLE, even after years of active synovitis. The shape of the joint deformities of the hands differs from that of rheumatoid arthritis in that occasionally a patient develops a deforming arthritis not because of joint erosion but as a result of capsular and ligamentous laxity. Tendon involvement may be prominent, leading in some cases to flexion contractures at the forearm and wrist.

Myositis is a common feature of SLE and should be suspected in any patient with active disease in whom there is eyelid discoloration or oedema. Rarely there may be a proximal myopathy; myasthenic features may be present and thymomas have been reported.

Skin manifestations

An erythematous macular eruption extending across the bridge of the nose to the malar areas on either side in a 'butterfly' distribution is the classical although uncommon manifestation of SLE (see Figure 3.28). The rash, which may only affect the eyelids, is characterised by erythema, scaling and scarring in which there may be minute purpuric or telangiectatic spots. Photosensitivity and livedo reticularis are common. Alopecia may occur in around 60 per cent of patients. Sometimes a new growth of hair occurs on the forehead (see Figure 3.29) and may occasionally provide the only clinical barometer of disease activity (Davis et al, 1973).

Ocular manifestations

Almost every structure in the eye can be involved in SLE. Whereas the inner eye is rarely involved in rheumatoid arthritis and the outer eye rarely involved in the seronegative arthritides and systemic vasculitis, SLE combines the findings of both groups even though the changes are rarely severe. This is of importance, because if fundus lesions or an anterior uveitis are seen in a patient with scleritis, it is likely that he has a disease akin to systemic lupus erythematosus.

Scleritis. Whilst there is nothing absolutely specific about the scleral changes found in SLE they do seem to follow some sort of pattern. Scleritis is not an uncommon presentation of SLE, the patient developing an anterior diffuse or nodular scleritis which recurs more and more frequently, each attack being more severe than the last. We have not seen an episcleritis in any patient with proven SLE. At a certain stage in the disease, probably when the renal and other systemic manifestations are becoming significant, the scleritis changes its character and becomes frankly necrotising, advancing from the original lesion in both directions circumferentially around the globe until it is stopped by treatment. Some patients present with a necrotising scleritis which is neither fulminating nor very severe, but will progress inexorably unless treated. Necrotising scleritis in SLE seems to be more difficult to control if treatment is delayed, but usually once systemic treatment is given, the eye remains under good control even though the systemic disease may progress. A uveitis and occasionally glaucoma, again not severe, usually accompany the scleritis and may be secondary to it. Renal complications are almost universal in patients who have scleritis.

Other ocular manifestations. Keratoconjunctivitis sicca occurs in about 25 per cent of patients with systemic lupus erythematosus, and conversely five per cent of patients with Sjögren's syndrome have been shown to have SLE. Keratoconjunctivitis sicca only appears in those who have the chronic benign disease and none of these patients has been found to have renal involvement.

Conjunctivitis. The conjunctiva is frequently affected, particularly when the lids are involved either with systemic lupus or discoid lupus erythematosus. At first both bulbar, fornix and tarsal conjunctiva are affected, there being no follicular or papillary reaction, or anything but a slight mucoid discharge. Later, either as a primary conjunctival lesion or by direct spread from the skin to the conjunctivae, an intense hyperaemia and a velvet-like oedema of the mucous membrane appear. This reaction may be diffuse or localised, but as the disease progresses these areas become violaceous and blue, eventually

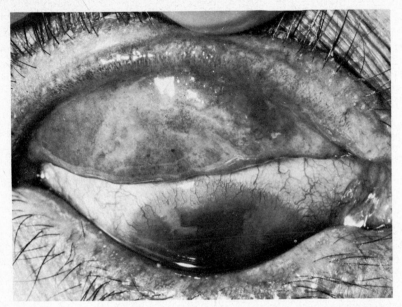

Figure 7.18. Conjunctival scarring in a patient with systemic lupus erythematosus.

resolving to leave white depressed scars (Figure 7.18). This violent immune reaction may well lead to considerable shrinkage of the conjunctivae (Duke Elder and Leigh, 1965).

Keratitis. Spaeth (1967) reported that 88 per cent of patients with SLE showed punctate epithelial corneal erosion, but Gold, Morris and Henkind (1972) only found this in 6.6 per cent. Whatever the incidence, when changes do occur, a very severe hyperkeratotic keratitis always develops. The corneal lesions stain with Bengal rose and fluorescein and have been described by Doesschate (1956) as looking like the well-worn surface of a skating rink. These lesions may eventually coalesce to form deep ulcers and an apparent discoid keratitis. Marginal ulceration and localised but intense infiltration and vascularisation may be so severe as to produce an entirely cloudy cornea.

Uveal and retinal changes. A primary anterior uveitis occurs in about one per cent of patients, and this usually takes the form of grey, white, or yellow foci of miliary type on both iris and choroid. Uveitis also occurs as a result of a concomitant scleral inflammation and although this may give rise to a secondary glaucoma it is never severe, rarely leading to synechiae formation and often so insignificant that it has to be specifically looked for. Reports vary as to the incidence of retinal involvement but the latest report by Gold, Morris and Henkind (1972) indicates that some retinal changes occur in about 20 per cent of patients. The fundus changes in systemic lupus consist primarily of superficial retinal haemorrhages, cotton wool spots and oedema of the discs and surrounding retina. Although these appearances are similar to hypertensive retinopathy, they are not necessarily mere reflections of a concomitant hypertension, but are a distinct part of the disease. Superficial fluffy cotton wool spots representing microinfarcts of the retina can occur at any stage during the disease without hypertension, although they are not usually seen except in severely ill people.

Other reported fundus findings include macular stippling, central retinal vein occlusion, papilloedema, retinal vasculitis and retinal scarring. All are uncommon. If fluorescein angiography is performed in these patients, retinal microangiopathy is commonly found, even though the ophthalmoscopic appearance of the fundus is apparently normal.

Cardiovascular features

Pericarditis frequently occurs during acute exacerbations of the disease and echocardiography should always be performed as pericarditis may easily be missed. It has become increasingly recognised that myocardial disease is common in SLE and although this commonly produces little more than slight cardiac enlargement, it may sometimes lead to arrhythmias and even signs of cardiac failure. Hypertension occurs frequently and usually, but not always, denotes severe renal involvement. Endocarditis involving the right side of the heart (Libman–Sacks endocarditis) is usually haemodynamically insignificant and is not easily diagnosed in life. Murmurs are frequently heard in SLE often in the absence of any anatomical proof of endocarditis and are an unreliable guide to its diagnosis.

Raynaud's phenomenon is common, although not as prominent as in scleroderma. Digital ulceration and atrophic skin changes may occur. While many of the visceral changes in SLE are themselves due to vasculitis, more obvious evidence of blood vessel disease may be present. A vasculitis may produce a scleritis, digital gangrene, bowel perforation and chronic leg ulceration. Thrombophlebitis also occurs and may be recurrent or migratory.

Respiratory system

Pleurisy is common and pleuritic pain may remain a problem long after all other evidence of disease activity has regressed. Recurrent pneumonitis with scanty physical signs but with radiological evidence of patchy plate-like atelectasis or diffuse basal infiltration may occur and lead to gradual elevation of both hemidiaphragms and restrictive lung defects.

Haematological features

A mild normochromic normocytic anaemia and elevation of the erythrocyte sedimentation rate are common. Absolute lymphocytopenia is a frequent finding and may be of diagnostic value. An acquired haemolytic anaemia with a positive Coombs test may antedate the other manifestations of the disease by many years. This responds well to corticosteroids but not to splenectomy.

A low platelet count with or without platelet agglutinins is common and may be sufficiently low to cause all the signs and symptoms of idiopathic thrombocytopenic purpura. Response to splenectomy is good.

Lymphadenopathy is common; the pathological changes are those of reactive hyperplasia. Occasionally patients present with marked lymphadenopathy. Splenomegaly, while not uncommon, is rarely gross.

Renal system

Sixty per cent of patients have renal involvement and its presence significantly affects the patient's prognosis (Harvey et al, 1954; Dubois, 1966; Estes and Christian, 1971). The extent and severity of the renal lesion mirror the severity of the disease. If renal involvement cannot be detected two years after diagnosis, then it is unlikely to develop and the prognosis for prolonged life is accordingly better. The pathogenesis of the renal lesion is thought to be that of immune complex deposition (Agnello, Koffler and Kunkel, 1973), giving rise to low serum complement which is due to deposition of complement and antigen–antibody complexes upon the capillary basement membrane. These complexes are composed of DNA and anti-DNA antibodies. According to current concepts of immune complex disease, renal involvement probably occurs in the majority of cases, but it is now known that patients may recover completely from many forms of renal injury. For example, mesangial deposition of immunoglobulin may be a reversible change.

Central nervous system

Recent studies of SLE have demonstrated the frequent occurrence of neuropsychiatric involvement (Estes and Christian, 1971; Bennett et al, 1972; Baker, 1973). The commonest abnormalities were disorders of mental function and seizures; other manifestations include cranial nerve signs, chorea, tremor and headache. Although frequently overlooked, psychological abnormalities may lead to suicidal depression and psychosis. It has also been recognised recently that CNS disease may carry an even worse prognosis than the renal involvement and this is becoming the major clinical problem in SLE.

In summary, therefore, young female patients with fever, alopecia lymphadenopathy, arthritis, a skin rash, serositis, splenomegaly, Raynaud's phenomenon and evidence of renal involvement are likely to have SLE. The ocular features may antedate the other manifestations of SLE and should therefore be looked upon with suspicion, particularly when they occur for the first time in a young female. Other unusual presentations include convulsions, idiopathic thrombocytopenic purpura, acquired haemolytic anaemia or even a positive Coombs test and drug sensitivity reactions.

Discoid lupus erythematosus

Discoid lupus erythematosus is a chronic skin disease characterised by erythema, scaling, plugging of the sebaceous glands and scarring, often on the cheeks and bridge of the nose. There may be marked alopecia. It is generally benign but a small proportion of patients do develop systemic disease (Beck and Rowell, 1966). Conversely, it is not uncommon for patients with SLE to have discoid skin lesions. Furthermore, a variety of serological abnormalities may be found in otherwise benign discoid lupus, for example antinuclear factor tests may be positive in one-third of cases (Shrank and Doniach, 1963). Although the likelihood of discoid lupus erythematosus becoming systemic is small, there is at present no way of forecasting this event in the individual patient.

Drug-induced lupus

For some time confusion has existed regarding the relationship of drug-induced lupus to SLE and the increasing usage of drugs is often suggested as the cause of the apparent increase in frequency of SLE. A large number of drugs may, in certain individuals, give rise to a syndrome closely resembling SLE, with rashes, fever, arthritis, polyserositis and pulmonary manifestations. The long list of drugs includes hydralazine, procainamide, practolol, the hydantoins, the sulphonamides, isoniazid and oral contraceptives.

Anti-DNA antibodies are usually present in low titre (Hughes, 1971) and renal disease is absent in the majority of cases. Furthermore the disease is usually reversible on stopping the drugs though some cases of hydralazine-induced lupus have had more prolonged courses. Winfield and Davies (1974) studied anti-DNA antibody in procainamide-induced lupus; they were able to show that whereas about 50 per cent of patients with symptomatic pro-cainamide-induced lupus exhibited anti-denatured DNA, none had anti-native DNA. Variations in drug metabolism have been shown to be related to the induction of antinuclear antibody (ANA). It has been demonstrated that individuals who are slow acetylators of hydralazine (Perry et al, 1970) and isoniazid (Price Evans et al, 1972) have a higher incidence of ANA than individuals taking these drugs who are fast acetylators. Whilst it has been suggested that the drugs act as catalysts in patients who already have a lupus diathesis, there is little evidence of this, and it is generally considered that it is a drug hypersensitivity reaction, clinically and aetiologically distinct from SLE.

Mixed connective tissue disease

In a small group of patients the features of SLE, myositis and systemic sclerosis occur in sequence or concurrently. Sharp et al (1972) have proposed the term mixed connective tissue disease for this group. The sera of these patients have three distinguishing immunological features:

1. The absence of anti-DNA antibodies.
2. The strongly positive 'speckled' pattern of ANF tests.
3. Antibodies in high titre to extractable nuclear antigen, an as yet incompletely characterised RNA protein.

These patients generally have a good prognosis and a low incidence of renal disease.

Immunological features of SLE

LE cells

The LE cell factor is an IgG antibody to native DNA histone. The sequence of events resulting in the LE cell has been illustrated in Figure 3.33. The ANA penetrates the damaged cell membrane of the leucocyte and induces nuclear destruction, shown by swelling, and the normal chromatin pattern of the nucleus is lost. The leucocyte dies and the altered nucleus is extruded and then surrounded by a 'rosette' of polymorphonuclear leucocytes, one of which engulfs the extruded nucleus forming the LE cell. This must not be confused with the 'tart' cell which is simply a polymorphonuclear leucocyte which has engulfed an undamaged extruded nucleus and which has no clinical significance.

The test is positive in up to 75 per cent of SLE patients. Positive, though weak reactions are found in a number of other conditions, particularly rheumatoid arthritis, Sjögren's disease, chronic liver disease, and other connective tissue diseases.

Antinuclear factors

The demonstration of ANFs by immunofluorescence (Holborow, Weir and Johnson, 1957) provides the most widely used screening test for SLE. The test is very sensitive and a negative test almost always excludes a diagnosis of SLE (uraemia may render an ANF result negative). However, positive tests are found in a long list of other conditions.

Anti-DNA antibodies

In 1957 a number of groups reported the findings of antibodies against native (double-stranded) DNA in the serum of patients with SLE (Cepellini, Polli and Celada, 1957; Miescher and Strässle, 1957; Robbins et al, 1957; Seligmann and Milgrom, 1957). It became apparent that the antibodies were a heterogenous group, binding to a variety of sites on the DNA molecule (Cohen et al, 1971). In particular, antibodies against native DNA were found to be almost always specific for SLE.

The measurement of DNA antibodies by immunoassay has proved a major advance in the management of SLE. Problems remain in standardisation of the DNA and in the exclusion of denatured DNA fragments or strands. Whilst small amounts of native DNA antibody may be detectable in a variety of conditions, the clearcut differential between results obtained in active SLE and in controls has made the test a standard procedure in the diagnosis and management of SLE. In the majority of patients with SLE, fluctuations in DNA-binding parallel clinical activity.

Prognosis

Unless there is severe renal and CNS involvement, the outlook in SLE is now much improved. There is, for example, no contraindication to pregnancy in an SLE patient who is in reasonable remission and who has good renal function.

SERONEGATIVE CONDITIONS

Included in this group are the diseases listed under 'seronegative conditions' on page 208. Eye disease is found in ankylosing spondylitis, psoriatic arthritis, Reiter's disease, ulcerative colitis, Crohn's disease and Behçet's syndrome. The only eye complication described in Whipple's disease is peripheral retinal vasculitis. All these diseases are characterised by seronegativity in respect of rheumatoid factor, axial skeletal involvement, an asymmetrical peripheral arthritis, and in some instances a definite but incomplete form of inheritance. They have now been firmly associated with one another and linked together as a group by transplantation antigen or histocompatibility antigen (HLA) testing.

Professor V. Wright and his group at Leeds have described clinical and familial linkages between ankylosing spondylitis and other types of seronegative arthritis and have called them the seronegative spondoarthritides (Moll et al, 1974). These diseases have a number of common features:

1. Negative serological tests for rheumatoid factor.
2. Absence of rheumatoid nodules.
3. Inflammatory peripheral arthritis.
4. Radiological sacroiliitis.
5. Evidence of clinical overlap between members of the group.
6. Tendency to familial aggregation.

As far as the eye signs of this group are concerned, the uveal tract is commonly involved, the external eye, cornea and sclera are rarely involved, and the retina and vasculature are practically never involved.

It is the clinical and familial cross associations and the difference in prognosis and treatment, and not just that they do not have rheumatoid factor or antinuclear factor in the serum, which justify grouping these conditions together. The term seronegative spondoarthritis is in this sense a specific term and should not be used as a diagnostic pigeonhole just because these conditions are seronegative.

The general prognosis for this group of conditions is better than for rheumatoid arthritis, its management is different and the knowledge that uveitis and sacroiliitis can occur prevents each being treated in isolation and avoids the errors of labelling back pain as lumbar disc disease.

Awareness of the frequency of familial associations may one day help the patient or undiagnosed relative.

Contrasting Features of Seropositive and Seronegative Arthritis

The clinical features between seropositive and seronegative groups tend to be distinct (Table 7.6); however, some overlap between these groups can occur.

Radiological examination of the affected joints helps to differentiate the groups since bony ankylosis, marginal periostitis, asymmetry and lack of osteoporosis are more commonly found in the seronegative group. These differences suggest separate underlying pathological processes between the two groups.

Table 7.6. *Features of seronegative and seropositive arthritis*

	Seronegative	Seropositive
Peripheral arthritis	Asymmetrical	Symmetrical
Spinal involvement	Ankylosis	Cervical subluxation
Cartilagenous joints	Commonly affected (especially sacroiliac joints)	Rarely affected
Tissue typing	HLA-B27	No association known
Eye involvement	Anterior uveitis, conjunctivitis	Scleritis, keratitis, keratoconjunctivitis sicca
Skin involvement	Epidermal dysmaturation (psoriasis, keratoderma blennorrhagica), mucosal ulceration, erythema nodosum	Cutaneous nodules, vasculitis
Heart involvement	Fibrosis of aortic root, aortic regurgitation, conduction defects	Pericarditis
Pulmonary involvement	Chest wall ankylosis	Alveolitis, nodules, effusions
Gastrointestinal involvement	Ulceration of small or large intestine	Drug-induced symptoms
Genitourinary involvement	Urethritis/prostatitis, genital ulceration	

HLA System

Recently the concept of the seronegative arthritides as a group has been emphasised by the discovery of an increased incidence of the transplantation antigen HLA-B27 in these conditions. The HLA system comprises a series of antigens (probably proteins) which are found on the surface membranes of a wide variety of human cells. Current knowledge suggests that there are two or possibly three closely linked autosomal genes which code for these antigens. The two well characterised genes are known as first and second

HLA loci. Each haplotype will have a first and second locus antigen, and each diploid cell will express two antigens from the first and two antigens from the second locus. When an individual is tissue typed for HLA antigens there will be four of these antigens to be identified. If two genes are closely linked on a chromosome then they will tend to stay together within a family tree because there are relatively few genetic recombinations. However, in the population at large there are many more opportunities for recombination and the two closely linked genes of a family will not remain so in a population. Nevertheless, in some situations closely linked genes do occur in a population in a higher frequency than one would expect. An example of this is HLA-1 and HLA-8 antigens (from first and second HLA loci respectively). This is known as linkage disequilibrium and occurs because for some reason the population contains more people than expected with the two genes on the same chromosome. It is possible that this combination produces some selective advantage. When looking for HLA markers for a disease, they can only be found if the gene involved in the disease is closely linked on the same chromosome to the HLA gene. In the case of ankylosing spondylitis the HLA antigen B27 (second locus antigen) was found in up to 96 per cent of cases compared to seven per cent of the population. If HLA-B27 were directly involved in the disease, one would expect 100 per cent association. The fact that it is slightly less than this would suggest that there is a gene in close linkage disequilibrium to the HLA-B27 which is involved in ankylosing spondylitis.

This is important because it implies involvement of a specific genetic factor in the disease and also explains why an association of less than 100 per cent might merely reflect the distance between the two loci, which are still, however, in linkage disequilibrium. Hence even a weak association of a disease with an HLA antigen might be an indication that there is a gene near the HLA region involved in the pathogenesis of the disease.

At present it is not known how the association with HLA-B27 influences pathogenesis. Animal experiments suggest that HLA antigens may be directly involved in disease processes in one of three ways: by acting as receptors for viruses or other infective agents, by incorporation into the coats of foreign agents, or by molecular mimicry. The latter means that the HLA antigens are similar to the antigenic determinants of foreign agents so that the host cannot produce a suitable immune response. Alternatively the HLA antigens may not be directly involved, but their importance may lie in their close association with the immune response genes that segregate in the same genetic region.

HLA association with the seronegative arthritides

With the identification of the strong association of HLA-B27 with ankylosing spondylitis (Brewerton et al, 1973; Schlosstein et al, 1973) as mentioned above, the other inflammatory polyarthritides have been investigated. In Reiter's disease the incidence is almost as high as that of ankylosing spondylitis (Table 7.7), especially in the cases of chronic Reiter's disease (Brewerton et al, 1973b).

The conditions associated with seronegative arthritis all show an increased incidence of the HLA-B27 antigen when there is a polyarthropathy. The correlation is much stronger when there is spinal involvement. An interesting group is the reactive arthritis associated with a known infection, e.g. yersinia (Aho et al, 1973), salmonella, and shigella (Aho et al, 1973), where there is about a 90 per cent correlation with HLA-B27 (Brewerton, 1975). This is the first example of an infection producing an arthritis associated with this specific genetic marker. This antigen is not in increased frequency in seropositive arthritis, gout, osteoarthritis or in the non-rheumatic diseases studied.

Table 7.7. *Percentage incidence of HLA-B27 in seronegative arthritis*

	With arthropathy	Without arthropathy
Normal population (NP)	–	7%
Ankylosing spondylitis	96%	–
Reiter's syndrome	75% (65–95%)	–
Psoriasis	37%	7% as NP
Ulcerative colitis ⎫ Crohn's disease ⎭	67% if sacroiliitis 7% if peripheral	7% as NP
Still's disease	25%	–
Yersinia dysentery	90%	–
Anterior uveitis	98%	40%

One hundred adults with acute anterior uveitis were investigated. Associated disease was diagnosed in 33 and HLA-B27 was present in 29. HLA-B27 was also present in 29 out of 60 patients who had never had rheumatic symptoms and had no evidence of other disease (Brewerton, 1973a). Men and women were about equally affected. The significance of this finding in the pathogenesis of anterior uveitis is not known. A similar study was undertaken in scleritis, a condition in which familial associations are very unusual, and no increase in any antigen was found (Joycey, 1976, unpublished observations).

Despite the correlation of HLA-B27 with seronegative arthritis, population studies indicate that only about five per cent of men and 0.6 per cent of women with the HLA-B27 antigen will develop clinical ankylosing spondylitis. Hence its usefulness is limited at the moment to diagnostic and prognostic investigation.

Overlapping Clinical Features of the Seronegative Arthritides

These have already been briefly mentioned in Table 7.6 and mainly comprise the propensity for ankylosing axial skeletal involvement, an asymmetrical pattern of peripheral arthropathy, psoriasiform lesions, inflammation of the uveal tract, an aortitis caused by fibrosis of the aortic root, and buccal, intestinal and genital ulceration. Any one patient, or in fact any one disease, does not necessarily show all these features. For example, the clinical and histological picture of keratoderma blennorrhagica in Reiter's disease is very similar to that of pustular psoriasis. However, there is no association between psoriasis and anterior uveitis which can occur in Reiter's disease, ankylosing spondylitis and enteropathic arthropathy.

Similarities also exist between ulcerative colitis and Crohn's disease. Both have asymmetrical non-destructive lower limb synovitis and they share many other features, such as ocular inflammation, erythema nodosum, buccal ulceration and thrombophlebitis. Behçet's syndrome shares many of these features and indeed colonic involvement, similar to ulcerative colitis, may occur. In addition, Behçet's syndrome has many points in common with Reiter's disease, including anterior uveitis (although possibly of different type), genital and buccal ulceration and bowel involvement. A further link is the association of inflammatory bowel disease, usually ulcerative colitis, in 17 per cent of ankylosing spondylitis patients. Extending this further, there seems to be an excess of ulcerative colitis in psoriatic arthritic patients and also an excess of psoriasis in ulcerative colitis and Crohn's disease.

Familial Association

There is now evidence that not only do these diseases have familial aggregation, but that other seronegative arthritides occur within this family group. For example, relatives of patients with psoriatic arthritis can have psoriatic arthritis, ankylosing spondylitis or Reiter's disease.

The Individual Seronegative Arthritides

Until now the emphasis has been on considering the unifying features of seronegative arthritis. The diseases within this group, however, are all sufficiently distinct to warrant individual description. All these conditions are diagnosed on clinical and radiological evidence as laboratory investigations are of limited help, although the sedimentation rate provides an indication of disease activity.

Ankylosing Spondylitis

Although Hippocrates described a condition identical to the modern disease, it was not until the separate descriptions of von Bechterew (1893), Strumpell (1897) and Marie (1898) that the disease was widely recognised. The prevalence among men is reported as 1 in 200, and among women as 1 in 2000.

The early histological changes in the synovial joints resemble rheumatoid arthritis but with less prominent lesions of the surface layers. However, the most important features are in the cartilagenous joints. Bony ankylosis is more frequent and the sacroiliac joints often become fused. The apophyseal joints are involved and the discs show replacement of the nucleus pulposus, the annulus fibrosus and parts of the vertebral body by vascular fibrous tissue without any evidence of marked inflammatory changes. In the spine, Ball (1971) has drawn attention to the importance of lesions of ligamentous attachment to bone (the 'enthesis') and considers this to be characteristic of ankylosing spondylitis. The disease is characterised by bilateral sacroiliitis.

As the disease extends up to the intravertebral joints, there is 'squaring' of the vertebral bodies and calcification of the annulus fibrosus giving the characteristic syndesmophytes which fuse to form the classic 'bamboo spine'. This is due to inflammation of the anterior corners of the vertebrae which extend into the outer layers of the annulus fibrosus.

Calcification and ossification run vertically in contrast to spondylosis where calcification takes place horizontally to form osteophytes. Calcification of the spinal ligaments can also occur. At this stage there is osteoporosis of the vertebrae and fractures of the spine; after minor trauma can occur. Other cartilaginous joints such as the sternomanubrial joint and the symphysis pubis can be affected with erosions, sclerosis and bony ankylosis.

The interpretation of the early radiological changes of sacroiliitis are subject to a great degree of observer error and only the later changes of bone sclerosis, erosion and fusion are of real diagnostic value.

The disease usually begins between the ages of 16 and 40 years. Its onset is gradual and often accompanied by constitutional disturbances. The initial symptom is usually low back pain, often worse at night, with morning stiffness and stiffness after immobility. Diagnosis is often delayed, symptoms being ascribed to lumbar disc disease. Thoracolumbar pain is often a helpful diagnostic feature. In spondylitis spinal mobility is limited in all directions in contrast to disc prolapse when lateral flexion is usually normal. Peripheral joints are involved in about one-quarter of patients and involvement of the hip is important because of the functional implications. Sometimes pain and tenderness at sites of tendinous insertions, e.g. the heels, pelvic brim and ischial tuberosities, can be a prominent feature.

The lumbar spine becomes flattened and the normal lordosis is lost relatively early. Spinal mobility is restricted in all directions. Involvement of the costovertebral joints accounts for the thoracic pain and limitation of chest expansion.

In an advanced case, the diagnosis is easy, as posture, gait and limitation of back movement are typical. However, only a minority of patients exhibit marked kyphosis and spinal rigidity and the scatter of the chest and spinal mobility in spondylitic patients is considerable, with an extensive overlap into the normal range.

Ocular complications

Iritis occurs at some time in the life of almost all these patients and is frequently the presenting feature, antedating the joint symptoms by as much as 12 years or occurring when the disease is entirely quiescent. It is so common that it might be regarded as a clinical feature of the disease rather than a complication of it. In 20 per cent of the patients it is the most disabling feature of the disease, not so much because it is severe but because it is recurrent and often bilateral, with either the disease or the treatment upsetting the patient's vision for much of his life. The anterior uveitis, the severity of which is unrelated to the severity of the arthritis, is of the acute exudative type, presenting with hyperaemia of the conjunctiva with a circumlimbal congestion of the anterior ciliary vessels, photophobia, pain and visual loss if there is much exudation in the anterior chamber. Keratic precipitates, if present at all, are very fine.

Anterior synechiae will occur if treatment is not prompt, but most patients know the symptoms and are able to abort an attack with immediate application of steroid drops and dilation of the pupil by some sort of mydriatic. Provided these patients are under intermittent supervision to see that they do not develop steroid reactions or the cataract and glaucomatous complications of the disease, this routine often saves much morbidity and everyone's time. Unless the attacks are very severe the iritis usually clears up without any residual damage to the eye, even though many attacks may have occurred over a period of years. Although it is unusual, severe intractable uveitis can occur which eventually leads to phthisis bulbi or blindness.

Scleral inflammation

Scleritis can also occur in ankylosing spondylitis; like the uveitis it can precede the joint symptoms by many years. It can also occur without any evidence of uveitis. Whilst there was only one overt case in our published series of 207 patients (Watson and Hayreh, 1976), seven other cases were found on careful clinical examination and we have since seen scleritis on several other occasions. Invariably it has been of the anterior diffuse type, not severe, and although recurrent has never progressed to a necrotising scleritis. Episcleritis does not seem to occur as such although the limbal episcleral plexus is extremely congested when the anterior uveitis is severe. There is no infiltration of the episcleral tissue.

Other complications

Aortitis and myocarditis can cause death, as can uraemia from amyloidosis. The spinal cord may be compressed by atlantoaxial subluxation or the fracture of the rigid spine. Occasionally the cauda equina can be compressed by the overgrowth of the bone in the sacroiliac region. Chest infections may occur due to poor chest expansion and recently rare apical pulmonary changes simulating tuberculosis have been described (Campbell and MacDonald, 1965).

Prognosis

With adequate treatment the prognosis is excellent and 85 per cent of these patients never lose a day from work. After the painful phase, the back may be stiff but disability is minimal unless hip involvement is present. Only five per cent of patients have an unfavourable course from the onset.

Psoriatic Arthropathy

Both psoriasis and rheumatoid arthritis occur in about two per cent of the population and hence there can be a coincidental association of these conditions. However, the arthropathy which develops most commonly in psoriasis is distinct. It seems to affect the sexes equally.

Again, the histological synovial changes resemble rheumatoid arthritis, but the joints involved and the pattern of destruction are different. While any joint can be affected, the most characteristic are the distal interphalangeal joints of the hands and feet. Radiological features of psoriatic arthritis are erosions in the distal interphalangeal joints with ankylosis, reabsorption of the terminal phalanges, and marginal bone overgrowths at the tendon insertions. When this last feature is associated with osteolysis of the middle phalanx the radiological 'pencil-in-cup' deformity appears. If osteolysis progresses to 'telescoping' of the phalanges, the condition is known as arthritis mutilans (Figure 7.19).

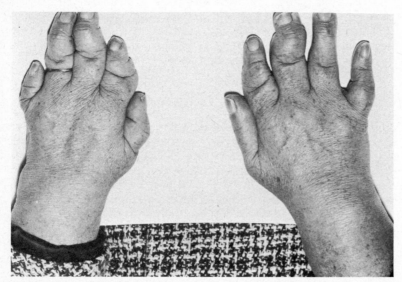

Figure 7.19.   Hands in psoriatic arthritis showing 'telescoping' of fingers due to bone destruction. This deformity is unusual in rheumatoid arthritis.

Sacroiliitis is found in up to 30 per cent of cases in which erosions, sclerosis and ankylosis may occur and is particularly common in patients with the severe arthritis mutilans form of disease. Unlike ankylosing spondylitis, the involvement of the sacroiliac joints is usually asymmetrical. Paravertebral calcification and occasional large syndesmophytes may be seen. The incidence of fully developed ankylosing spondylitis is higher in psoriatics and relatives than might be expected in the general population. Hyperuricaemia can occur in up to 20 per cent of psoriatics and the arthropathy should not be confused with gout.

The onset of arthritis, which usually follows a long history of psoriasis, can be acute, insidious, monoarticular or polyarticular, but occasionally it precedes the skin lesions. There does not appear to be a correlation between the severity of the skin lesions and the development of the arthropathy, although the activity of the skin and joint lesions may be synchronous. The nails, which are usually involved in those with joint lesions, can be pitted. The nail plates are thickened, discoloured and ridged, and the end of the nail is split.

The activity and ultimate deformity caused by the disease are usually less than rheumatoid arthritis and remissions are more frequent.

Ocular manifestations

Eye disease is uncommon in psoriasis, but more often involves the outer eye than the inner eye. Anterior uveitis, if it occurs, is mild with a fine coating of keratic precipitates (KP) on the posterior corneal surface.

A mild anterior diffuse scleritis is seen from time to time and it is indistinguishable from any other type. All patients with scleral disease should be asked whether they have any skin rashes because the psoriatic patient is so used to his skin troubles that he never associates the two conditions and in consequence never volunteers the information about the rashes.

Reiter's Syndrome

This disease was mentioned several times before Hans Reiter's 1916 description of a Prussian cavalry officer serving on the Balkan Front who, following an episode of bloody diarrhoea, developed an acute febrile illness characterised by arthritis, urethritis and conjunctivitis. Although the 'post-sexual' form of the disease is more common in Britain, the post-dysenteric form predominates in Continental Europe. The incidence of Reiter's syndrome in dysenteric patients has been estimated as 0.24 per cent and only 0.8 per cent of patients with nonspecific urethritis develop Reiter's disease.

The diagnostic triad in Reiter's disease consists of urethritis, conjunctivitis and arthritis. Even though one of these may be absent, the disease may still be diagnosed and it should be noted that urethritis can occur in the post-dysenteric form of the disease. Other well-recognised features include oral and genital ulceration, the skin lesions of keratoderma blennorrhagica and pain in the heels, which is frequently associated with calcaneal spurs. The arthritis varies in severity from a mild, transient synovitis to a chronic destructive arthritis.

The sex incidence is striking in that Reiter's disease occurs about 20 times more frequently in men than in women.

Urethritis is usually the first feature to appear and in some cases can occur up to one month after sexual exposure or the attack of diarrhoea. The discharge which is often mild, thin, watery or mucopurulent, but rarely blood-stained, is accompanied by dysuria, frequency and suprapubic discomfort which testify to bladder involvement. Prostatitis and involvement of the seminal vesicles are frequent. Usually there are no sequelae, but cases of hydronephrosis as a late complication of diminished bladder capacity have occurred. Chlamydial organisms can be isolated from this type of urethritis and although in a number of patients these organisms together with T-strain mycoplasma have been isolated from synovial fluid, the conjunctiva and urethra, the significance is uncertain.

Mucocutaneous lesions in the glans penis commonly accompany the discharge and form a characteristic feature of the disease, often coalescing to form circinate patches. Identical lesions found on the mouth in ten per cent of patients are painless and subside spontaneously (Figure 7.20).

The typical cutaneous lesions of Reiter's disease is keratodermia blennorrhagica (Figure 7.21). Appearing initially as a red macular eruption, it becomes hyperkeratotic and histologically identical to pustular psoriasis. The eruptions can occur anywhere on the body, but are seen most characteristically on the palms of the hands and soles of the feet. The crust is eventually shed leaving no scar. If the nails become involved, a yellow waxy mass forms under the nail which may force it right off.

Frequent transient abnormalities of cardiac conduction which may extend to complete heart block may occur alone or as part of cardiac disease accompanied by pericarditis and aortic valve disease. Transient pulmonary shadowing has been described (Cratter and Moskovitz, 1962).

The arthritis tends to involve large weight-bearing joints. Reiter's disease may on occasion be monoarticular but this is uncommon and is usually asymmetrical involving fingers and toes. In a typical case, arthritis which may be of sudden onset and be very severe, may last for weeks to months. If incorrectly treated permanent joint damage may result. A feature of the arthritis is its tendency to recur and over 60 per cent of cases have two attacks or more. Symptom-free intervals of ten years or more are not uncommon but in a small number of patients no clearcut remission occurs.

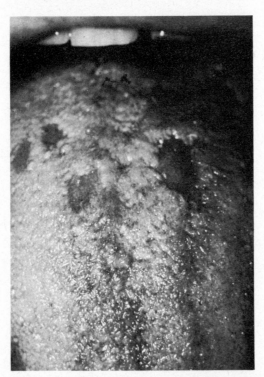

Figure 7.20.   Ulceration of the tongue in a patient with Reiter's disease. These ulcers are similar to those found on the penis.

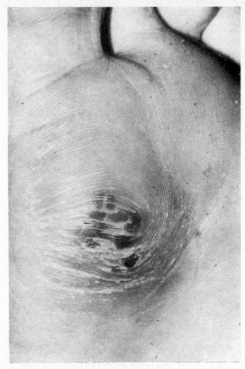

Figure 7.21.   Keratodermia blennorraghica of Reiter's disease histologically identical to pustular psoriasis.

Radiological examination in the early weeks may reveal no abnormality, or at the most some juxta-articular osteoporosis. Periostitis is a characteristic finding and should be sought, especially in the metatarsals and in the phalanges of the feet; the new bone formation has an exuberant fluffy appearance. Plantar calcaneal spurs occur in 20 to 45 per cent of cases. Unilateral or bilateral changes are seen in the sacroiliac joints, the frequency increasing to 50 per cent after five years and changes of ankylosing spondylitis may be seen in the spine.

Both the skin lesions and the arthropathy may resemble psoriasis and cases have been described when apparently typical Reiter's disease has progressed to typical psoriatic arthropathy. The link is emphasised by family studies, where among the male relatives of patients with Reiter's disease, the prevalence of psoriasis is 13 per cent.

Ocular involvement

Conjunctivitis

Among the connective tissue diseases, Reiter's disease and psoriasis are the only conditions in which conjunctivitis is a complication. About one-third of the patients develop a mild bilateral mucopurulent conjunctivitis appearing within four weeks of the onset of the disease. The conjunctiva is hyperaemic with little or no follicular or papillary reaction in the bulbar, tarsal and fornix conjunctivae. Although chlamydia have been grown from the conjunctival sac from time to time, the conjunctivitis of Reiter's disease has none of the follicular reaction seen from chlamydial infection of trachoma and inclusion conjunctivitis. The discharge when present is yellow, and though not particularly tenuous in consistency it may be copious in amount. The conjunctivitis is usually transient, but if it persists the bulbar conjunctiva develops a mild overall congested appearance as though the patient had been in a smoky atmosphere (Figure 7.22) and the eye is extremely uncomfortable (Figure 7.23). Treatment with antibiotics has no effect on the conjunctivitis.

Scleral and episcleral involvement

Inflammation of these tissues occurs but rarely. Reiter's disease is yet another example of the difference between inflammation of the conjunctiva and the episclera: two tissues which appear so similar are juxtaposed yet inflammation of one seems to exclude inflammation of the other.

Both simple and nodular episcleritis and diffuse anterior scleritis have been seen during the course of the disease but only in the later stages and in patients with severe ocular involvement. Patients with scleritis will often admit to having had nonspecific urethritis in the past when directly questioned and some also have changes in the sacroiliac joints, but whether they have had some form of Reiter's disease in the past is difficult to determine.

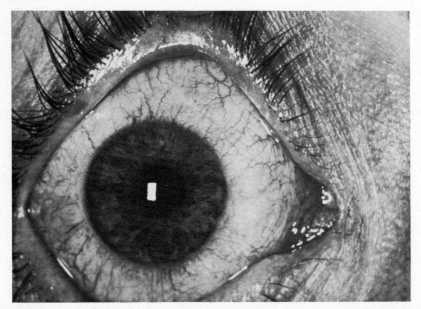

Figure 7.22. Reiter's disease. The conjunctiva is hyperaemic. There is no discharge, papillae or follicle formation.

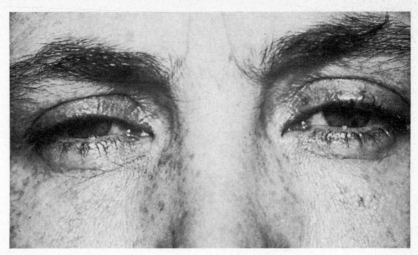

Figure 7.23. The typical appearance of a patient with Reiter's disease in which, because of the severe conjunctivitis and discomfort, the lids are held half shut and the blink rate is much reduced.

Keratitis

Less commonly the cornea becomes involved and then only when the conjunctivitis is severe. The keratitis usually consists of punctate epithelial erosions which may occasionally coalesce to leave a large ulcer. The stroma below and adjacent to the erosions may occasionally opacify but this change is never permanent. A mild uveitis may accompany the keratitis.

Uveitis

Uveitis when it occurs as the primary ocular lesion may be very severe, resembling that found in ankylosing spondylitis, with much exudate in the anterior chamber, dense synechiae and fine keratic precipitates. The uveitis is readily treatable with steroids but has a marked tendency to recur even though all the other signs and symptoms of the systemic disease may have disappeared. Secondary glaucoma can develop from pupil block and needs to be treated accordingly (Figure 7.24).

Reiter's disease should be suspected as a cause of recurrent uveitis and if searched for will probably be found (Catterall, 1961).

Other changes

Optic neuritis, retinitis and posterior uveitis have been recorded in Reiter's syndrome, but these complications are very rare and it is uncertain whether the posterior sclera is involved (Alagna, 1952; Mattsson, 1955).

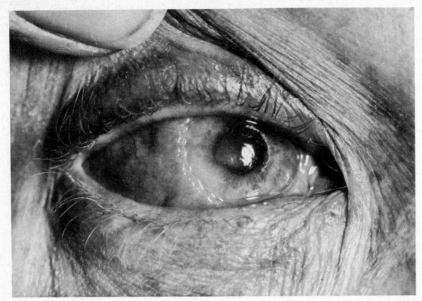

Figure 7.24. Acute anterior uveitis which developed three months after the onset of Reiter's disease in the same patient. The pupil is bound down, there is iris bombé and secondary glaucoma.

Arthritis of Chronic Inflammatory Bowel Disease

Joint manifestations in ulcerative colitis (Wright and Watkinson, 1965) and Crohn's disease (Haslock and Wright, 1973) take two distinct forms: an episodic synovitis mainly involving large weight-bearing joints or ankylosing spondylitis.

Synovitis occurs in about 12 per cent of patients with ulcerative colitis and 21 per cent of those with Crohn's disease. The synovitis correlates with exacerbations of ulcerative colitis and is more likely to occur when the bowel disease is extensive or when complications such as perianal suppuration occur. A total proctocolectomy abolishes the synovitis completely. The relationship is less clearcut in Crohn's disease and surgery never offers radical cure, but nevertheless synovitis correlates with bowel activity. The synovium shows nonspecific inflammatory changes and irrespective of the number of recurrences joint destruction does not occur.

Ankylosing spondylitis or sacroiliitis occurs in 17 per cent of cases and frequently antedates the bowel symptoms. Radical excision of the colitic colon does not provide a cure for the spondylitis and the iritis (Jayson et al, 1970). The involvement of the peripheral joints may lead to confusion with enteropathic synovitis but the presence of sacroiliac and spinal disease, the lack of association of joint and bowel symptoms, and the presence of radiological changes in the involved joints all help in differentiation.

Family studies show an increased evidence of sacroiliitis and ankylosing spondylitis in relatives, and this reinforces the view that the spondylitis is a hereditary accompaniment, rather than a complication of the bowel disease.

Ocular manifestations

Fifty-two per cent of those patients with bowel disease who develop ankylosing spondylitis are liable to develop an anterior uveitis, although this is not as severe as that seen with ankylosing spondylitis occurring on its own (Wright, 1965). At some stage during the disease, many patients will develop transient attacks of episcleritis and we have seen one patient with a recurrent nodular necrotising scleritis similar to that described by Jameson, Evans and Eustace (1973). Recently the patient seen in Figures 7.25 and 7.26 presented with a 15-year history of recurrent bowel ulceration and the sudden onset of a severe anterior necrotising scleritis in both eyes. Treatment with steroids stopped the condition from advancing further and a graft was placed over the defect. The patient found that thereafter the dose of steroids which kept the bowel symptoms under control was sufficient to prevent further inflammation in the eye. Billson et al (1967) found that in a survey of 465 patients with ulcerative colitis seven had episcleral and scleral involvement and five had iritis. Ellis and Gentry in 1964 also found five patients whose eye disease involved cornea, sclera and iris. The scleritis associated with Crohn's disease cannot be distinguished from that due to other causes and responds to treatment in a similar nonspecific manner.

Behçet's Syndrome

Behçet's syndrome has much in common with Reiter's syndrome, being characterised by ulcers of the mouth and genitalia, together with uveitis and hypopyon (Mason and Barnes, 1969). Joint involvement of varying severity occurs in 60 per cent of the patients, knees and ankles being the most frequently affected. However, unlike Reiter's syndrome the consequences are more severe and may include cranial nerve palsies, meningoencephalitis, organic mental syndromes, pseudobulbar palsy, hemiplegia and paraplegia. The disease, which is chronic in nature (men in the third decade being the most frequently involved), is characterised by recurrent attacks in which all or some of the symptoms may occur independently of each other. The oral ulcers, which are identical to 'aphthous ulcers' both in clinical appearance and histologically, are large and painful with a yellow base and a red halo around them. Each batch of ulcers may last any time from a few days to three weeks, recurring at intervals.

The genital ulcers occur on the scrotum or the shaft of the penis (rarely on the glans). In the female the lesions occur throughout the genital tract but are most commonly found on the labia and vaginal wall. These ulcers coalesce and may become destructive or serpiginous, resembling a cancerous process. No effective treatment is known.

Ocular involvement

Once the eye has become involved, blindness appears inevitable however vigorous the treatment and expert the care. The disease is always bilateral

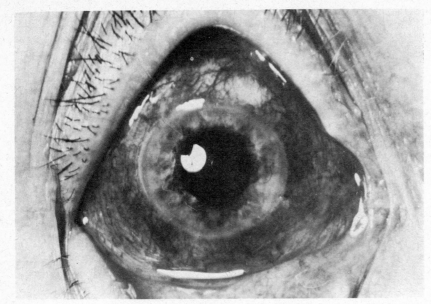

Figure 7.25.   Necrotising anterior scleritis with an avascular area above in a patient with long-standing Crohn's disease.

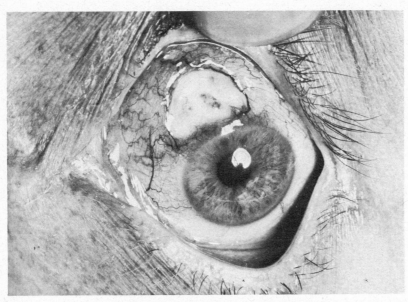

Figure 7.26.   The other eye of the same patient with total loss of scleral tissue. Progression ceased with treatment.

and the onset is often simultaneous in both eyes. The whole eye appears to be involved in the inflammatory process and although this usually manifests itself as a hypopyon, posterior uveitis, retinitis and perivasculitis have been known to precede the hypopyon. Appearances resembling classic retinitis pigmentosa have also been seen. Difficulty in viewing the fundus because of the anterior uveitis may have resulted in less attention being paid to these complications than they merit and may account for the hypopyon sometimes appearing without severe congestion of the anterior segment of the eye.

The uveitis settles spontaneously whether treated or not, but recurs at intervals of a few weeks to several years, causing synechiae formation and secondary glaucoma, and in the posterior segment retinal destruction, macular changes and optic neuritis. Eventually as the ciliary body is destroyed the eye becomes phthisical.

A keratitis has been described consisting of superficial punctate lesions, ulceration and red-stained opacities, but it is not clear whether these are the result of the intraocular inflammation or a separate lesion (Fruhwald, 1956).

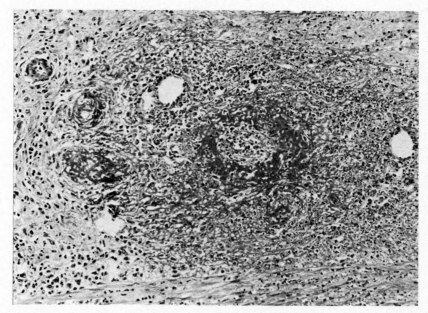

Figure 7.27.   Behçet's disease. A fibrinoid necrosis of a vessel wall typical of an allergic vasculitis.
Courtesy of Dr D. Wight, Cambridge.

Scleritis is not common, but we have recently seen two patients of Turkish origin who had developed genital ulceration and joint symptoms. They then developed a typical anterior diffuse scleritis of moderate severity in the absence of any other eye signs other than a few large cells circulating in the anterior chamber. The scleritis was treated with oxyphenbutazone and rapidly resolved but within six weeks they both developed a hypopyon with very little ciliary infection and no episcleral inflammation. Although the hypopyon resolved with local steroids, it did not appear that it was necessarily the result of treatment because the response was not dramatic.

Pathologically the eyes show a chronic inflammatory change of a granulomatous type which is most marked around vessels, particularly those of the uveal tract, and this has resulted in necrosis of the surrounding tissues. Inclusion bodies have been found in scrotal lesions by Behçet (1937) and others, but none has been found in the eye although Sezer (1953) produced a chorioretinitis, uveitis and hypopyon in rabbits inoculated with the contents of allantoic lesions derived from subretinal fluid and vitreous of patients with Behçet's disease. Although these results have not been convincingly repeated, it would appear that the signs of the disease are due to a viral infection and the response to this agent which may be in part an allergic vasculitis (Figure 7.27).

VASCULITIS

In this group of conditions in which the sclera is commonly involved, the primary cause of the eye changes appears to be a vasculitis. As a result either of vascular occlusion, increased permeability or immune complex deposition, irritative granulomatous or frankly destructive lesions occur. All these conditions are characterised by inflammation of the blood vessels, chiefly the medium or small-calibre arteries but sometimes very large arteries, all of which show fibrinoid necrosis in the vessel wall with some degree of associated granulomatous formation. There appears to be a spectrum of disease ranging from polyarteritis at one end, in which there is little or no granulomatous change but much change in the arteries, to Wegener's granulomatosis, in which there is a very large amount of granulomatous reaction but relatively little vasculitis. Joint involvement takes the form of an arthralgia, rather than an arthritis, the changes being extremely transitory and rarely, if ever, permanent.

Zeek (1952, 1953) has suggested the following classification of these conditions, based on clinical and pathological observations, which is now widely adopted:

1. Classical polyarteritis nodosa.
2. Hypersensitivity angiitis.
3. Arteritis occurring with rheumatic fever.
4. Allergic granulomatous angiitis including Wegener's granulomatosis.
5. Giant cell arteritis.
6. The vasculitis associated with the other connective tissue diseases: rheumatoid arthritis, systemic lupus, etc.

To this list we wish to add Cogan's syndrome and erythema nodosum.

Scleritis has never been described with rheumatic fever, but several patients who have developed episcleritis and scleritis have given a history of having had this condition in the past.

The syndromes are in general separable on the basis of clinical and histological features and by the distribution of lesions in the vascular system. The findings in individual cases may vary considerably, however, and diagnosis may prove impossible during life. For instance, Pitkeathly (1970) has described three patients with aortic incompetence and scleritis but with no evidence of rheumatoid arthritis. Blatz (1957) cited 18 patients who had necrotising scleritis and a presumed but unproven vasculitis. An attempt at separation is however of value, since there are appreciable differences in prognosis and appropriate therapy.

Polyarteritis Nodosa (PAN) and Hypersensitivity Angiitis

This is an affection mainly of the medium-sized arteries. Fibrinoid necrosis usually occurs at the bifurcation of a medium-sized vessel into its small branches or in isolated segments of medium and small vessels. The changes start in the media of the vessel and weakening of the vessel wall may result in aneurysm formation although this is less common than thrombotic occlusion. Healing takes place by scarring which often occludes the vessel causing infarction of the tissue beyond the obstruction, thus causing many of the manifestations of the disease. Practically every system in the body can be involved, the commonest being the central nervous system, the heart, kidneys and gastro-intestinal tract. Although histologically the vascular lesions in hypersensitivity angiitis which result from adverse reaction to drugs start in and around the smallest branches of the blood vessels and affect the intima and subendothelial ground substance, the lesions produced are very similar to those found in polyarteritis nodosa. The lesions affect smaller vessels and not specifically at bifurcations. The kidneys and gut are affected to a lesser extent, and the lungs more obviously. It possesses a much more favourable prognosis than PAN. Hypersensitivity to drugs, especially sulphonamides, appears to have been a major cause of polyarteritis in the past; the disease sometimes subsides following drug withdrawal (Citron, 1970).

It has been shown that a high proportion of patients with PAN have circulating hepatitis-associated Australia antigen in their blood (Gocke et al, 1970; Heathcote et al, 1972). Complexes of Australia antigen with immuno-globulin and complement have been shown to be deposited in blood vessel walls and renal glomeruli and associated at the sites of deposition with polyarteritis and glomerulonephritis (Nowoslawski et al, 1972).

Arteritis very similar to that seen in polyarteritis nodosa may occur in patients with systemic lupus erythematosus, which may be associated with the deposition of DNA–immunoglobulin complexes in the vessel wall. This observation has started a dispute as to whether the fibrinoid found in blood vessels is degraded nuclear protein or immunoglobulin (Vazquez and Dixon, 1957).

Clinical features

Unlike the other connective tissue diseases PAN is more common in men. It is characterised by intense inflammation of all three layers of the small and medium-sized arteries, together with the formation of multiple aneurysms. General malaise may be marked, particular features being myalgia, testicular pain and arthralgia. A variety of skin rashes occurs and purpura and peripheral

gangrene are common (Figures 7.28 and 7.29). Despite the many clinical manifestations of PAN a number of presentations recur:

1. Pyrexia of unknown origin and weight loss.
2. Nephritis.
3. Acute abdomen (haemorrhage, pancreatitis, small bowel ulceration, superior
   mesenteric artery occlusion).
4. Hypertension (rapid).
5. Asthma and focal pulmonary infiltrates.
6. Myocardial infarctions.
7. Peripheral neuropathy (mainly motor).
8. Muscle pain, tenderness and wasting.

Cardiac involvement occurs in up to 80 per cent of these patients. Persistent
tachycardia is an important finding and myocardial infarction may result from
vasculitis. The incidence of pulmonary involvement depends on one's definition
of the disease. Some separate those with pulmonary infiltrates, eosinophils
and asthma from the remainder. These findings occur in about one-fifth of
those with PAN.

Involvement of the kidney is the commonest cause of death in PAN and there
are a variety of pathological changes, including renal infarcts. Hypertension
is a difficult problem and occurs in up to 60 per cent of patients.

Abdominal pain is a major complaint and may result from a variety of
causes. Peripheral neuropathy occurs in one-half to two-thirds of these patients,
mononeuritis multiplex and mononeuropathy accounting for more than half.

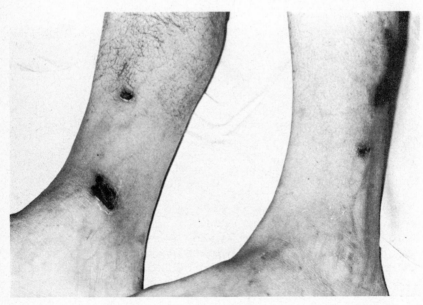

Figure 7.28.　Necrotic skin areas which are small and well circumscribed in polyarteritis nodosa.

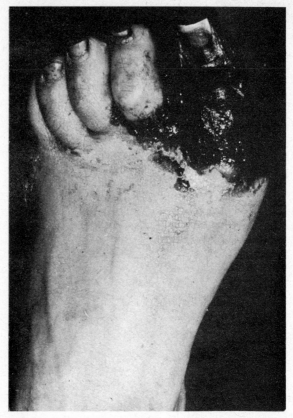

Figure 7.29. Involvement of a larger artery in polyarteritis nodosa leading to gangrene of the great toe.

Ocular involvement

Eye changes occur in 20 per cent of patients with polyarteritis nodosa and hypersensitivity angiitis.

Scleral and corneal changes

In hypersensitivity angiitis, all types of episcleritis and both anterior and posterior scleritis can occur depending on the severity of the underlying process and may precede the systemic manifestations by several years (Deutsch, 1966; Guseva and Shubina, 1973). The changes in classical polyarteritis nodosa are similar in the early and less severe forms of the disease but polyarteritis nodosa not infrequently presents as a necrotising scleritis requiring extremely vigorous treatment for its control (Cogan, 1975) (Figure 7.30).

When changes occur in the larger vessels at the limbus, quite characteristic

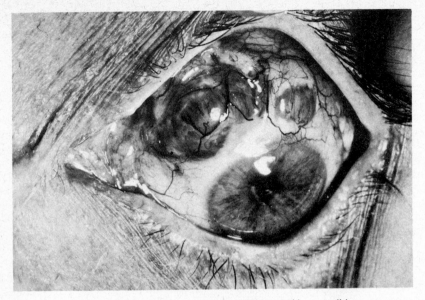

Figure 7.30.   Severe necrotising scleritis caused by vasculitis.

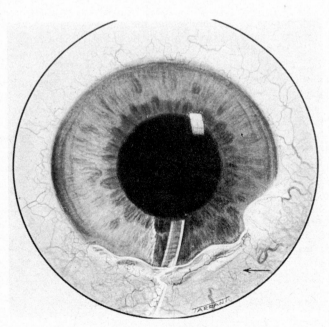

Figure 7.31.   Periarteritis nodosa. Deep guttering ulcer involving the corneoscleral margin. The scleral edge is well demarcated.

changes follow in the adjacent cornea and sclera. The eye becomes extremely painful, areas of the limbal arcade become avascular and simultaneously guttering of the peripheral cornea appears (Figure 7.31). These gutters have sharp edges and invade the scleral margin, the cornea remaining almost normal thickness. In certain areas just prior to the breakdown of the corneal stroma the deep stroma becomes densely infiltrated with grey opacities, the cornea becomes soft over these and the stroma becomes absorbed. The epithelium remains intact. If left untreated the gutter becomes circumferential and extremely deep but with treatment the opacities disappear and where no absorption of corneal tissue has taken place the cornea returns to normal or, at worst, retains a slight grey nebula. Where destruction has taken place, this will gradually fill in with fibrous tissue over the next few months, usually leaving a shallow but smooth-edged peripheral corneal gutter. The episcleral tissue overgrows any avascular areas. Perforation is very rare but if the cornea has become very thin then a lamellar annular graft can be used. Continuous treatment does not appear to inhibit healing.

Histologically the blood vessels in this area show the changes found in polyarteritis elsewhere (Sheehan et al, 1958), fibrinoid necrosis of the media extending through all the coats of the vessels which may be occluded altogether by oedema leading to thrombosis. The media is infiltrated with a pleomorphic inflammatory cellular infiltrate consisting largely of polymorphonuclear leucocytes. These cells spread out to the margin of the damaged corneal and scleral tissue where the collagen tissue begins to be destroyed. The first change which can be detected adjacent to these cells is that the collagenase coating which normally covers the mucopolysaccharide of the corneal collagen fibres disappears, indicating that the collagenase has been activated and is starting to destroy the underlying tissue. Whilst the disease is active no attempt at healing occurs, the defect being covered only by corneal epithelium.

The guttering seen in polyarteritis nodosa differs from that seen in Mooren's ulcer and rheumatoid arthritis uncomplicated by a vasculitis in that it is exceptionally painful, the edges are sharply cut off and the central cornea remains almost unaffected, is never eroded and rarely becomes oedematous.

In spite of the fact that the vessels of the whole of the uveal tract are known to be involved and the uveal tract infiltrated with inflammatory cells, uveitis is rarely seen clinically, and when it occurs is almost always posterior.

The commonest ocular change is in the retinal circulation where a retinopathy, indistinguishable from a severe hypertensive retinopathy, is produced, but again appears to be caused by vasculitis of the retinal vessels rather than as a result of systemic hypertension. Ford and Seikert (1965) found retinal lesions in 32 per cent of 114 patients with periarteritis. There is always a fluorescein leakage on angiography and sometimes a blood leak will give rise to intraretinal and subhyaloid haemorrhages. When the vasculitis involves the disc, papilloedema and central retinal arterial occlusion may result.

Treatment and prognosis

Prednisone is the drug of choice, although the results are often disappointing, especially in those with neuropathy. While immunosuppressives have been successful in treating Wegener's granulomatosis, their effectiveness in PAN must await greater experience.

The prognosis depends on the site and intensity of the vasculitis, but more favourable figures—70 per cent five-year survival and 50 per cent ten-year survival—are now being achieved.

Wegener's Granulomatosis

This is a rare condition where granulomatous angiitis involves arteries and veins throughout the respiratory tract and kidneys causing severe necrosis, ulceration and tissue gangrene. The ophthalmic manifestations include orbital lid oedema, nasolacrimal duct obstruction, conjunctival chemosis, sclerokeratitis, anterior uveitis and a retinal vasculitis with cotton wool exudates.

Wegener in 1936 realised that nasal granuloma and pulmonary arteritis probably formed a distinct symptom complex which was a clinical offshoot of polyarteritis nodosa.

The three pathological diagnostic criteria are (Godman and Churg, 1954):

1. Necrotising granulomatous lesions of the respiratory tract.
2. Generalised necrotising angiitis.
3. Renal involvement with necrotising glomerulitis.

The condition is commonest in the fourth and fifth decades and was until recently almost invariably fatal, running a rapidly progressive course over a period of a few months. The most common causes of death are renal failure and respiratory insufficiency.

The aetiology is obscure. Among the various causes suggested are infection (Mills, 1958), although no single microbial agent has been isolated, and auto-immunity (Blatt et al, 1959). Recently it has been suggested that the disease may be associated with a partial cell-mediated immunodeficiency (Shillitoe et al, 1974).

Wegener's granulomatosis shares many clinical and pathological features with polyarteritis nodosa, and the differential diagnosis, which can be difficult, may have to be made by lung or renal biopsy.

Treatment with corticosteroids and immunosuppressive drugs in combination has been associated with prolonged remission.

Ocular complications

Forty-three per cent of patients with this condition have some eye involvement (Straatsma, 1957). There is either direct involvement, characteristically a necro-tising angiitis, scleritis and peripheral keratitis, or invasion of the posterior segment by granulation tissue.

When the eye is involved by direct spread of the granuloma from the para-nasal sinuses, the patient has proptosis which may be very severe, limitation of movement of the globe and a rapid reduction in vision either due to the involvement of the optic nerve or more usually to an exudative retinal detach-ment resulting from a posterior scleritis. However, the eye may be involved without orbital involvement. The anterior sclera is almost always involved by a massive necrotising scleritis which advances with alarming rapidity unless treated very vigorously.

A marginal guttered peripheral keratitis exactly like that seen in polyarteritis nodosa almost always accompanies the scleral disease (Figures 7.32 and 7.33) which is histologically the same as that pattern seen in inflammatory scleral disease of any other origin in that there is a very obvious vasculitis of the major vessels and a granulomatous reaction in which giant cells are prominent (Frayer, 1960). Histologically, the perilimbal corneal ulcer is well demarcated, the stromal collagen being destroyed to the level of Descemet's membrane. The edges of the ulcer contain epithelioid and giant cells and the adjacent sclera is infiltrated with masses of lymphocytes, plasma cells and epithelioid cells (Frayer, 1960; Ferry and Leopold, 1970). Rarely a superficial or mid-stromal keratitis may occur without other eye changes.

The proptosis, which is a common clinical feature, is due to the invasion of first the orbit and later the sclera by granulomatous tissue. The sclera is destroyed from outside inwards; the episcleral covering becomes infiltrated and destroyed and the underlying collagen attacked by the granulation tissue, which contains many eosinophils, lymphocytes and monocytes. The histological picture differs from that usually seen in scleral inflammatory disease in that the invasion is from the outside rather than from foci within the sclera; very large areas of sclera are involved, giant cell, eosinophil and epithelioid cells being the prominent features. The associated mild vasculitis involves the larger vessels of the orbit and optic nerve as well as the intraocular vessels. Straatsma (1957) has also noted this clinically as cotton wool spots and narrowed arteries in spite of a normal blood pressure. Shindo (1965) also reported a very intense papilloedema as an early presenting feature.

In the occasional patient who has recovered or gone into remission, the scleral lesions have responded with healing of the defects, even though the cornea is scarred and the sclera thin.

Giant Cell Arteritis and Polymyalgia Rheumatica

Whilst scleral disease is an unusual complication of giant cell arteritis, when it occurs it is exceptionally resistant to standard therapeutic measures. The diagnosis needs to be considered in elderly patients with resistant scleral disease, who have a high erythrocyte sedimentation rate.

Giant cell (temporal or cranial) arteritis and the closely related condition of polymyalgia rheumatica have received increasing attention in recent years. Polymyalgia is often a manifestation of giant cell arteritis and some feel that all patients with polymyalgia rheumatica probably have arteritis (even if not clinically demonstrable). Evidence for this concept is not completely convincing, however. The clinical presentation of both can be often readily recognised, but a number of clinical features, many of a nonspecific nature, and the absence of physical signs may make diagnosis difficult. In view of the nonspecific laboratory findings, attempts to define precise clinical criteria have been made (Healey, Parker and Wilske, 1971).

Horton and his colleagues are usually credited with the first description

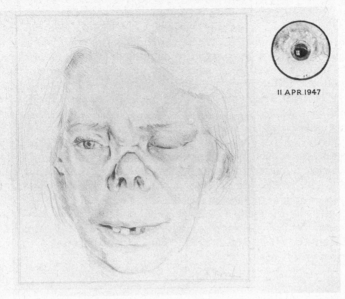

II APR 1947

Figure 7.32. A 58-year-old female with Wegener's granulomatosis and peripheral corneal guttering similar to that seen in polyarteritis nodosa. The left eye is proptosed and the root of the nose destroyed.

Courtesy the late H. B. Stallard.

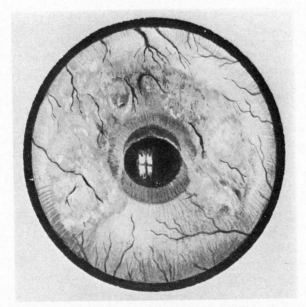

Figure 7.33. Seven months later both the guttering and the scleral involvement have extended considerably.

of giant cell arteritis. In 1932 they published a paper entitled 'An undescribed form of arteritis of the temporal vessels', and they suggested the name temporal arteritis. However, in 1890 Jonathan Hutchinson, a surgeon at the London Hospital, described a 'peculiar form of thrombotic arteritis of the aged, which is sometimes productive of gangrene'. An elderly porter at the hospital is described as having 'red streaks' on his head, which prevented him from wearing his hat. These proved to lie over his temporal arteries, which were inflamed and swollen on both sides. At first feeble pulsation could be detected but this ceased and the redness subsided. The old man lived for several years without any other manifestation of arterial disease. The arteritis was at first thought to be a benign condition, limited to the temporal arteries, but there was evidence of more extensive involvement in reports by Paviot and colleagues in 1934, and by Barnard in 1935. However, it was not until 1946 that Cooke and his co-workers emphasised its widespread nature.

Polymyalgia rheumatica was probably first described by Bruce in 1888 in a paper entitled 'Senile rheumatic gout'. The clinical manifestations were well described by Barber in 1957, and he also suggested the name which is now commonly used.

Incidence

Although several attempts have been made to determine the incidence of giant cell arteritis reliable data have proved difficult to obtain. Figures vary between 10 per 100 000 and 2.9 per 100 000 (Hauser et al, 1971).

The temporal arteries of all adults who died in hospital in Malmo throughout one year were examined by Östberg (1971) and although active temporal arteritis was not found, evidence of previous arteritis was found in one per cent of the specimens. It was found that in 75 per cent of these subjects there had been either biopsy evidence or a clinical history suggestive of temporal arteritis. This study suggests that giant cell arteritis may be underdiagnosed but further studies are required. The variety of symptoms and lack of specificity of signs and symptoms make such studies difficult.

Paulley and Hughes (1960) described giant cell arteritis as an 'arteritis of the aged', and with this disease and with polymyalgia rheumatica the age group most commonly involved is that between 65 and 70 years. However, younger patients can have these disorders and Mowat and Hazleman (1974) found that 35 per cent of their patients were under the age of 60 years. Bruk (1967) has suggested that the disease is more severe and that the incidence of arteritis is higher in those over the age of 60, but this has not been substantiated. Both conditions are more common in women.

Familial aggregation of polymyalgia rheumatica and giant cell arteritis has been reported by several workers (Barber, 1957; Hamrim, 1972).

Clinical features

There is an increasing tendency to consider giant cell arteritis and polymyalgia rheumatica as closely related conditions and it is difficult to maintain a practical distinction between them by clinical or histological criteria. Patients originally suffering from polymyalgia rheumatica have later had symptoms of cranial arteritis and in a number of patients with typical myalgia and those symptoms from the temporal region, biopsies have shown arteritic changes. Fauchald, Rygvold and Oystese (1972) studied 94 patients and found histological evidence of giant cell arteritis in 61. Systemic involvement was similar in the groups with or without clinical and/or biopsy evidence of arteritis. Of those with myalgia alone 40 per cent had a positive biopsy and of those with a proven arteritis only 11 did not have myalgia. The musculoskeletal symptoms are almost always bilateral and the onset can be sudden with pain and tenderness of muscle on periarticular structures. Patients may be so disabled in the early stages that they become dependent on others (Mowat and Hazleman, 1974). In this series of 59 patients evidence of an inflammatory synovitis was present in 15. The histology of the synovium showed nonspecific changes.

The systemic features of the disease can be vague and easily overlooked: they include fever, anorexia and weight loss. Conversely, they can be striking and may suggest neoplasia. Patients may present with a pyrexia of unknown origin. Despite a typical pattern of musculoskeletal symptoms and the presence in many of significant systemic features, there is often considerable delay before diagnosis—a mean of 6.2 months in one series (Mowat and Hazleman, 1974).

A hidden malignancy can mimic the symptoms of polymyalgia rheumatica and such patients do not usually respond to corticosteroids. Von Knorring and Somer (1974) have emphasised that the possibility of an underlying tumour must be considered even in long-standing cases of polymyalgia rheumatica although at present there is no evidence to suggest that malignancy is more common in these patients. The deterioration in health or a poor initial response to steroids must always be taken seriously and a search for an occult neoplasm must be made.

Abnormalities of thyroid and liver function have also been well described. Thomas and Croft (1974) in a retrospective survey of 59 cases of giant cell arteritis found five patients with thyrotoxicosis and this provides further evidence of an immunological basis for the disease. Raised serum values for alkaline phosphatase were found in 20 per cent of patients with polymyalgia rheumatica (Glick, 1972) and increased 5-nucleotidase values and/or mitochondrial antibodies were found in 50 per cent of the patients with a raised alkaline phosphatase. Long and James (1974) reported on a liver biopsy which showed portal and intralobular inflammation with focal liver cell necrosis and a small epithelioid cell granuloma.

There is often little to find on examination of patients with polymyalgia rheumatica, although anaemia and weight loss are quite frequent. The muscles may be tender and stiffness may limit joint range, but there is no muscle weakness.

The widespread nature of the vasculitis has been previously mentioned and a careful history and clinical examination will often aid diagnosis. Examination of the major vessels for tenderness or bruit, particularly over the subclavian vessels, may prove useful (Bruk, 1967). (These are presumably due to arteritis as they disappear with treatment.) An early sign of arteritis is increased sensitivity of the carotid sinus. Light pressure will often lead to transient asystole for two or more beats, and it is therefore advisable for the patient to be lying down. Ischaemia of the masseter muscles and involvement of the tongue may cause pain and even ischaemic necrosis. Tenderness in areas distant from arteries can be present even when the vessels are clinically normal (Ross Russell, 1959).

Ocular involvement

The ocular complications are not only devastating but are also largely preventable. Giant cell arteritis is associated with visual problems in 40 to 50 per cent of patients (Hunder, Disney and Ward, 1969; Hamilton, Shelley and Tumulty, 1971), and is due to involvement of branches of the ophthalmic artery, particularly posterior ciliary arteries.

Visual loss is usually profound, sudden and dramatic because of obstruction of the central retinal or posterior ciliary arteries or a branch of them. However, occasionally a patient will complain of transient blurring of vision or transient unilateral homonomous altitudinal hemianopia and such a symptom must be regarded very seriously, treatment being instituted with a high dosage of systemic steroid before any investigations other than an ESR are performed. Prompt action has saved many eyes; it should be remembered that if one eye is affected the other is likely to follow suit within five days.

When the central retinal artery or the main trunk of the ophthalmic artery is involved, the clinical picture is the same as that of a central retinal artery obstruction from any cause in that the retina is pale, oedematous with a cherry red spot at the macula. When the posterior ciliary arteries behind the disc are obstructed, the disc is swollen and there may be adjacent intraretinal haemorrhages when the occlusion first takes place (Figure 7.34), the oedema gradually subsiding to reveal a waxy grey disc. In this case the vascular supply to the nerve head is cut off even though the central retinal artery remains patent. If the arterial supply to the posterior part of the nerve is cut off, then an ischaemic neuropathy results. The eye looks normal but the vision is still lost.

Occlusion or inflammation of the anterior ciliary vessels gives rise to either anterior segment necrosis with a heavy uveitis and discoloured iris, or a scleritis. The long posterior ciliary arteries have been shown to be involved histologically by Daiker and Keller (1971).

The scleritis takes the form of a necrotising anterior scleritis which remains localised to one area of the globe, usually adjacent to or underlying one of the rectus muscles (Figure 7.35). One patient of ours with this condition uses the state of her eye as an indication of the level of her ESR and regulates her dose of steroids accordingly. (She is remarkably accurate.) Usually the scleritis is very difficult to bring under control and may be the source of considerable disability to the patient.

The uveitis associated with temporal arteritis has many of the features of anterior segment ischaemia. Horven (1973) has observed that patients with ophthalmic involvement may have a decreased amplitude of the ocular pulse pressure, indicating derangement of ocular blood flow; bruits may also be heard over an involved eye. Burian (1963) has shown that the A-wave in the ERG is very large in both affected and unaffected eyes and this falls to normal when treatment is instituted.

Cranial nerve palsies occur in 15 to 20 per cent of the patients and ischaemia of the muscles has been said to cause periorbital pain. Because of the concomitant involvement of the intracranial vasculature some patients are totally unaware that they have become blind, and being convinced that they can still see are a menace to themselves and others. Conversely, many patients for the same reason do not worry about their blindness as much as might be expected.

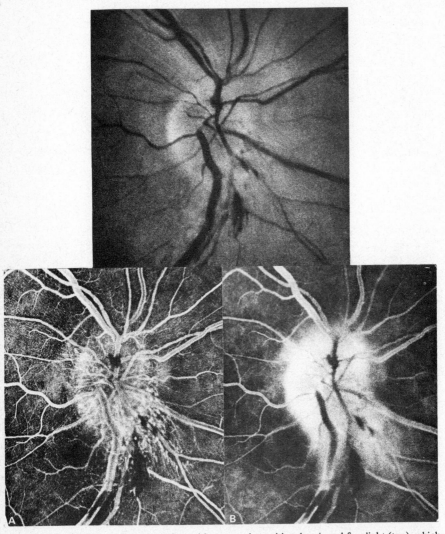

Figure 7.34. The optic disc in a patient with temporal arteritis taken in red-free light (top), which shows oedema of the disc and haemorrhages at the lower nasal margin. The fluorescein angiogram confirms the swollen disc which shows early filling (A) and late fluorescence (B).
Courtesy of Dr Alan Bird.

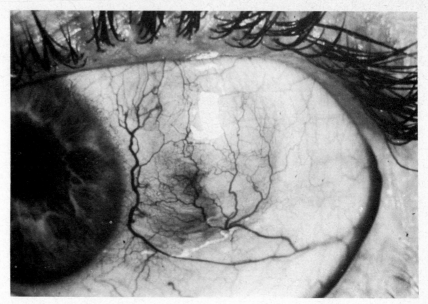

Figure 7.35.   Scleritis in temporal arteritis which is persistent and remains localised to one area of the globe.

Hunder, Disney and Ward (1969) have suggested that ten per cent of patients with polymyalgia rheumatica who develop arteritis will have visual loss. This probably errs very much on the conservative side, being low due to patient selection and early treatment with corticosteroids. We agree with Henkind and Gold (1973) that they should be treated as having temporal arteritis because recovery of useful vision seldom returns once affected. Although corticosteroids offer protection from involvement of the opposite eye and further progress of the systemic disease they have no effect upon established visual failure.

Laboratory investigation

The erythrocyte sedimentation rate is usually markedly elevated in almost all these patients and provides a useful means of monitoring treatment, although it must be appreciated that some elevation of the ESR may occur in otherwise healthy elderly people. Establishing a raised ESR is the key investigation although normal ESR may be found very occasionally in patients with active, biopsy-proven disease (Bruk, 1967).

Anaemia, usually of a mild hypochromic type, is common and resolves without specific treatment but a marked normoblastic anaemia occasionally occurs and may be the presenting symptom (Healey and Wilske, 1971). Protein electrophoresis may show a nonspecific rise in the alpha 2-globulin with less frequent elevation of alpha 1 and gammaglobulins and Fauchald, Rygvold and Oystese (1972) noted high gammaglobulin values in those with biopsy evidence of arteritis.

Temporal artery biopsy is of assistance when there is doubt as to the diagnosis but it only positive at sites of active arteritis. Temporal arteriography provides an additional diagnostic tool and may assist in selecting the optimal site for biopsy (Gillanders, Strachen and Blair, 1969).

If there are any eye signs treatment should never be delayed to await a biopsy result.

Pathology

Reports on the histology of giant cell arteritis have been published by several workers (Harrison, 1948; Bevan, Dunnill and Harrison, 1968). The arteritis is histologically a panarteritis with giant cell granuloma formation, often in close relationship to a disrupted internal elastic lamina (Figure 7.36). Large

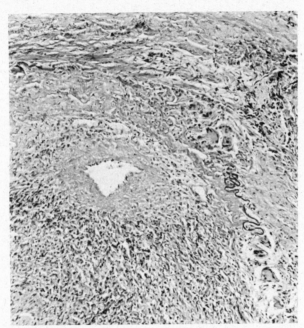

Figure 7.36.   Histology of giant cell arteritis showing disruption of internal elastic lamina.

and medium-sized arteries are usually affected but even the relatively small ciliary arteries and their terminal branches can be affected. The involvement is patchy and 'skip lesions' are often found. The gross features are not characteristic; the vessels are enlarged and nodular and have little or no lumen. Thrombosis is the exception and plays little part in the development of the lesion. The lumen is narrowed by intimal proliferation and this is identical to that of ordinary atherosclerosis. It seems probable that this is a nonspecific response and in vitro studies using radioactive sulphate (Balmforth, 1964) have shown fixation of the isotope by elongated mesenchymal cells lying adjacent to the damaged internal elastic lamina.

In the larger vessels, the adventitia is usually invaded by mononuclear and occasionally polymorphonuclear inflammatory cells, often cuffing the vasa vasorum, and here fibrous proliferation is frequent. The medial changes are dominated by the giant cells, which vary from small cells with two to three nuclei up to masses of 100 containing many nuclei. Here there is invasion by mononuclear cells resembling histiocytes. Fibrinoid necrosis is infrequently found. A definitive progression of changes can be demonstrated from the active infiltrative phase to the scarred artery with little cellular infiltrate (Kimmelstiel, Gilmour and Hodges, 1950). At first the most severe changes are centred on the internal elastic lamina which becomes swollen and fragmented (Parker, Healey and Wilske, 1972), and portions of this can be demonstrated within giant cells with surrounding plasma cell and lymphocytic infiltration. That the disease may have its origin as a lesion of the elastic lamina has been suggested and will be discussed later.

Histological changes also occur in temporal arteries with advancing age and they differ only in degree from those encountered in giant cell arteritis; it can sometimes be difficult to distinguish between the two (Ainsworth, Gresham and Balmforth, 1961). However, an inflammatory cell infiltrate does not occur except in relationship to large plaques of atherosclerosis.

The widespread nature of the vasculitis has been well documented, and involvement of the aorta and its branches, the abdominal vessels and the heart have all been described. The pulmonary and renal vessels and the small arterioles are generally not involved and this may be useful in differentiating between this condition and polyarteritis nodosa. Although there is a high incidence of involvement of the head and neck vessels in giant cell arteritis, it is interesting that the intracranial vessels are seldom involved (Crompton, 1958; Kjeldsen and Reske-Nielsen, 1968). Wilkinson and Russell (1972) studied the head and neck vessels and they demonstrated a close correlation between the susceptibility to arteritis and the amount of elastic tissue present in the arterial wall. Aneurysm formation is rare and this has been attributed to the protective role of the intimal proliferation (Harrison, Harrison and Kopelman, 1955).

There is little to support a concept of primary muscle disease in polymyalgia rheumatica. Serum aldolase and creatine phosphokinase are normal and there is no abnormality on electromyography (Bruk, 1967). Muscle biopsy has shown only mild atrophic changes and there is no evidence of inflammatory changes (Hamilton, Shelley and Tumulty, 1971; Brooke and Kaplan, 1972). Histochemical examination of muscle has demonstrated some abnormalities of the motor nerve terminals and end plates which have been interpreted as consistent with a neuropathy (Isaacs and Frere, 1973). However, it has been suggested by other workers that these changes are nonspecific.

Immunological processes have only recently been implicated in the pathogenesis of these conditions and Hazleman, MacLennan and Esiri (1975) have suggested that giant cell arteritis may arise as an immune reaction to the internal elastic lamina which has been damaged with advancing age. Certainly a widespread vasculitis would explain many of the features of polymyalgia rheumatica; Hunder, Disney and Ward (1969) found arteritis in 50 per cent of temporal biopsies and Fauchald, Rygvold and Oystese (1972) found arteritis in 20 temporal artery biopsies from 49 patients who had myalgia alone. Other workers are not convinced that the musculoskeletal symptoms are always due to arteritis and certainly arteries in painful areas may be normal. Many patients with temporal arteritis do not have associated myalgia and also when arteritis occurs in proximal vessels there is not always associated myalgia.

Giant cell arteritis is almost always limited to vessels with an internal elastic lamina. An electron-microscopic study (Parker, Healey and Wilske, 1972) showed fragmentation of the elastic lamina with mononuclear cell accumulation compatible with cell-mediated injury. The anterior ciliary vessels and peripheral retinal vessels, which have little or no elastic lamina, are very occasionally affected. Fragments of elastic tissue can be demonstrated within giant cells and Smith (1969) showed that giant cells engulf fibrillar material thought to be altered internal elastic membrane. Immunofluorescent techniques have revealed the presence of immunoglobulin and complement adjacent to the elastic lamina (Liang et al, 1974), and it is possible that elastic tissues are antigenic and that the deposited immunoglobulins are antibodies to this component of the arterial wall. However, another explanation could be that circulating immune complexes penetrate a damaged endothelium. The antigenic properties of elastin have been demonstrated by Papajiannis, Spina and Gotte (1970) when an injection of heterologous elastin produced an inflammatory reaction consisting of giant cells. Jackson, Sandberg and Cleary (1966) demonstrated precipitating antibodies to alpha-1 elastin.

Treatment

Treatment of patients with eye involvement with corticosteroids is urgent and obligatory if only to prevent similar changes in the opposite eye, which will be involved within five days if treatment is not undertaken (Egge, 1966). An initial loading dose of 80 to 120 mg of prednisolone is given and this dose reduced as soon as the ESR begins to fall. The dosage is now titrated against the ESR, the aim being to keep the ESR below 25 mg in one hour with the minimum dosage of steroid possible. It is important to remember that the ESR can be moderately high in this age group from other causes. If the ESR does not fall, the clinical symptoms are used as assessment of activity. Of 104 patients treated by Hollenhorst (1960) using this regime, only one lost vision after treatment was started.

Most of the symptoms of polymyalgia rheumatica are improved with salicylates or other anti-inflammatory agents. However, these drugs do not control the underlying arteritis and may allow vascular and ocular complications to develop. Corticosteroids dramatically relieve the myalgic symptoms and also suppress the arteritis and because of the difficulty in establishing the presence of vasculitis it is usually advocated that corticosteroids be used in almost every case of polymyalgia rheumatica. In an attempt to exclude arteritis in polymyalgia rheumatica, Hunder (1974) advocates generous biopsies of both temporal arteries plus a biopsy of the occipital artery if this is abnormal. If these biopsies are normal and there is no clinical evidence of arteritis, he feels that the changes of arteritis are small and that corticosteroids need not be given. Using this approach he has found that 50 per cent of patients can be treated satisfactorily with anti-inflammatory drugs alone. This approach has not found general acceptance and should be used with circumspection if there is any evidence of ocular disease.

It is rarely necessary to exceed 20 mg of prednisolone daily to control the myalgic symptoms but symptoms and signs of arteritis may require dosages exceeding 60 mg of prednisolone daily. The dramatic response to steroid therapy supports the diagnosis. The constitutional symptoms — muscle pain and stiffness — disappear within days although the ESR falls more slowly. Patients must be reviewed regularly for exacerbations of the disease or for the development of arteritis and the steroid dosage adjusted accordingly. In an attempt to avoid the side-effects of systemic steroids, particularly in susceptible elderly patients, Hunder and colleagues (1974) carried out a trial of alternate daily corticosteroid therapy. They concluded that these regimes did not control symptoms satisfactorily and could not be recommended for treatment of patients with severe disease.

Natural history

Patients treated with non-steroidal drugs usually recover without significant disability within two to four years (Gordon, 1960; Davison, Spiera and Plotz, 1966). It is debatable whether corticosteroids shorten the course of the disease; they probably suppress symptoms and signs whilst the disease runs its self-limiting course. In patients treated with corticosteroids it is often difficult to know when the disease is under control as many patients have symptoms from degenerative joint disease. Dixon (1969) has commented that these patients do not tend to develop the complications of steroid therapy that occur in similarly aged patients with rheumatoid arthritis. It should be emphasised that patients require subsequent follow-up as further episodes of disease activity can occur. Mowat and Hazleman (1974) reported an apparent second episode of typical polymyalgia rheumatica 12 months after corticosteroids had been discontinued. Fauchald, Rygvold and Oystese (1972) recommend continuing treatment for a minimum of two years since 13 of their patients who had been treated for an average of 16 months relapsed after steroid withdrawal. In three cases relapse occurred after more than one year. They report that there may be a persistent elevation in gammaglobulins and ESR may also be helpful. They show how biopsy studies demonstrate evidence of active arteritis ten years after completion of treatment.

Cogan's Syndrome

In 1945 Cogan described a syndrome consisting of an interstitial keratitis associated with profound deafness, vertigo and tinnitus. Several cases have been reported of this syndrome in association with periarteritis nodosa (Gilbert and Talbot, 1969) and very similar cases have been seen with scleritis or uveitis as an additional sign. It is probable that most examples of this syndrome are due to a vasculitis affecting the small vessels of the inner ear and eye.

The patients usually present with an inflamed eye, together with a rapid decrease in visual acuity.

Central yellowish opacities are noted in the deep stroma of the cornea, and neovascularisation occurs deep in the stroma, close to Descemet's membrane (Figure 7.37). A mild uveitis may be present with fine keratin precipitates on the posterior corneal surface in the region of the keratitis which lasts many months. As the inflammatory signs fade, the typical corneal changes of an interstitial keratitis remain, and these are indistinguishable from

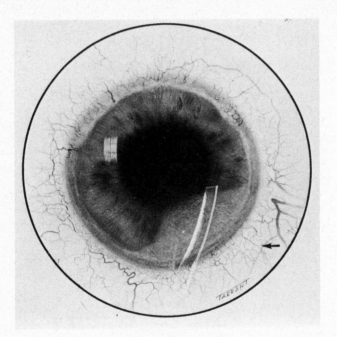

Figure 7.37. Deep infiltrate on Descemet's membrane of the cornea in a patient with Cogan's syndrome.

those found in old congenital syphilis. Deep stromal infiltrates remain in the cornea; the overall grey opacity is interrupted by clear intervals around the now empty old vessels. Although deafness usually occurs at the same time as the corneal or scleral involvement, it may precede the other signs by many months. When scleritis occurs as part of the syndrome it always seems to be of the nodular anterior variety and has always started close to the insertion of the medial and lateral rectus muscles.

Hypersensitivity Vasculitis

Henoch–Schönlein purpura (anaphylactoid purpura)

This is an allergic vasculitis of unknown cause in which preceding haemolytic streptococcal infection is no longer thought to be implicated. It can occur at any age but is particularly common in young children, especially boys. The peak age of onset is between two and five years. The onset is acute with fever, headache and a rash. Initially, macules or urticarial papules occur on the buttocks and the extensor aspects of the limbs. These become flat and purpuric and may coalesce or even ulcerate. Localised oedema of the face, scalp, hands and feet occurs. In young children it can mimic arthritis. Haemorrhage into the gut wall can cause colic, melaena or haematemesis. A flitting arthritis is common. The joint pain may be out of all proportion to the physical signs. A mild focal glomerulonephritis producing proteinuria and microscopic haematuria occurs in 50 per cent of cases (Meadow et al, 1972). Occasionally it progresses to the nephrotic syndrome and very rarely to renal failure. The disease usually settles in 4–6 weeks without sequelae, but may recur. Renal involvement, if not present initially, rarely develops in a second attack.

The eponymous title Henoch–Schönlein purpura derives from Henoch's original description of the colicky abdominal pain attributable to bleeding into, and oedema of, the intestinal wall and to the description of the articular manifestations by Schönlein. However, the condition was probably first described by William Heberden (Rook, 1958).

The joint symptoms consist of attacks of transient synovitis, leaving no residua, usually affecting the knee joints. Corticosteroid may be used to treat oedema and gastrointestinal symptoms. Simple episcleritis may accompany the onset of this condition or develop at any time during the course of the illness and may recur without any recrudescence of the other physical signs. Scleritis has never been described in this condition.

OTHER CONNECTIVE TISSUE DISORDERS IN WHICH THE SCLERA IS INVOLVED

Erythema Nodosum

Whilst erythema nodosum is a sign of other coexisting conditions, it warrants separate description because a nodular episcleritis so often appears at the same time as the skin lesions. The lesions occur most commonly in young and middle-aged females, particularly on the exterior surface of the legs and arms. The nodules, which are very often painful and involve the whole thickness of the skin, are between 1 and 7 mm in size; the centre of the nodule is purple and the periphery bright red. The eruption, which appears suddenly with fever, malaise and joint pains, disappears spontaneously. Although in many instances the cause is unknown, the following conditions are associated with erythema nodosum: tuberculosis, streptococcal and fungal infections, sarcoidosis, and drug allergy, particularly to sulphonamides.

Nodular episcleritis is commonly found at the same time as the eruptions appear under the skin, and resolves spontaneously as the nodules disappear. Scleral nodules, anterior uveitis and corneal involvement do sometimes appear during the course of the disease with which the erythema nodosum is associated. Whether the eye changes are related to the erythema nodosum or to the underlying disease is uncertain but they seem to require treatment directed specifically at them, rather than treatment of the general condition.

Relapsing Polychondritis

Jaksch-Wartenhorst in 1923 described a patient with polyarthritis and fever, who two months later developed pain in both ears which became swollen and later deformed. Three months later the nose collapsed giving a saddle-nose deformity and shortly afterwards the patient became deaf. These symptoms are now recognised as the cardinal features of the disease.

Relapsing polychondritis is a relatively uncommon disorder in which recurrent inflammation occurs in cartilage and other tissues with a high concentration of glycosaminoglycans. Inflammation of the pinnae and nasal cartilages is the commonest feature but the sclera, eustachian tubes, larynx, trachea, bronchi and costochondral junctions are frequently involved. Other features include arthropathy, intraocular inflammation, inner ear involvement, aortitis and fever. The majority of reported cases have had an illness confined to one or several of these features, but some have been associated with generalised vasculitis or collagen disorders such as rheumatoid arthritis (Dolan, Lemmon and Teitelbaum, 1966; Anderson, 1967).

Hughes et al (1972) listed the commonest presenting features in 98 cases (Table 7.8).

Table 7.8.   *Presenting features of relapsing polychondritis*

Symptom	No.
Inflammation of ear cartilage	31
Arthropathy	22
Inflammation of nasal cartilage	16
Laryngotracheal involvement	13
'Episcleritis'[a]	8
'Conjunctivitis'[a]	3
'Iritis'[a]	2
Low back pain	2
Vertigo	2
Painful exophthalmos and diplopia	1
Otitis media	1
Fever	1

[a] Hughes et al (1972) reported episcleritis and conjunctivitis as a complication, but we have not seen this. It may be that their cases were also of mild anterior diffuse scleritis.

Hughes et al (1972) have shown that at an early stage of the disease all classes of glycosaminoglycans are lost from the interstitial tissues of cartilage and vessels and this is evidence against a primary biochemical defect. Similarly there is evidence that autoimmunisation does occur but its pathogenetic significance remains to be demonstrated.

Pain, swelling and tenderness of subcutaneous cartilagenous structures, particularly the nose and panni, are common and lead to collapse of the nose and deformity of the ears, leading to suspicion of the presence of Wegener's granulomatosis (Figure 7.38). Inflammation of the tracheal rings also occurs and is a common cause of death from tracheal collapse and airway obstruction. Surgery to the nose, eye, or affected cartilage should be avoided as disastrous bleeding can occur.

Although tests for rheumatoid factor are negative, radiographs of the hands and feet may easily be mistaken for those of rheumatoid arthritis.

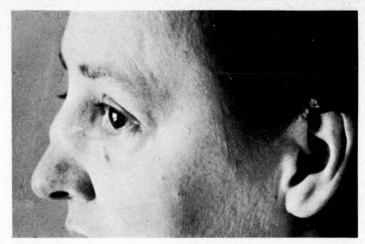

Figure 7.38. Loss of cartilage from the tip of the nose and the ear in a patient with relapsing polychondritis.
Courtesy of Alan Lyne, Peterborough.

Ocular complications are extremely common and are seen in up to 60 per cent of the patients, a scleritis and accompanying uveitis being by far the commonest and frequently the first presenting feature (Figure 7.39). Patients may have an episcleritis or true scleritis which may be diffuse, anterior, not necrotising and responding readily to treatment, or may be frankly necrotising.

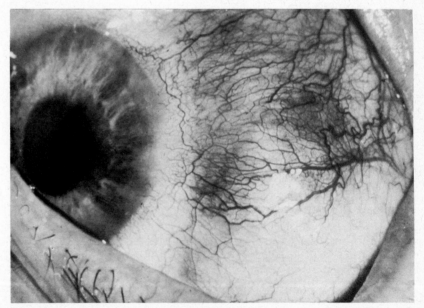

Figure 7.39a. Anterior diffuse scleritis in a patient with relapsing polychondritis. There is marked scleral oedema and increased transparency indicating an early necrotising disease.

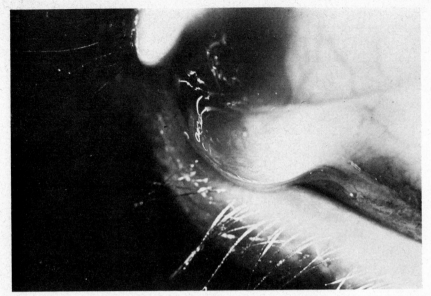

Figure 7.39b. Sarcoid nodule which appeared to arise in the deep conjunctival tissue and extended to involve the episclera and superficial sclera.

We have recently seen two patients who have developed severe necrotising scleritis. One of these has lost the whole thickness of the sclera on the nasal side and has required high steroid dosage for its control. The peripheral cornea can be involved, consisting of sharply demarcated gutters which look very like those seen in periarteritis nodosa. Uveitis may occur alone (Pearson, 1960; Kaye and Sones, 1964; Rucker and Ferguson, 1965) and McKay, Watson and Lyne (1974) have reported cases which presented with extraocular muscle palsies and proptosis. A posterior scleritis with involvement of the choroid and exudative retinal detachment is common (Anderson, 1966). Of the six cases reported by this author, five had evidence of posterior scleritis as we now define it, with exudative retinal detachments, swollen discs and areas of choroidoretinal scarring. One of these patients, who was mistakenly thought to have Coats' disease, had an exudative retinal detachment. The eye, which was obtained postmortem, showed granuloma formation in the sclera and adjacent choroid in the area where the retina was detached. Three of his cases showed evidence of vasculitis (one proved by conjunctivo-episcleral biopsy), two dying of rupture of intracranial and aortic aneurysms.

Sarcoidosis

Sarcoidosis is found in about four per cent of patients with granulomatous uveitis (Woods, 1961) but, conversely, uveitis is observed in about 25 per cent of patients with sarcoidosis. James (1974) has listed the clinical and laboratory associations in patients with ocular sarcoidosis (Table 7.9). It will

Table 7.9.   *Clinical and laboratory associations in patients with sarcoidosis*

Clinical associations	No. of patients	Percentage incidence
Females	100	68
Aged 20–50	112	76
Intrathoracic	111	75
Reticuloendothelial	65	44
Skin plaques (Figure 7.40)	53	36
Erythema nodosum	38	26
Nervous system	22	15
Parotids	14	12
Lacrimals	10	8
Bone cysts	12	8
Positive Kveim–Siltzbach test	105/132	80
Negative tuberculin test	83/124	66
Hypercalcaemia	20/99	20

be seen from this table that three-quarters of patients with ocular sarcoidosis are aged 20 to 50 years old, only three per cent are under 20 years and only 20 per cent over 50 years. James suggests the following diagnostic routine:

1. Full general medical examination to determine whether the disease is of acute or insidious onset. The prognosis is better and the response to corticosteroids good when the disease is of acute onset.

2. Biopsy of any enlarged lacrimal glands or obvious conjunctival follicles.

3. Chest radiography, since this is abnormal in three-quarters of patients with ocular sarcoidosis.

4. Kveim–Siltzbach and Mantoux skin tests, for these frequently provide diagnostic help.

5. Serum calcium (transient elevations are fairly common in sarcoidosis).

Sarcoidosis is best defined in terms of its pathology as a disease characterised by the presence in all of several affected organs of epithelioid cell tubercles without caseation (Scadding, 1970). The sarcoid tubercle consists of a rounded collection of large epithelioid cells without caseation. Lymphocytes tend to be sparse and concentrated at the periphery of the tubercle and giant cells may occur. Often the granulomas resolve completely but occasionally they become chronic and fibrotic, often leading to functional impairment.

The incidence of the disease in Britain is about 3 per 100 000 per year, being maximal in the age group 23 to 35 years (British Thoracic and Tuberculosis Association, 1969). It is especially prevalent in Negroes in the U.S.A. Women are affected more than men. The aetiology has not been established.

A common feature of sarcoidosis is multiple organ involvement, contrasting with the mildness or absence of symptoms. The most commonly involved organs are the lungs and the eye. Sarcoidosis is the commonest cause of erythema nodosum in the 20 to 40 years age group in Britain and this is not uncommonly the presenting symptom in Britain, although it is rarely so in the U.S.A.

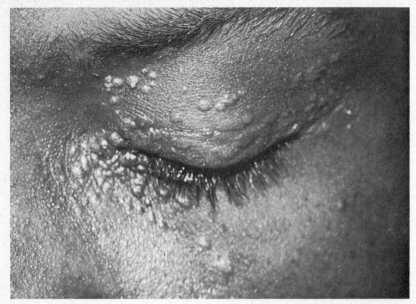

Figure 7.40.   Sarcoid nodules on the skin of the eyelid in a patient who also had a nodular scleritis and anterior uveitis.

Thoracic involvement

Bilateral hilar lymph node enlargement is often asymptomatic and resolves spontaneously within two years in some 90 per cent of patients. Pulmonary infiltration is the most important manifestation of sarcoidosis, since it may result in severe incapacity or death (Scadding, 1961). About two-thirds of patients undergo a complete spontaneous resolution of the pulmonary shadows, usually within two years.

Eye involvement

Anterior uveitis

Uveitis of the chronic granulomatous type occurs in about 33 per cent of patients with sarcoidosis (Figure 7.41) (Perkins, 1958). Both acute and chronic anterior iridocyclitis are seen in this condition. Acute anterior uveitis is less common, nonspecific, affecting both eyes, of sudden onset, and readily treatable with local steroid therapy. The chronic anterior uveitis is more typically found and is almost untreatable (James et al, 1964). The onset is insidious, affecting both eyes, and accompanied by minimal inflammatory signs. Typically waxy pink nodules appear over the surface of the iris and gradually coalesce. The cells present in the anterior chamber aggregate on the cornea and lens and in the angle, leading to glaucoma, cataract and phthisis bulbi.

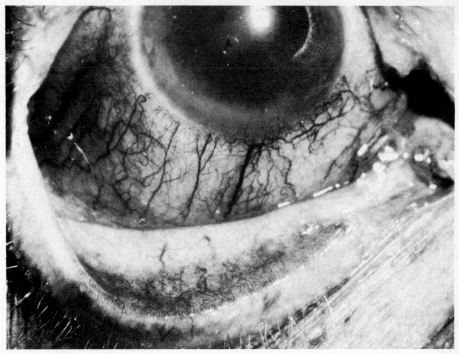

Figure 7.41.   Uveitis and diffuse anterior scleritis in a patient with sarcoidosis.

Posterior uveitis

Whilst involvement of the posterior segment is unusual, a waxy choroiditis, often related to blood vessels is so typical as to be diagnostic. A periphlebitis may be present at the same time and probably represents the drainage of the products of inflammation from the active lesion through the perivascular space (Figure 7.42, a and b). The fundus is often difficult to see because of the vitreous haze which usually accompanies the inflammation. Central nervous system involvement is found in 30 per cent of patients with posterior uveitis and sarcoidosis (Ricker and Clark, 1949).

Lacrimal gland involvement

This may occur either separately or as part of the conjunctival involvement in which case the tear secretion is very much reduced even though the gland may retain normal, causing a severe keratoconjunctivitis sicca. If the salivary glands become enlarged at the same time, this is known as Mikulicz's syndrome and if, in addition, the nervous system (usually the seventh cranial nerve) is involved, this becomes known as Heerfordt's syndrome (uveoparotid fever).

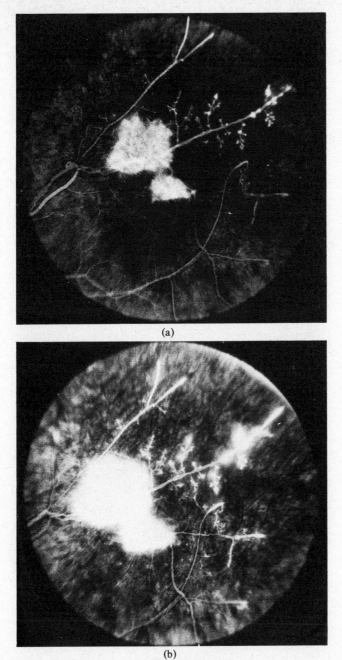

(a)

(b)

Figure 7.42.   Fluorescein angiogram of a 20-year-old patient with sarcoidosis who presented with an acute paraplegia. (a) Early arterial phase showing loss of capillary pattern and occlusion of the peripheral vessels which are clubbed. New vessel fronds are forming. (b) Late venous phase showing massive leakage of dye from the new vessels.
Courtesy of M. Sanders, London.

Conjunctival lesions

Conjunctival lesions occur in 14 per cent of patients with sarcoidosis; this may take the form of a diffuse infiltrate and subsequent scarring or nodule formation, usually in the lower fornix; these nodules sometimes occur on the bulbar conjunctiva in the limbal area where they are easily mistaken for a nodular episcleritis. The typical histological features are present in the conjunctival nodules; biopsy rarely confirms a diagnosis of sarcoidosis unless these nodules are very large and obvious.

Cornea

Although the cornea is usually involved as a result of accompanying uveitis, stromal keratitis can occur without any further ocular signs and when it does it tends to progress gradually throughout the whole of the cornea which may eventually need corneal grafting. Vascularisation may or may not occur in these lesions but never precedes the corneal changes.

Scleral and episcleral lesions

Episcleral lesions occurring in sarcoidosis are transient recurring episodes of inflammation which arise at the same time as the skin lesions, erythema nodosum or other systemic manifestations. Localised lesions on the sclera can be direct

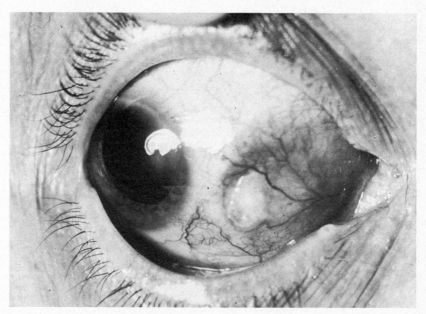

Figure 7.43.   Sarcoid nodule of the sclera.

extensions of uveal or conjunctival lesions, but diffuse scleral nodules can occur which are independent of any other intraocular inflammation (Ide and Inoue, 1968) (Figures 7.39a, 7.41 and 7.43). These lesions gradually disperse over a period of several months, recurring only if the systemic condition deteriorates. James et al (1964) described scleral 'plaques' which appeared to have been nodules in the sclera of three of 132 patients with eye disease and sarcoidosis. They all had erythema nodosum, lymphadenopathy, hilar adenopathy, pulmonary mottling and a positive Kveim test.

Optic nerve

Tumours at the optic nerve head and optic neuritis have been described but are rare.

Arthritis

A transient arthralgia is common in this disease and arthritis may occasionally be a major manifestation and may precede the other features of the disease. Arthritis of acute onset is polyarticular, usually affecting the peripheral joints and is associated with a good prognosis.

A chronic destructive arthritis may also occur. This is more common in Negroes and is usually accompanied by other signs of sarcoid. Synovial membrane biopsy may uncommonly reveal granuloma; radiological changes appear late and are thereafter of limited diagnostic value. The joint space is narrowed and mottled rarefactions and multiple 'punched out' cystic areas may be seen in the metacarpals and phalanges.

Diagnosis and treatment

Sarcoidosis is most reliably confirmed either by histology of biopsy material or by a Kveim test. Convenient sources of biopsy material are enlarged superficial lymph nodes, skin lesions and follicular conjunctival lesions. Less simple biopsy techniques include biopsy of sclera, liver or lung or of lymph nodes removed by scalene node biopsy or mediastinoscopy.

The Kveim test involves intradermal injection of an antigen consisting of a suspension of human sarcoid tissue. The site of injection is marked and biopsy carried out a month later. This reveals a characteristic granuloma in about 80 per cent of active cases of sarcoidosis. The test is less often positive in older fibrotic cases. The main disadvantages of this test are the scarcity of validated antigens, the frequency of negative reactions in long-standing cases and the occasional occurrence of false positive reactions.

There is a defect in cell-mediated immunity in this disease and this can be demonstrated by the paucity of skin reactions of the delayed type to PPD, mumps and *Candida albicans* (Topilsky et al, 1972).

Whilst corticosteroid therapy usually given systemically is mandatory for active uveitis, most other manifestations of sarcoidosis are best left untreated, since spontaneous resolution occurs in most cases. Controlled studies have shown that the corticosteroid suppression of the disease in the prefibrotic stage of pulmonary involvement does not improve the long-term outlook (Young et al, 1970).

Amyloidosis

The clinical features of this disorder are a consequence of the replacement and destruction of vital organs by the extracellular deposition of a proteinaceous substance known as amyloid. This material can be recognised by its homogeneous eosinophilic appearance with light microscopy, and by its staining properties with alkaline congo red and certain metachromatic dyes.

Amyloidosis is relatively rare as a clinically significant disease. Nevertheless, because of its association with a number of diseases involving the immune system and deposition of amyloid as part of the ageing process, amyloidosis has attracted the interest of clinicians, immunologists and pathologists since its discovery 125 years ago.

Electron-microscopy studies have shown that the apparently homogeneous amyloid material consists of characteristic long fibrils. These have a diameter of 100 to 150 Å and are made up of two longitudinal subunits or filaments 40 to 60 Å in diameter.

Classification

The following major forms of amyloidosis are recognised:

1. Primary amyloidosis and the type associated with plasma cell neoplasms.
2. Secondary amyloidosis.
3. A variety of familial forms, e.g. familial Mediterranean fever.
4. Amyloidosis associated with ageing.
5. Amyloidosis of certain endocrine glands.

It is generally possible to classify a particular patient on the basis of the presence or absence of other associated diseases and the tissue distribution of the amyloid deposits. However, it is now recognised that the organ distribution is not clearly defined between primary and secondary types in view of the frequent occurrence of deposits in atypical sites (Symmers, 1956).

Secondary amyloidosis

This is the most common form of amyloidosis and suppurative conditions such as osteomyelitis and bronchiectasis were the most frequent chronic underlying illness. With the decline of these illnesses, rheumatoid arthritis now ranks as the commonest cause and the incidence has been estimated to range from 20 to 60 per cent (Calkins and Cohen, 1960). In secondary amyloidosis deposits are most common in the eyes, kidneys, spleen, liver and adrenals and only rarely involve the heart and gastrointestinal tract.

Primary amyloidosis

This condition and the type associated with plasma cell and lymphocytic neoplasma are now recognised more frequently because of the wider use of tissue biopsies and the routine performance of immunochemical analysis of serum and urine. It has been suggested that idiopathic primary amyloidosis and myelomatosis are clinical expressions of the same abnormality of the plasma cells and that patients with primary amyloidosis ultimately develop clinical evidence of a plasma cell dyscrasia.

Though at one time it was suggested that only some 15 per cent of patients with myelomatosis had amyloidosis there is increasing evidence to link these two conditions (Osserman, Takatsuki and Talal, 1964). The concept that the elaboration of Bence Jones protein is associated with the development of amyloidosis has been strengthened by the finding that the amino acid sequence of fragments of amyloid protein is homologous with a part of the kappa type of light chain (Glenner, Ein and Terry, 1972).

The distribution of amyloid involves tongue, heart and skeletal muscle and gastrointestinal tract, but can also involve the same organs as the secondary type. These patients often present to rheumatologists because of a carpal tunnel syndrome, periarticular thickening or synovial infiltration.

The polyarthritis due to the deposition of amyloid in or around joints can mimic rheumatoid arthritis with symmetrical swelling of joints due to invasion of synovial tissue. The tendons and their sheaths may be affected. The diagnosis should be suspected in a middle-aged patient who, in addition to joint symptoms, presents with profound weakness and features suggesting deposits in sites other than joints.

The presence of amyloidosis should be expected whenever one encounters hepatosplenomegaly, unexplained renal disease, macroglossia, unexplained neuromuscular disease, congestive heart failure or malabsorption. A biopsy of an involved organ or, if not possible, a rectal biopsy is likely to yield positive results in 80 per cent of patients with amyloidosis.

The urine should be tested for Bence Jones protein, though occasionally the serum proteins will show an increase with a typical 'M' component, or the bone marrow plasmacytosis may be the first finding.

Nature of amyloid fibrils

In general, amyloid fibrils are composed of two major types of proteins which exist either singly or in combination. One of these, present as the major and often sole constituent in amyloid of the primary and myeloma-associated types, consists of fragments of immunoglobulin light chains. This group of proteins, first identified by Glenner, Ein and Terry (1972) is now called AL (amyloid L-chain) protein and is usually associated with a similar L-chain-containing immunoglobulin in the serum. Although it is clear that these immunoglobulins constitute most if not all of the protein in this type of amyloid fibril, it is not yet certain whether the fragments are synthesised as such, or if they are the result of degradation of an intact L-chain. The latter appears more likely.

Amyloid fibrils from patients with the secondary type of amyloidosis consist primarily of another protein that is unrelated to any known immunoglobulin. Using antisera to this component, it has been possible to detect in serum an antigenically related larger component known as SAA (serum A-related) protein which it is hoped will ultimately be shown to be the precursor of the tissue component.

Although this advance in our knowledge has at present few clinical implications, it seems likely that they will soon be of value. For instance, antisera specific for the conformational antigens of the fibrils may prove useful as sensitive diagnostic reagents in examining biopsies, and may allow us to classify patients more accurately.

Pathogenesis

Amyloidosis is associated with exposure to a large antigenic load. In the pre-antibiotic era, by far the highest incidence of amyloidosis was seen in association with chronic states of infection, states presumably associated with prolonged immunological stimulation. Amyloid occurs in horses subjected to prolonged immunisation for the commercial production of antisera. Furthermore, amyloidosis can be produced by repeated injections of casein into mice.

Recent studies indicate that the deposition of amyloid may be accompanied by depressed T-cell function (Scheinberg and Cathcart, 1974), can be accelerated by immunosuppressive agents, and often accompanies naturally occurring immunodeficiency states (Mandema et al, 1968).

Franklin and Zucker-Franklin (1972) have suggested that amyloid appears to be deposited in situations in which the immune system is overwhelmed by an antigenic load or in which it undergoes neoplastic transformation. These findings suggest that, if the stimulus is removed, amyloid production may stop but the situation may be irreversible. Although some instances of disease regression after care of the underlying condition have been reported, the resistance of amyloid to proteolysis hinders the ready removal of material (Sorenson and Binington, 1964).

Kedar, Ravid and Sohar (1974) have recently reported that colchicine can prevent the appearance of amyloidosis in mice given casein. Although the exact mechanism of action of colchicine is unknown, this finding warrants a trial of this drug in human amyloidosis.

Ocular complications

The conjunctiva is the most frequently affected tissue in the eye, the affection occurring alone and as part of a generalised amyloidosis. The lesions start in the fornix and conjunctiva, spreading later to involve the bulbar conjunctiva as well. The tumour-like masses found may become enormous so that the patient is unable to lift the lid (Figure 7.44). The only effective treatment is incision and mucous membrane grafting.

The cornea may be involved either as part of a generalised amyloidosis of the conjunctiva, in which case the lesion resembles a band-shaped keratopathy, or if it results from prolonged and recurrent inflammation of the cornea, lumps appear on the corneal surface as in Salzmann's dystrophy.

Amyloid changes also follow intraocular inflammation involving iris, stroma and choroid. Russell bodies, dense accumulations of plasma cells, may be found on the iris or floating free in the aqueous in chronic uveitis. The rare primary familial amyloidosis which affects vascular and mucous tissues also involves the eye in ten per cent of patients leading to proptosis, ptosis

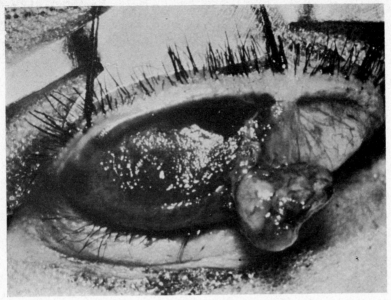

Figure 7.44. Tumour-like masses of amyloid of the conjunctiva of the upper lid.

and to infiltration of conjunctiva, cornea, sclera and choroid. When involved, the vitreous looks like glass wool (Paton and Duke, 1966) and may be so opaque as to obscure vision.

No specific scleral lesion has been described in amyloidosis even in patients in whom the sclera has later been found to be infiltrated.

Weber–Christian Disease

This condition is also known as relapsing febrile nodular non-suppurative panniculitis (MacDonald and Feiwel, 1968). It is of unknown cause and focal inflammatory lesions appear in the panniculus adiposus associated with fever. It is more common in adults; rarely is it associated with other connective tissue diseases and there are none of the 'markers' of an autoimmune process.

The lesions in the panniculus pass through three stages: first there is focal degeneration and necrosis of the fatty tissue with an aggregation of inflammatory cells; these are replaced by macrophages and at this stage the lesion contains many foam cells; finally the cellular infiltrate disappears and fibrosis follows.

The disease is marked by the appearance of nodules, 2 cm or more in diameter, in the subcutaneous fat, particularly of the arms, thighs, chest wall and buttocks. At first they are rounded and tender; later the skin becomes adherent, reddened and often oedematous. Finally the nodule resolves to leave a saucer-like depression of fat atrophy, often with a faint brown staining of the skin. The nodules tend to occur in crops and in the early stages they are accompanied by fever and malaise. Similar nodules occur in the scleral tissue (Freidman and Henkind, 1974).

There is no specific treatment; corticosteroids will usually control the acute symptoms but appear to have no sustained beneficial effect. Although long remissions occur, relapses are frequent.

REFERENCES

Agnello, V., Koffler, D. & Kunkel, H. G. (1973) Immune complex system in the nephritis of systemic lupus erythematosus. *Kidney International*, 3, 90–99.

Aho, K., Ahvonen, P., Lassus, A. et al (1973) HL-A27 in reactive arthritis. A study of yersinia arthritis and Reiter's disease. *Arthritis and Rheumatism*, 17, 521–526.

Ainsworth, R. W., Gresham, G. A. & Balmforth, G. V. (1961) Pathological changes in temporal arteries removed from unselected cadavers. *Journal of Clinical Pathology*, 14, 115–119.

Alagna, G. (1952) Su di una rara complicanza oculare nella sindrome di Reiter. *Archivio di Ottalmologia*, 56, 5–26.

Ansell, B. M. (1974) Acute arthritis in children. *Current Medical Research and Opinion*, 2, 594.

Ashton, N. & Hobbs, H. E. (1952) Effect of cortisone on rheumatoid nodules of the sclera (scleromalacia perforans). *British Journal of Ophthalmology*, 36, 373–384.

Bacon, P. A. & Gibson, D. G. (1974) Cardiac involvement in rheumatoid arthritis: an echo-cardiographic study. *Annals of the Rheumatic Diseases*, 33, 20–24.

Baker, M. (1973) Psychopathology in systemic lupus erythematosus. I. Psychiatric observations. *Seminars in Arthritis and Rheumatism*, 3, 95–110.

Ball, J. (1971) Enthesopathy of rheumatoid and ankylosing spondylitis. *Annals of the Rheumatic Diseases*, 30, 213–223.

Balmforth, G. V. (1964) *Temporal arteritis: a Clinical and Laboratory Study.* M.D. Thesis, University of London.

Barber, H. S. (1957) Myalgic syndrome with constitutional effects: polymyalgia rheumatica. *Annals of the Rheumatic Diseases*, 16, 230–237.

Barnard, W. G. (1935) Tuberculous arteritis. *Journal of Pathology and Bacteriology*, 40, 433–436.

Barnes, C. G., Turnbull, A. L. & Vernon-Roberts, B. (1971) Felty's syndrome. A clinical and pathological survey of 21 patients and their response to treatment. *Annals of the Rheumatic Diseases*, 30, 359–374.

Beck, J. S. & Rowell, N. R. (1966) Discoid lupus erythematosus. *Quarterly Journal of Medicine*, 35, 119–136.

Beck, J. S., Anderson, J. R., McElhinney, A. J. et al (1962) Antinuclear antibodies. *Lancet*, ii, 575–577.

Behçet, H. (1937) Ueber rezidivierende, aphthose, durch ein Virus verursachte Geschwüre am Mund, am Auge und der Genitalien. *Dermatologisches Wochenschrift*, 105, 1152–1157.

Bennett, G. A., Zeller, J. W. & Bauer, W. (1940) Subcutaneous nodules of rheumatoid arthritis and rheumatic fever. *Archives of Pathology*, 30, 70–89.

Bennett, R., Hughes, G. R., Bywaters, E. G. et al (1972) Neuropsychiatric problems in systemic lupus erythematosus. *British Medical Journal*, iv, 342–345.

Bergaust, B. & Abrahamsen, A. M. (1969) Relapsing polychondritis. *Acta Ophthalmologica*, 47, 174–181.

Bevan, A. T., Dunnill, M. S. & Harrison, M. J. (1968) Clinical and biopsy findings in temporal arteritis. *Annals of the Rheumatic Diseases*, 27, 271–277.

Billson, F. A., deDombal, F. T., Watkinson, G. et al (1967) Ocular complications of ulcerative colitis. *Gut*, 8, 102–106.

Blatt, I. M., Seltzer, H. S., Rubin, P. et al (1959) Fatal granulomatosis of the respiratory tract. *Archives of Otolaryngology*, 70, 707–757.

Blatz, G. (1957) A case history of scleromalacia associated with rheumatism and Mönckeberg's sclerosis. *Klinische Monatsblatter für Augenheilkunde*, 131, 396–400.

Bloch, K. J. & Bunim, J. J. (1963) Sjögren's syndrome and its relation to connective disease. *Journal of Chronic Diseases*, **16**, 915–927.

Bloch, K. J., Buchanan, W. W., Wohl, M. J. et al (1965) Sjögren's syndrome, clinical, pathological serological study of 62 cases. *Medicine,* **44**, 187–231.

Brewerton, D. A. (1975) Histocompatibility and rheumatic disease. *Annals of the Rheumatic Diseases*, Supplement, **1–34**.

Brewerton, D. A., Caffrey, M., Nicholls, A. et al (1973a) Reiter's disease and HL-A27. *Lancet,* **ii**, 996–998.

Brewerton, D. A., Caffrey, M., Nicholls, A. et al (1973b) Acute anterior uveitis and HL-A27. *Lancet,* **ii**, 994–996.

British Thoracic and Tuberculosis Association Research Sub-Committee (1969) Geographical variation in the incidence of sarcoidosis in Great Britain: comparative study in four areas. *Tubercle,* **50**, 211–232.

Brooke, M. H. & Kaplan, H. (1972) Muscle pathology in rheumatoid arthritis, polymyalgia rheumatica and polymyositis: a histochemical study. *Archives of Pathology,* **94**, 101–118.

Bruce, W. (1888) Senile rheumatic gout. *British Medical Journal,* **ii**, 811–813.

Bruk, M. I. (1967) Articular and vascular manifestations of polymyalgia rheumatica. *Annals of the Rheumatic Diseases,* **26**, 103–116.

Buchanan, W. W., Cox, A. G. & Harden, R. M. (1966) Gastric studies in Sjögren's syndrome. *Gut,* **7**, 351–354.

Burian, H. M. (1963) Electroretinography in temporal arteritis. *American Journal of Ophthalmology,* **56**, 796–800.

Butler, J. J. (1969) Non-neoplastic lesions of lymph nodes of man to be differentiated from lymphomas. *National Cancer Institute Monograph,* **32**, 233–255.

Bywaters, E. G. L. (1967) A survey of Still's disease. *Annals of the Rheumatic Disease,* **26**, 185.

Cairns, J. E. (1968) Trabeculectomy. *American Journal of Ophthalmology,* **66**, 673–679.

Calkins, E. & Cohen, A. S. (1960) Diagnosis of amyloidosis. *Bulletin of the Rheumatic Diseases,* **10**, 215–218.

Campbell, A. H. & MacDonald, C. B. (1965) *British Journal of Diseases of the Chest,* **59**, 90.

Caplan, A. (1953) Certain unusual radiological appearances in the chests of coal miners suffering from rheumatoid arthritis. *Thorax,* **8**, 29–37.

Catterall, R. D. (1961) Significance of non-specific genital infection in uveitis and arthritis. *Lancet,* **ii**, 739–741.

Cepellini, C., Polli, C. & Celada, F. (1957) A DNA reacting factor in serum of a patient with lupus erythematosus diffusus. *Proceedings of the Society for Experimental Biology and Medicine,* **96**, 572–574.

Chamberlain, M. A. & Bruckner, F. E. (1970) Rheumatoid neuropathy: clinical and electrophysiological features. *Annals of the Rheumatic Diseases,* **29**, 609–616.

Christenson, L. (1951) The pathology of collagen disease applied to the eye. *Transactions of the American Academy of Ophthalmology and Otolaryngology,* **55**, 536–542.

Citron, B. P., Halpern, M., McCarron, M. et al (1970) Necrotising angiitis associated with drug abuse. *New England Journal of Medicine,* **283**, 1003–1011.

Clawson, B. J. & Wetherby, M. (1932) Subcutaneous nodules in chronic arthritis. *American Journal of Pathology,* **8**, 283–293.

Cogan, D. G. (1945) Syndrome of non-syphilitic interstitial keratitis and vestibuloauditory symptoms. *Archives of Ophthalmology,* **33**, 144–149.

Cogan, D. G. (1955) Corneo-scleral lesions in periarteritis nodosa and Wegener's granulomatosis. *Transactions of the American Ophthalmological Society,* **53**, 321–344.

Cohen, A. S., Hughes, G. R., Noel, G. L. et al (1971) Character of anti DNA antibodies. *Clinical and Experimental Immunology,* **8**, 551–561.

Collins, D. H. (1937) The subcutaneous nodule of rheumatoid arthritis. *Journal of Pathology and Bacteriology,* **45**, 97–115.

Cooke, W. T., Cloake, P. C. & Govan, A. D. (1946) temporal arteritis: a generalised vascular disease. *Quarterly Journal of Medicine*, **15**, 47–75.

Cratter, R. A. & Moskovitz, R. W. (1962) *Diseases of the Chest*, **42**, 433.

Cruikshank, B. (1954) The arteritis of rheumatoid arthritis. *Annals of the Rheumatic Diseases*, **13**, 136–146.

Daiker, B. & Keller, H. H. (1971) Riesenallarteriitis mit endookulärer Ausbreitung und Hypotonia bulbi dolorosa. *Klinische Monatsblatter für Augenheilkunde*, **158**, 358–372.

Davis, P., Atkins, B., Josse, R. G. et al (1973) Criteria for classification of systemic lupus erythematosus. *British Medical Journal*, **iii**, 88–89.

Davison, S., Speira, H. & Plotz, C. M. (1966) Polymyalgia rheumatica. *Arthritis and Rheumatism*, **9**, 18–36.

Dawson, M. H. (1933) Comparative study of subcutaneous nodules in rheumatic fever and rheumatoid arthritis. *Journal of Experimental Medicine*, **57**, 845–858.

Deutsch, A. R. (1966) Early ocular manifestations of periarteritis nodosa. *Journal of the Tennessee State Medical Association*, **59**, 992–995.

Dixon, A. St-J. (1969) Polymyalgia rheumatica. *Journal of the Royal College of Physicians*, **4**, 55–61.

Doesschate, J. (1956) Corneal complications in lupus erythematosus discoides. *Ophthalmologica*, **132**, 153–156.

Doig, J. A., Whaley, K., Dick, W. C. et al (1971) Otolaryngeal aspects of Sjögren's syndrome. *British Medical Journal*, **iv**, 460–463.

Dolan, D. L., Lemmon, G. B. & Teitelbaum, S. L. (1966) Relapsing polychondritis. Analytical literature review and studies on pathogenesis. *American Journal of Medicine*, **41**, 285–299.

Dubois, E. L. (1966) *Lupus Erythematosus: Discoid and Systemic*. New York: McGraw Hill.

Dubois, E. L. & Tuffanelli, D. L. (1964) Clinical manifestations of systemic lupus erythematosus. Computer analysis of 520 cases. *Journal of the American Medical Association*, **190**, 104–111.

Duke Elder, S. & Leigh, A. G. (1965) *System of Ophthalmology*. Vol. 8, pp. 1036–1042 (a); p. 1099 (b). London: Kimpton.

Eber, C. T. (1934) Fistula at limbus (scleromalacia perforans). *American Journal of Ophthalmology*, **17**, 921–923.

Edström, G. & Osterlind, G. (1948) Case of nodular rheumatic episcleritis. *Acta Ophthalmologica*, **26**, 1–6.

Egge, K., Midtbo, A. & Westby, R. (1966) Arteritis temporalis. *Acta Ophthalmologica*, **44**, 49–56.

Ellis, P. P. & Gentry, J. H. (1964) Ocular complications of ulcerative colitis. *American Journal of Ophthalmology*, **58**, 779–785.

Estes, D. & Christian, C. L. (1971) The natural history of systemic lupus erythematosus by prospective analysis. *Medicine*, **50**, 85–95.

Fauchald, P., Rygvold, O. & Oystese, B. (1972) Temporal arteritis and polymyalgia rheumatica. Clinical and biopsy findings. *Annals of Internal Medicine*, **77**, 845–852.

Feltkamp, T. E. & van Rossum, A. L. (1968) Antibodies to salivary duct cells and other autoantibodies in patients with Sjögren's syndrome and other idiopathic autoimmune diseases. *Clinical and Experimental Immunology*, **3**, 1–16.

Ferry, A. P. (1969) Histopathology of rheumatoid episcleral nodules: an extra articular manifestation of rheumatoid arthritis. *Archives of Ophthalmology*, **82**, 77–78.

Ferry, A. P. & Leopold, I. H. (1970) Marginal (ring) corneal ulcer as a presenting manifestation of Wegener's granuloma. *Transactions of the American Academy of Ophthalmology and Otolaryngology*, **74**, 1276–1782.

Fienberg, R. & Colpoys, F. L. (1951) Involution of rheumatoid nodules treated with cortisone and of non-treated rheumatoid nodules. *American Journal of Pathology*, **27**, 925–949.

Ford, R. G. & Seikert, R. G. (1965) Central nervous system manifestations of periarteritis nodosa. *Neurology*, **15**, 114–122.

Franceschetti, A. & Bischler, V. (1950) La sclerite nodulaire nécrosante et ses rapports avec la scleromalacia. *Annales d'Oculistique*, **183**, 737–744.

François, J. (1951) Scleromalacia perforans, arthritis deformans and pemphigus. *Transactions of the Ophthalmological Societies of the United Kingdom*, **71**, 61–75.

François, J. (1970) Ocular manifestations in the collagenases. *Advances in Ophthalmology*, **23**, 1–54.

Franklin, E. C. & Zucker-Franklin, D. (1972) Current concepts of amyloid. *Advances in Immunology*, **15**, 249–304.

Fraunfelder, F. T. & Watson, P. G. (1976) Evaluation of eyes enucleated for scleritis. *British Journal of Ophthalmology*, **60**, 227–230.

Frayer, W. C. (1960) Histopathology of perilimbal ulceration in Wegener's granulomatosis. *Archives of Ophthalmology*, **64**, 58–64.

Freidman, A. H. & Henkind, P. (1974) Unusual causes of episcleritis. *Transactions of the American Academy of Ophthalmology and Otolaryngology*, **78**, 890–895.

Fruhwald, R. (1956) Syndroma Ernst Fuchs. *Dermatologische Wochenschrift*, **134**, 841–844.

Gilbert, W. S. & Talbot, S. J. (1969) Cogan's syndrome: signs of periarteritis nodosa and cerebral venous sinus thrombosis. *Archives of Ophthalmology*, **82**, 633–636.

Gillanders, L. A., Strachen, R. W. & Blair, D. W. (1969) Temporal arteriography: a new technique for the investigation of giant cell arteritis and polymyalgia rheumatica. *Annals of the Rheumatic Diseases*, **28**, 267–269.

Glenner, G. G., Ein, D. & Terry, W. D. (1972) The immunoglobulin origin of amyloid. *American Journal of Medicine*, **52**, 141–147.

Glick, E. N. (1972) Raised serum alkaline-phosphatase levels in polymyalgia rheumatica. *Lancet*, **ii**, 328.

Gocke, D. J., Hsu, K., Morgan, C. et al (1970) Association between polyarteritis and Australia antigen. *Lancet*, **ii**, 1149–1153.

Godman, G. C. & Churg, J. (1954) Wegener's granulomatosis: pathology, and review of literature. *Archives of Pathology*, **58**, 533–553.

Gold, D. H., Morris, D. A. & Henkind, P. (1972) Ocular findings in systemic lupus erythematosis. *British Journal of Ophthalmology*, **56**, 800–804.

Gordon, I. (1960) Polymyalgia rheumatica: a clinical study of 21 cases. *Quarterly Journal of Medicine*, **29**, 473–488.

Gougerot, H. (1926) Insuffisance progressive et atrophie de glands salivaires et muqueuses de la bouche, des conjunctives etc. *Bulletin de Médecine*, **40**, 360–368.

Guseva, I. L. & Shubina, L. F. (1973) Ocular changes in periarteritis nodosa. *Oftalmologicheskii Zhurnal*, **28**, 300–302.

Hamilton, C. R., Shelley, W. M. & Tumulty, P. A. (1971) Giant cell arteritis: including temporal arteritis and polymyalgia rheumatica. *Medicine*, **50**, 1–27.

Hamrin, B. (1972) Polymyalgia arteritica. *Acta Medica Scandinavica*, Supplement, **533**, 1–131.

Harris, E. D. (1972) A collagenolytic system produced by primary cultures of rheumatoid nodule tissue. *Journal of Clinical Investigation*, **51**, 2973–2976.

Harrison, C. V. (1948) Giant cell or temporal arteritis. *Journal of Clinical Pathology*, **1**, 197–211.

Harrison, R. J., Harrison, C. V. & Kopelman, H. (1955) Giant cell arteritis with aneurysms: effect of hormone therapy. *British Medical Journal*, **ii**, 1593–1595.

Harvey, A. M., Shulman, L. E., Tumulty, P. A. et al (1954) Systemic lupus erythematosus: review of literature and clinical analysis of 138 cases. *Medicine*, **33**, 291–437.

Haslock, I. & Wright, V. (1973) The musculo-skeletal complications of Crohn's disease. *Medicine*, **52**, 217–225.

Hauser, W. A., Ferguson, R. H., Holley, K. E. et al (1971) Temporal arteritis in Rochester, Minnesota, 1951–1967. *Proceedings of the Mayo Clinic*, **46**, 597–602.

Hazleman, B. L., MacLennan, I. C. & Esiri, M. M. (1975) Lymphocyte proliferation to artery antigen as a positive diagnostic test in polymyalgia rheumatica. *Annals of the Rheumatic Diseases*, **34**, 122–127.

Healey, L. A. & Wilske, K. R. (1971) Anaemia as a presenting manifestation of giant cell arteritis. *Arthritis and Rheumatism*, **14**, 27–31.

Healey, L. A., Parker, F. & Wilske, K. R. (1971) Polymyalgia rheumatica and giant cell arteritis. *Arthritis and Rheumatism*, **14**, 138–141.

Heathcote, E. J., Dudley, F. J. & Sherlock, S. (1972) Association of polyarteritis and Australia antigen. *Gut*, **13**, 319.

Henkind, P. & Gold, D. H. (1973) Ocular manifestations of the rheumatic diseases. *Rheumatology Annual Review*, **4**, 13–59.

Henoch, E. H. (1874) Uber der Zusammenhang von Purpura und Intestinalstorungen. *Berliner Klinische Wochenschrift*, **5**, 517–519.

Holborow, E. J., Weir, D. M. & Johnson, G. D. (1957) A serum factor in lupus erythematosus with affinity for tissue nuclei. *British Medical Journal*, **ii**, 732–734.

Hollenhorst, R. W., Brown, J. R., Wagener, H. P. et al (1960) Neurologic aspects of temporal arteritis. *Neurology*, **10**, 490–498.

Horton, B. T., Magath, T. B. & Brown, G. E. (1932) Undescribed form of arteritis of temporal vessels. *Proceedings of the Staff Meetings of the Mayo Clinic*, **7**, 700–701.

Horven, I. (1973) Dynamic tonometry. IV. The corneal indentation pulse in giant cell arteritis. *Acta Ophthalmologica*, **48**, 710–718.

Hughes, G. R. (1971) Significance of anti DNA antibodies in systemic lupus erythematosus. *Lancet*, **ii**, 861–863.

Hughes, G. R. (1974) Systemic lupus erythematosus. *British Journal of Hospital Medicine*, **12**, 309–319.

Hughes, R. A., Berry, C. L., Seifert, M. et al. (1972) Relapsing polychondritis. Three cases with a clinico pathological study, and literature review. *Quarterly Journal of Medicine*, **41**, 363–380.

Hunder, G. G. (1974) Polymyalgia rheumatica. *Journal of Rheumatology*, **1**, 140–142.

Hunder, G. G., Disney, T. F. & Ward, L. E. (1969) Polymyalgia rheumatica. *Proceedings. Mayo Clinic*, **44**, 849–875.

Hunder, G. G., Sheps, S. G., Allen, G. L. et al (1974) Alternate day corticosteroid therapy in giant cell arteritis. *VIth Pan-American Congress on Rheumatic Disease*.

Hurd, E. R., Snyder, W. B. & Ziff, M. (1970) Choroidal nodules and retinal detachments in rheumatoid arthritis. *American Journal of Medicine*, **48**, 273–278.

Hutchinson, J. (1890) On a peculiar form of thrombotic arteritis of the aged which is sometimes productive of gangrene. *Archives of Surgery*, **1**, 323–329.

Ide, T. & Inoue, K. (1968) Case of unilateral episcleral sarcoid tubercle. *Folia Ophthalmologica Japonica*, **19**, 632–636.

Isaacs, H. & Frere, G. (1973) Nonspecific arthralgia and myalgia with subclinical neuropathy: histochemical and histological study. *South African Medical Journal*, **47**, 1581–1587.

Jackson, D. S., Sandberg, L. B. & Cleary, E. G. (1966) Antigenic properties of soluble elastins and their use in detecting soluble elastin in ligament extracts. *Nature*, **210**, 195–196.

Jaksch-Wartenhorst, R. (1923) Polychondropathia. *Wiener Archiv fur Innere Medizin*, **6**, 93–100.

James, D. G. (1974) Multisystem ocular syndromes, *Journal of the Royal College of Physicians*, **9**, 63–78.

James, D. G., Anderson, R., Langley, D. et al (1964) Ocular sarcoidosis. *British Journal of Ophthalmology*, **48**, 461–470.

Jameson Evans, P. & Eustace, P. (1973) Scleromalacia perforans associated with Crohn's disease. *British Journal of Ophthalmology*, **57**, 330–335.

Jayson, M. I. & Jones, D. E. (1971) Scleritis and rheumatoid arthritis. *Annals of the Rheumatic Diseases*, **30**, 343–347.

Jayson, M. I., Salmon, P. R. & Harrison, W. J. (1970) Inflammatory bowel disease in ankylosing spondylitis. *Gut*, **11**, 506.

Kanski, J. (1976) *Transactions of the Ophthalmological Societies of the United Kingdom*, **96**, in press.

Kedar, J., Ravid, M. & Sohar, E. (1974) Colchicine inhibition of casein-induced amyloidosis in mice. *Israel Journal of Medical Sciences*, **10**, 787–789.

Kiehle, F. A. (1937) Scleromalacia. *American Journal of Ophthalmology*, **20**, 565–570.

Kimmelsteil, P., Gilmour, M. T. & Hodges, H. H. (1950) Degeneration of elastic fibers in granulomatous giant cell arteritis. *Archives of Pathology*, **54**, 157–168.

Kirk, J. & Cosh, J. (1969) The pericarditis of rheumatoid arthritis. *Quarterly Journal of Medicine*, **38**, 397–423.

Kjeldsen, M. H. & Reske-Nielsen, E. (1968) Pathological changes in the central nervous system in giant cell arteritis. *Acta Ophthalmologica*, **46**, 49–56.

Klein, M., Calvert, R. J., Joseph, W. E. et al (1955) Rarities in ocular sarcoidosis. *British Journal of Ophthalmology*, **39**, 416–421.

Klemperer, P., Pollack, A. D. & Baehr, G. (1942) Diffuse collagen disease: acute disseminated lupus erythematosus and diffuse scleroderma. *Journal of the American Medical Association*, **119**, 331–332.

Klinge, F. (1930) Das Gewebsbild des fieberhaften Rheumatismus; das rheumatische Frühinfiltrat. *Virchow's Archiv fur Pathologische Anatomie*, **278**, 438–461.

Kolmokova, A. E. (1965) Changes occurring in the interstitial substance of the eye in rheumatism. *Vestnik Oftalmologii*, **78**, 76–79.

Lackington, M. C., Charlin, V. C. & Gormas, B. A. (1951) Keratoconjunctivitis sicca y artritis rheumatoidea. *Revue de Medicine Chile*, **79**, 133–137.

Larson, D. L. (1961) *Systemic Lupus Erythematosus*. Boston: Little Brown.

Leber, T. (1882) Ueber die Entstehung der Netzhautablosung. *Berichte Deutsch Ophthalmologische Gessellschaft*, **14**, 165–166.

Lenoch, F., Brémova, A., Kankova, D. et al (1964) The relation of Sjögren's syndrome to rheumatoid arthritis. *Acta Rheumatologica Scandinavica*, **10**, 297–304.

Liang, G. C., Simkin, P. A., Hunder, G. G. et al (1974) Familial aggregation of polymyalgia rheumatica and giant cell arteritis. *Arthritis and Rheumatism*, **17**, 19–24.

Long, R. & James, O. (1974) Polymyalgia rheumatica and liver disease. *Lancet*, **i**, 77–79.

Lowney, E. D. & Simons, H. (1963) Rheumatoid nodules of the skin: their significance as an isolated finding. *Archives of Dermatology*, **88**, 853–858.

Lyne, A. J. (1970) 'Contact lens' cornea in rheumatoid arthritis. *British Journal of Ophthalmology*. **54**, 410–415.

Lyne, A. J. & Pitkeathley, D. A. (1968) Episcleritis and scleritis: association with connective tissue disease. *Archives of Ophthalmology*, **80**, 171–176.

Lyne, A. J. & Rosen, E. S. (1968) Still's disease and rheumatoid nodules of the sclera. *British Journal of Ophthalmology*, **52**, 853–856.

MacDonald, A. & Feiwel, M. (1968) A review of the concept of Weber-Christian panniculitis with a report of five cases. *British Journal of Dermatology*, **80**, 355–361.

MacKenzie, W. (1830) *A Practical Treatise on the Diseases of the Eye*. pp. 406–410. London: Longman.

Mandema, E., Ruinen, L., Shutter, J. H. et al (1968) *Amyloidosis*. Amsterdam: Excerta Medica Foundation.

Manschot, W. A. (1960) The eye in relation to collagen disease. *Transactions of the Ophthalmological Societies of the United Kingdom*, **80**, 137–151.

Marie, P. (1898) Sur la Spondylose Rhizomelique. *Revue de Medicine*, **18**, 285–315.

Mason, R. M. & Barnes, C. G. (1969) Behçet's syndrome with arthritis. *Annals of the Rheumatic Diseases*, **28**, 95–103.

Mathias, D. W. (1955) Scleromalacia perforans associated with retinitis pigmentosa and rheumatoid arthritis. Report of a case. *American Journal of Ophthalmology*, **39**, 161–166.

Mattsson, R. (1955) Recurrent retinitis in Reiter's disease. *Acta Ophthalmologica*, **33**, 403–408.

McGavin, D. D., Williamson, J., Forrester, J. V. et al (1976) Episcleritis and scleritis—a study of their clinical manifestations and association with rheumatoid arthritis. *British Journal of Ophthalmology*, **60**, 192–226.

McKay, D. A., Watson, P. G. & Lyne, A. S. (1974) Relapsing polychondritis and eye disease. *British Journal of Ophthalmology*, **58**, 600–605.

Meadow, S. R., Glasgow, E. F., White, R. H. et al (1972) Schönlein–Henoch nephritis. *Quarterly Journal of Medicine*, **41**, 241–258.

Miescher, P. & Strässle, R. (1957) New serological methods for the detection of the L.E. factor. *Vox Sanguinis*, **2**, 283–287.

Mills, C. P. (1958) Malignant granulomas of the nose and paranasal sinuses. *Journal of Laryngology*, **72**, 849–887.

Moll, J. M., Haslock, I., Macrae, I. et al (1974) Associations between ankylosing spondylitis, psoriatic arthritis, Reiter's disease, intestinal arthropathies and Behçet's syndrome. *Medicine,* **53**, 343–364.

Moore, J. G. & Sevel, D. (1966) Corneo-scleral ulceration in periarteritis nodosa. *British Journal of Ophthalmology,* **50**, 561.

Morgan, W. S. & Castleman, B. (1953) Clinicopathologic study of 'Mikulicz's disease'. *American Journal of Pathology,* **29**, 471–503.

Mowat, A. G. (1971) Anaemia in rheumatoid arthritis. In *Modern Trends in Rheumatology* (Ed.) Hill, A. G. London: Butterworth.

Mowat, A. G. & Hazleman, B. L. (1974) Polymyalgia rheumatica: a clinical study with particular reference to arterial disease. *Journal of Rheumatology,* **1**, 190–202.

Mulock-Houwer, A. W. (1927) Keratitis filamentosa and chronic arthritis. *Transactions of the Ophthalmological Societies of the United Kingdom,* **47**, 88–96.

Mundy, W. L., Howard, R. M., Stillman, P. H. et al (1951) Cortisone therapy in a case of rheumatoid nodules of the eye in chronic rheumatoid arthritis. *Archives of Ophthalmology,* **45**, 531–538.

Nowoslawski, A. & Brzosko, W. J. (1967) Immunopathology of rheumatoid arthritis. II. The rheumatoid nodule. *Pathological Europaea,* **2**, 302–321.

Nowoslawski, A., Krawczynski, K., Brzosko, W. J. et al (1972) Tissue localisation of Australia antigen immune complexes in acute chronic hepatitis and liver cirrhosis. *American Journal of Pathology,* **68**, 31–56.

Oast, S. P. (1937) Scleromalacia perforans. *Archives of Ophthalmology,* **17**, 698–701.

Oliner, L., Taubenhaus, M., Shapira, T. M. et al (1953) Non-syphilitic interstitial keratitis and bilateral deafness (Cogan's syndrome) associated with essential polyangiitis (periarteritis nodosa). *New England Journal of Medicine,* **248**, 1001–1008.

Osserman, E. F., Takatsuki, K. & Talal, N. (1964) Multiple myeloma. I. The pathogenesis of amyloidosis. *Seminars in Haematology,* **1**, 3–85.

Ostberg, G. (1971) Temporal arteritis in a large necropsy series. *Annals of the Rheumatic Diseases,* **30**, 224–235.

Papajiannis, S. P., Spina, M. & Gotte, L. (1970) Sequential degradation and phagocytosis of heterologous elastin. *Archives of Pathology,* **89**, 434–439.

Parker, F., Healey, L. A. & Wilske, K. R. (1972) Electron microscopy of giant cell ateritis: unique changes in internal elastic lamina. *Arthritis and Rheumatism,* **15**, 449.

Paton, D. & Duke, J. R. (1966) Primary familial amyloidosis. Ocular manifestations with histopathological observations. *American Journal of Ophthalmology,* **61**, 736–747.

Paulley, J. W. & Hughes, J. P. (1960) Giant cell arteritis, or arteritis of the aged. *British Medical Journal,* **ii**, 1562–1567.

Paviot, J., Chevallier, R., Guichard, A. et al (1934) Algie sympathique cranio-faciale a type migraineux avec dilatation des artères temporales, au cours d'un rhumatisme cardiaque solitaire. *Lyons Médicine,* **154**, 45–51.

Perkins, E. S. (1958) The aetiology and treatment of uveitis. *Transactions of the Ophthalmological Societies of the United Kingdom,* **78**, 511–522.

Perry, H. M., Tan, E. M., Carmody, S. et al (1970) Relationship of acetyl transferase activity to antinuclear antibodies and toxic symptoms in hypertensive patients treated with hydralazine. *Journal of Laboratory and Clinical Medicine,* **76**, 114–125.

Petrohelos, M. A. & Wolter, J. R. (1956) Necroscleritis nodosa. *Archives of Ophthalmology,* **55**, 221–228.

Pitkeathley, D. A. (1970) Scleritis and aortic incompetence. Two manifestations of connective tissue disease. *Annals of the Rheumatic Diseases,* **29**, 477–482.

Price Evans, D. A., Bullen, M. F., Houston, J. et al (1972) Antinuclear factors in rapid and slow acetylator patients treated with isoniazid. *Journal of Medical Genetics,* **9**, 53–56.

Ramsay, A. M. (1909) *Diasthesis and Ocular Disease.* pp. 37. London: Balliere Tindall & Cox.

Reiter, H. (1916) Über eine bischer unerkannte Spirochäten Infektin. *Deutsche Medizinische Wochenschrift,* **42**, 1535–1536.

Ricker, W. & Clark, M. (1949) Sarcoidosis: clinicopathological review of 300 cases including 22 autopsies. *American Journal of Clinical Pathology,* **19**, 725—749.

Robbins, W. C., Holman, H. R., Deicher, H. et al (1957) Complement fixation with cell nuclei and DNA in lupus erythematosus. *Proceedings of the Society for Experimental Biology and Medicine,* **96**, 575—579.

Rook, A. (1958) William Heberden's cases of anaphylactoid purpura. *Archives of Disease in Childhood,* **33**, 271.

Rucker, C. W. & Ferguson, R. H. (1965) Ocular manifestations of relapsing polychondritis. *Archives of Ophthalmology,* **73**, 46—48.

Russell, R. W. (1959) Giant cell arteritis. A review of 35 cases. *Quarterly Journal of Medicine,* **28**, 471—489.

Scadding, J. G. (1961) The prognosis of intrathoracic sarcoidosis in England. Review of 136 cases after five years observation. *British Medical Journal,* **iii**, 1165—1172.

Scadding, J. G. (1970) The definition of sarcoidosis. *Postgraduate Medical Journal,* **46**, 465—467.

Schaller, J. G., Johnson, G. D. & Holborow, E. J. (1974) The association of antinuclear antibodies with the chronic iridocyclitis of juvenile rheumatoid arthritis. *Arthritis and Rheumatism,* **17**, 409.

Scheinberg, M. A. & Cathcart, E. S. (1974) Casein induced experimental amyloidosis. III. Response to mitogens, allogenic cells and graft-versus-host reactions in the murine model. *Immunology,* **27**, 953—963.

Schlosstein, L., Terasaki, P. I., Bluestone, R. et al (1973) High association of an HL-A antigen, W27 with ankylosing spondylitis. *New England Journal of Medicine,* **288**, 704—706.

Schonlein, J. L. (1837) Peliosis rheumatica. *Allgemeine und Specielle Pathologie und Therapie,* **2**, 48—49.

Seligmann, M. & Milgrom, F. (1957) Mise en évidence par la fixation du complement de la réaction entre acide des oxyribonucleique et serum de maladies atteints de lupus erythemateux dissemine. *Compte Rendu Hebdomadaire des Séances de l'Academie des Sciences,* **245**, 1472—1475.

Sezer, F. N. (1953) Isolation of virus as a cause of Behçet's disease. *American Journal of Ophthalmology,* **36**, 301—315.

Sharp, G. C., Irvin, W. S., Tan, E. M. et al (1972) Mixed connective disease—an apparently distinct rheumatic disease syndrome associated with a specific antibody to an extractable nuclear antigen (ENA). *American Journal of Medicine,* **52**, 148—159.

Shearn, M. A. & Pirofsky, B. (1952) Disseminated lupus erythematosus—analysis of 34 cases. *Archives of Internal Medicine,* **90**, 790—807.

Sheehan, B., Harriman, D. G. & Bradshaw, J. P. (1958) Polyarteritis nodosa with ophthalmic and neurological complications. *Archives of Ophthalmology,* **60**, 537—547.

Shillitoe, E. J., Lehner, T., Lessoff, M. H. et al (1974) Immunological features of Wegener's granulomatosis. *Lancet,* **ii**, 81.

Shindo, S. (1965) Clinical and pathological studies of Wegener's disease. *Rinsho Ganka,* **19**, 25—33.

Shrank, A. B. & Doniach, D. (1963) Discoid lupus erythematosus. Correlation of clinical features with serum autoantibody. *Archives of Dermatology,* **87**, 677—685.

Siegel, M. & Lee, S. L. (1973) The epidemiology of systemic lupus erythematosus. *Seminars in Arthritis and Rheumatism,* **3**, 1—54.

Sjögren, H. (1933) Zur Kenntnis der Keratoconjunctivitis sicca. (Keratitis filiformis bei Hypo-funktion der Tränen drusen) *Acta Ophthalmologica,* Supplement, **2**, 1—151.

Smiley, W. K. (1974) The eye in juvenile rheumatoid arthritis. *Transactions of the Ophthalmological Societies of the United Kingdom,* **94**, 817—829.

Smith, K. R. (1969) Electron microscopy of giant cell (temporal) arteritis. *Journal of Neurology, Neurosurgery and Psychiatry,* **32**, 348—353.

Smoleroff, J. W. (1943) Scleral disease in rheumatoid arthritis. *Archives of Ophthalmology,* **29**, 98—108.

Sokoloff, L. (1963) The pathophysiology of the peripheral blood vessels in collagen disease. In *The Peripheral Blood Vessels* (Ed.) Orbison, J. H. & Smith, D. E. Baltimore: Williams and Wilkins.

Sokoloff, L., McCluskey, R. T. & Bunim, J. J. (1953) Vascularity of early subcutaneous nodule of rheumatoid arthritis. *Archives of Pathology*, **55**, 475–495.

Sorenson, G. D. & Binington, H. B. (1964) Resistance of murine amyloid fibrils to proteolytic enzymes. *Federation Proceedings*, **23**, 550.

Soriano, F. J. & Riva, A. (1937) Escleromalacia perforante. *Archivos de Oftalmologia de Beunos Aires*, **12**, 139–144.

Spaeth, G. L. (1967) Corneal staining in systemic lupus erythematosus. *New England Journal of Medicine*, **276**, 1168–1171.

Spector, W. G. & Heesom, N. (1969) The production of granulomata by antigen–antibody complexes. *Journal of Pathology*, **98**, 31–39.

Stephen, K. W., Chisholm, D. M., Harden, R. M. et al (1971) Diagnostic value of quantitative scintiscanning of the salivary glands in Sjögren's syndrome and rheumatoid arthritis. *Clinical Sciences*, **41**, 555–561.

Still, G. F. (1897) On a form of chronic joint disease in children. *Medico-Chirurgical Transactions*, **80**, 47–59.

Stillerman, M. L. (1951) Ocular manifestations of diffuse collagen disease. *Archives of Ophthalmology*, **45**, 239–250.

Straatsma, B. R. (1957) Ocular manifestations of Wegener's granulomatosis. *American Journal of Ophthalmology*, **44**, 789–799.

Strumpell, A. (1897) Bermerkungen über die chronische ankylosirende Entzündung der Wirbelsäule und der Hüftgelenke. *Deutsche Zeitschrift für Nervenheilkunde*, **11**, 338–342.

Swan, K. C. (1951) Some contemporary concepts of scleral disease. *Archives of Ophthalmology*, **45**, 630–644.

Symmers, W. St. C. (1956) Primary amyloidosis: review. *Journal of Clinical Pathology*, **9**, 187–211.

Talal, N. & Bunim, J. J. (1964) The development of malignant lymphoma in the course of Sjögren's disease. *American Journal of Medicine*, **36**, 529–540.

Thomas, R. D. & Croft, D. N. (1974) Thyrotoxicosis and giant cell arteritis. *British Medical Journal*, **ii**, 408–409.

Topilsky, M., Siltzbach, L. E., Williams, M. et al (1972) Lymphocyte response in sarcoidosis. *Lancet*, **i**, 117–120.

Tumulty, P. A. (1954) The clinical course of systemic lupus erythematosus. *Journal of the American Medical Association*, **156**, 947–953.

Tupikin, G. V. & Krikunov, V. P. (1972) Lesions of fundus vessels in patients with rheumatoid arthritis. *Voprosy Revmatizma*, **12**, 37–41.

Urrets Zavalia, A., Maldonado Allende, I. & Obregon Oliva, R. (1937) Skleromalazie im Verlauf einer chronischen Porphyrinurie. *Klinische Monatsblatter für Augenheilkunde*, **99**, 189–207.

Van der Hoeve, J. (1931) Scleromalacia perforans. *Nederlandsch Tijdschrift voor Geneeskunde*, **75**, 4733–4735.

Vasquez, J. J. & Dixon, F. J. (1957) Immunohistochemical analysis of lesions associated with fibrinoid change. *Archives of Pathology*, **66**, 504–517.

Verhoeff, F. H. & King, M. J. (1938) Scleromalacia perforans: report of a case in which the eye was examined microscopically. *Archives of Ophthalmology*, **20**, 1013–1035.

Victoria, V. & Fanjul, R. (1963) Escleromalacia perforante. *Revista Medica del Norte Argentino*, **1**, 1–6.

von Bechterew, W. (1893) Steifigkeit der Wirbelsäule und ihre Verkrümmung als besondere Erkrankungsform. *Neurologisches Centralblatt*, **12**, 426–434.

von Grosz, S. (1936) Aetiologie und Therapie der Keratoconjunctivitis sicca. *Klinische Monatsblatter für Augenheilkunde*, **97**, 472–485.

von Knorring, J. & Somer, T. (1974) Malignancy in association with polymyalgia rheumatica and temporal arteritis. *Scandinavian Journal of Rheumatism*, **3**, 129–135.

Walker, W. C. (1967) Pulmonary infections and rheumatoid arthritis. *Quarterly Journal of Medicine*, **36**, 239–251.

Walker, W. C. & Wright, V. (1969) Diffuse interstitial pulmonary fibrosis and rheumatoid arthritis. *Annals of the Rheumatic Diseases*, **28**, 252–259.

Watson, P. G. & Hayreh, S. S. (1976) Scleritis and episcleritis. *British Journal of Ophthalmology*, **60**, 163–191.

Wegener, F. (1936) Über generalisiebe septische Gefusserkrankunen. *Verhandlungen der Deutschen Pathologischen Gesellschaft*, **29**, 202–209.

Williamson, J. (1974) Incidence of eye disease in cases of connective tissue disease. *Transactions of the Ophthalmological Societies of the United Kingdom*, **94**, 742–752.

Wilkinson, I. M. & Russell, R. W. (1972) Arteries of the head and neck in giant cell arteritis. *Archives of Neurology*, **27**, 378.

Winfield, J. B. & Davis, J. S. (1974) Anti DNA antibody in procainamide induced lupus erythematosus. *Arthritis and Rheumatism*, **17**, 97–110.

Wolter, J. R. & Bentley, M. D. (1961) Scleromalacia perforans and massive granuloma of the sclera. *American Journal of Ophthalmology*, **51**, 71–80.

Woods, F. (1961) *Endogenous Inflammation of the Uveal Tract.* Baltimore.

Wright, R., Lumsden, K., Lusty, M. H. et al (1965) Abnormalities of the sacroiliac joints and uveitis in ulcerative colitis. *Quarterly Journal of Medicine*, **34**, 229.

Wright, V. & Watkinson, G. (1965) The arthritis of ulcerative colitis. *British Medical Journal*, **ii**, 670–675.

Young, R. L., Harkleroad, L. E., Lordon, R. E. et al (1970) Pulmonary sarcoidosis: a prospective evaluation of glucocorticoid therapy. *Annals of Internal Medicine*, **73**, 207–212.

Zeek, P. M. (1952) Periarteritis nodosa: a critical review. *American Journal of Clinical Pathology*, **22**, 770–790.

Zeek, P. M. (1953) Periarteritis nodosa and other forms of necrotising angiitis. *New England Journal of Medicine*, **248**, 764–772.

Zucker-Franklin, D. (1968) Electron microscopic studies of human granulocytes: structural variations related to function. *Seminars in Hematology*, **5**, 109–133.

CHAPTER EIGHT

Scleritis in Relation to Other Systemic Disorders

'A pox of this gout! or, a gout of this pox for one or the other plays the rogue with my great toe'.
Falstaff in *Henry IV, part ii* (Shakespeare).

If a systemic disease is uncovered when investigating a patient with scleritis, or scleritis appears during the course of an illness, it is usually one of the group of diseases now known as the connective tissue diseases. The sclera can, however, become affected either primarily or secondarily in other systemic diseases, either as a direct result of invasion by organisms which have caused the systemic signs, through a granulomatous or hypersensitivity reaction to those organisms, or because the condition is due to enzymatic defects with multiple manifestations of which the sclera is but one organ involved.

The commonest endogenous infections to involve the sclera are tuberculosis, syphilis, leprosy and the viral infections. As the scleritis produced by these conditions is identical to that which develops in the course of a connective tissue disease, it is most important to eliminate them from the differential diagnosis. Not only are the infections treatable with specific therapy, but if they are treated with anti-inflammatory agents alone, the causative organisms multiply, making the systemic disease worse.

BACTERIAL INFECTIONS

Tuberculosis

It used to be said that tuberculosis was the commonest cause of scleritis (Sorsby, 1963), almost always arising as an exogenous infection or in generalised systemic miliary tuberculosis. Indeed before this century this may well have been the case, but it has now become very rare.

Mycobacterium tuberculosis is a difficult organism to culture because of its waxy coat, and as it is acid-fast it has to be looked for with specific

Ziehl–Neelson staining in histological sections. To prove that any infection is due to this organism it is also necessary to produce the disease in the guinea-pig which is highly susceptible. Histologically the appearances suggestive of tuberculosis are of a granuloma composed of epithelioid cells and inflammatory cells, the centre of which shows caseation. The granulation tissue contains Langerhans' multinucleated giant cells. As the histological changes in nonspecific granulomatous scleral disease and tuberculosis are so similar, even to the formation of giant cells, it is most important that full identification of the cause is undertaken before ascribing the diagnosis of tuberculosis to any scleral change. Identification of the cause in this way has very rarely been reported. Brini (1953) grew *Mycobacterium tuberculosis* from a tuberculous ulcer of the sclera and we have recently grown this organism in guinea-pigs from a limbal perforating nodule which appeared to arise in the sclera at the limbus. Tuberculosis was considered as a cause because of the similarity to the case of Walker (1966), although the iris was not involved in our patient. Phillips, Williams and Maiden (1950) also excised scleral nodules which proved to be tuberculous granulomas (Andreani, 1954; Sarda, Mehrota and Adnani, 1969).

More often, the diagnosis of tuberculosis is presumed partly on the basis of finding giant cells in the histological section and partly on the presence of a strongly positive Mantoux test. Verhoeff writing in 1907 on 'Tuberculous scleritis, a commonly unrecognised form of tuberculosis', suggested that tuberculosis was a common cause but failed to grow tubercle bacilli from the sputum of any of his patients (although one had a strong family history); he found on histology a focal proliferation of epithelioid cells, among which an occasional giant cell occurred, surrounded by an infiltration of lymphoid and plasma cells. The vessels in the neighbourhood showed perivascular infiltration with chronic inflammatory cells and the subepithelial tissue showed a similar infiltration in a greater or lesser degree. Caseation was entirely absent. Numerous sections, specially stained for the purpose, were unsuccessfully examined for tubercle bacilli. He then commented that this result was not unexpected, since it is notoriously difficult to find the bacilli even in very active lesions!

The tubercle bacillus or tuberculous protein could be the trigger factor to a nonspecific granulomatous reaction, because it does seem that as a rule the organisms when enmeshed in the scleral collagen will not set up a chronic granulomatous reaction.

The sclera can be infected by direct injury (Bell, 1914) although in this report the infection probably established itself because of the presence of necrotic tissue in the area. It can also be attacked by direct spread of a tuberculous lesion in the conjunctiva (Das Gupta and Usman, 1949; Swan, 1951), may develop in the episclera to cause a nodular episcleritis (Sarda, Mehrota and Adnani, 1969), or may develop from conglomerate tubercle of the iris (Maitre-Jan, 1907; Finnoff, 1931).

Endogenous infection is much more common. These patients all have miliary tuberculosis, usually with pulmonary manifestations, and most are very ill and often have other miliary foci in the eye either on the retina, iris or ciliary body (Phillips, Williams and Maiden, 1950).

We have seen a 24-year-old female laboratory technician who fell into this category. She had became ill over the period of some six weeks with fever and loss of weight. The eye became red and sore three weeks after the illness began, and the vision became poor. Chest x-ray revealed miliary tuberculosis and acid-fast bacilli were found in the sputum. She was admitted to hospital for treatment with antituberculous therapy. Examination of the eye showed a nodular scleritis extending from 12 to 3 o'clock in one eye. The nodules were conglomerate and there was a very intense conjunctival and episcleral reaction around them (Figure 8.1). This feature was remarkable because it

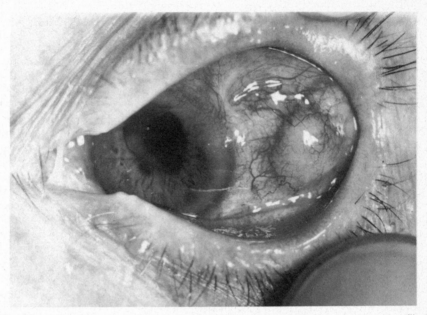

Figure 8.1. Conglomerate nodules in the sclera and anterior uveitis in a patient with miliary tuberculosis.

is most unusual for a reaction of this intensity to occur even in necrotising scleritis and particularly in such a young person. There was also an intense anterior and posterior uveitis and a small retinal miliary tubercle could be seen through the vitreous haze close to the disc. No local therapy other than atropine was given to the eye which improved over the next two weeks and within six weeks the scleritis had resolved. The vision returned to normal over the next eight weeks, but the conjunctival distention remained.

Untreated these nodules ulcerate centrally, turn yellow and extend on to the surface through the conjunctiva, eventually perforating the globe (Duke Elder and Leigh, 1965). Similar lesions have been produced by the injection of acid-fast bacilli into the vitreous of rabbits (Courtis, 1928; Dejean, 1953).

In patients in whom the scleritis occurs as part of their miliary disease, it is reasonable to assume that tuberculosis is the cause. Many other patients have been found to have strongly positive skin tests to tuberculous protein and to have calcified lesions in their lungs. There has been, however, no direct evidence to suggest that the scleritis seen in these patients was any different from that seen from other nonspecific causes. If, however, these patients are inadvertently treated with systemic steroid the eye may improve but the sputum may become full of acid-fast bacilli.

Tuberculosis or other reactions to the tubercle bacillus may coexist with connective tissue disease, the manifestations of one not necessarily being related to the other. The following two cases illustrate this:

Case study. Mrs L.B., aged 63, first sought ophthalmological advice in 1939 because her left eye had become inflamed during the previous two months. She was otherwise well. She had a sclerokeratitis in the left eye. Although she herself remained well, she continued to have attacks of scleritis over the next ten years, as a result of which the sclera became transparent but not thinned and the cornea progressively more opaque (Figure 8.2). All patients with scleritis in that era were presumed to have tuberculosis. She had a Mantoux reaction, positive at 1/10 000, but repeated sputum investigations were performed and were universally negative. She also had a period of sanatorium treatment without improvement. In 1955 she developed rheumatoid arthritis which was controlled thereafter with phenylbutazone and in 1959 she developed lesions on the face which were found by biopsy to be lupus, of a type of tuberculoid similar to that described by Krantz (1950) and Paufique, Audibert and Paupert-Ravault (1961).

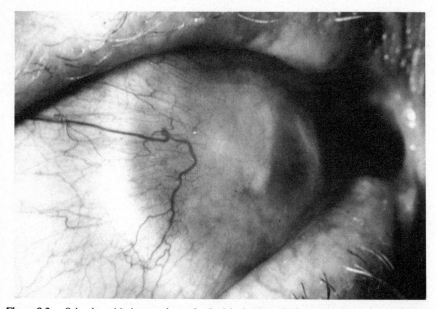

Figure 8.2. Sclerokeratitis in a patient who had had tuberculosis and had recurrent attacks of scleritis since the onset with gradual opacification of the cornea. She later developed lupus of the face and rheumatoid arthritis shortly before her death.

Simultaneously with the development of the facial lesions, the scleritis became very much more severe, failing to respond to any form of treatment. Repeated sputums were investigated and were negative. In spite of this in 1960 she was given antituberculous therapy which did not in any way alter the progress of the scleral disease. By this time the full circumference of the globe and the cornea was involved and both the lupus and the rheumatoid arthritis had progressed. She had developed nodules on the arms and marked deformity of the hands. She died suddenly of coronary occlusion. It would seem much more likely that her scleritis was associated with her rheumatoid disease rather than her tuberculous disease, although Type IV reactions are involved in both. Ellis and Holz (1953) have described a similar patient with rheumatoid arthritis who developed necrotising scleritis and later died of pulmonary tuberculosis.

Case study. Mrs E.B., 38 years old, had been known to have tuberculosis as a child and in 1965 developed a sudden pain in the right side of her chest radiating up to the shoulder. She had a constantly high temperature of 102°F during the day with severe sweating at night. First sputum was found to contain bacteria only, so she was treated with penicillin and sulphonamide to which she developed a marked allergic reaction. She had a maculopapular skin rash on arms and chest and enlargement of the liver. At this time she was also found to have tubercle bacilli in the sputum and x-ray of the chest showed expansion of the old tuberculous lesion. Concurrently with the sensitivity reaction to penicillin, she developed a bilateral anterior diffuse scleritis. The episclera and superficial sclera were biopsied and this showed a nonspecific granulomatous reaction. No acid-fast bacilli were found. Treatment with antituberculous drugs which were given to control the pulmonary tuberculosis had no effect on the scleritis, which has been kept reasonably well controlled with oxyphenbutazone during the succeeding ten years. She is still having occasional recurrences of the scleritis but this has not progressed markedly.

In the second patient it is probable that the scleral disease was related to the drug sensitivity reaction rather than to the original bacterial infections.

Phlyctenular disease is usually considered to be an allergic reaction to tubercular protein. The inflammation affects the corneoscleral margin and conjunctiva, but usually not the sclera. However, one case has been described in which the subconjunctival lesion had penetrated the sclera. This produced an extensive area of local necrosis and eventually led to perforation of the eye and permanent atrophy.

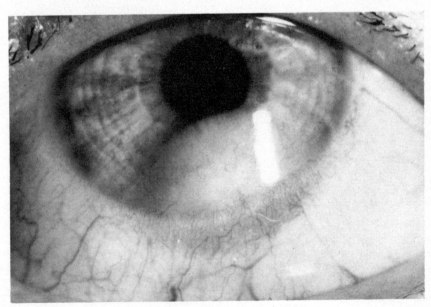

Figure 8.3.   Tuberculoma of the iris root and scleral margin.

Ulcerative and nodular tubercular conjunctival lesions always involve the underlying episclera and sometimes the overlying lids and skin. However, because they have involved the conjunctiva and caused ulceration, subsequent scarring can be readily distinguished from primary episcleral inflammations which never damage the conjunctiva. Tuberculomas arising from the iris or angle may occasionally spread forwards penetrating the sclera at the limbus (Walker, 1966). Figure 8.3 is a similar case; the granuloma in this instance was excised surgically together with a piece of affected iris. There has been no recurrence.

Leprosy

The greatest concentration of leprosy is in the Indian subcontinent (3 million), and scleritis is common in leprosy; in one leper hospital in India, of the 35 patients with eye involvement, 12 had some form of scleral disease.

This dreadful disease, which because of its characteristics tries the stamina of both patient and doctor alike, is caused by *Mycobacterium leprae*, a straight, gram-positive, acid-fast bacillus. It is still a common disease in tropical and subtropical zones and is imported from time to time into Europe and America. Europe has 52 000 cases (mainly in Southern Europe) and over 900 have been notified in England since 1951.

There are two clinically recognisable varieties of the condition, the tuberculoid and the lepromatous, depending on the tissue response to infection. Transmission remains something of a mystery. Leprosy is not highly infectious and it is thought that bacilli-laden nasal discharge is the main source of infection. Bacilli-ferous ulcerations, sweaty hairy skin and maternal milk may contain viable bacilli. Both types of the disease start with a prolonged period of general ill health, malaise and fever, the correct diagnosis is frequently missed for years and thereafter the course is determined by the patient's resistance to the infection. If resistance is marked, then the disease takes on a neurotropic pattern, producing a tuberculoid reaction with multiple peripheral nerve lesions commonly involving the VIIth cranial nerve. The consequent paralysis of one side of the face adds the problems of corneal exposure. The affection of the skin gives the widespread scaly eruption from which the condition takes its name.

In the lepromatous variety, which may coexist with the tuberculoid type, the changes are of a much longer duration with the production of chronic granulomas in virtually every tissue. These granulomas gradually eat away the surrounding structures to give rise to the horrific tissue deformities charac-teristic of the condition. Eye complications are common in this type of leprosy (90 per cent according to de Barros, 1939) but show marked racial variation, e.g. 90 per cent of patients with lepromatous leprosy develop eye complications in the Americas and Hawaii, but only 25 per cent in India, where European expatriates are more likely to develop these complications than native Indians (Duke Elder and Leigh, 1965).

The conjunctiva is never directly affected (de Barros, 1939), although leprosy bacilli can be found in the conjunctival secretions. It can, however, be invaded from the episclera. The cornea and sclera on the other hand are both commonly affected, bilaterally and systemically. The earliest corneal changes are a thickening of the corneal nerves, which become beaded, and the cornea becomes completely insensitive. White or grey punctate opacities in the epithelial and subepithelial layers of the cornea spread from the periphery until the whole of the cornea becomes involved, causing a gradual deterioration of vision. These lesions which are symptomless contain clumps of lepra bacilli which have migrated from the sclera. The opacities are therefore found throughout the thickness of the cornea peripherally but become more superficial centrally. The adjacent sclera and episclera are swollen and infiltrated but not congested (de Barros, 1939).

The lepromas which affect the episcleral and scleral tissues may be the result of direct extension from adjacent tissues including the lids and uveal tracts (Borthen and Lie, 1899), but usually arise de novo in either one of those tissues giving rise to a nodular scleritis or episcleritis similar to that seen in other granulomatous conditions.

Simple or nodular episcleritis

These lesions have a sudden acute onset and a transient course. The lesion itself is widespread and if it forms a nodule has a characteristically violaceous tint. Both episcleral plexuses are deeply congested. The lesions are said to be most common in the temporal sclera (de Barros, 1939) and often accompany erythema nodosum leprosum (Hibi and Shiozawa, 1955).

Nodular scleritis

Nodular scleritis is common in lepromatous leprosy but much less common in the tuberculous type. The onset can be acute with pain, discomfort and redness of the eye, again on the temporal side and symmetrical in both eyes, and the nodule may rapidly reach the size of a hazelnut, diminishing rapidly with treatment (Saxena, 1963). More often the lesions develop slowly over many years, with sudden exacerbations over three- to four-week periods, and are entirely painless and symptom-free. They start with fine dots and sheathing of the limbal vessels. Exudation occurs which gives rise to shining gelatinous yellowish nodules. They end by being similar in appearance to nodular scleritis of other types but being rather larger, more 'knobbly' and having a more marked yellow centre than those seen in other conditions (Figure 8.4). If a biopsy is taken, the nodule can be found to contain lepra bacilli and in this way it differs from all other forms of granulomatous scleritis. Unless the granuloma advances to involve the conjunctiva, it remains fairly mobile on the underlying tissue and normal in appearance.

If a lepromatous nodule arises close to the limbus, it has the appearance of a severe limbal vernal conjunctivitis. The cornea then becomes involved by direct extension producing an interstitial keratitis and phlyctenular keratitis.

The scleral lesions can also extend outwards and circumferentially and when this occurs the centre of the original nodule ulcerates leaving a patch of excessively thin sclera which, although it forms more slowly, is very like the necrotising scleral disease seen with the other granulomas. Perforation

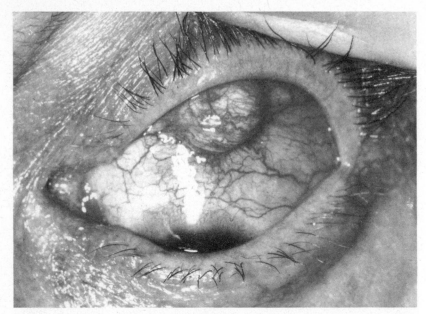

Figure 8.4.   Lepromatous nodule of the episclera and sclera in a patient with lepromatous leprosy.

of the cornea and limbus occurs, but scleral perforation is rare, usually following staphyloma formation.

Treatment is with the sulphone group of drugs which have to be given over a prolonged period and are continued for two years after all the signs have gone. This is supplemented by local steroid and occasionally subconjunctival intraorbital or systemic steroid if the eyes are affected. The sulphones are, however, toxic and some patients find them difficult to take. They may also induce a type of erythema nodosum reaction, in which case the eye signs are much more severe. A necrotising scleritis occurs with an intense uveitis which is very difficult to control and is quite different from the episcleral reaction seen with erythema nodosum which occurs in the natural course of the disease. The reason for this variation in reaction is unclear but may be due to the sudden release of toxic products from the destroyed bacilli.

Syphilis

In our experience syphilis is a surprisingly common cause of scleritis and investigation for syphilis should never be omitted when examining a patient with scleral disease. Syphilis is on the increase and so probably will be its scleral manifestations. Not infrequently scleritis is the presenting feature of the disease and has been found associated with both anterior and posterior scleritis and in two patients with necrotising disease.

Case study. A 19-year-old girl first attended our clinic in 1968 with a history of an inflamed left eye for one week. She was found to have scleral nodules at 3 o'clock and 6 o'clock in the left eye, accompanied by considerable oedema of the lids and conjunctivae (Figure 8.5). Four days later the other eye became involved with a similar nodule at 9 o'clock. Treatment with local steroids was given while investigations were undertaken and both eyes responded.

She was found to have a strongly positive Wassermann reaction (WR) and cardiolipin WR was strongly positive as was the *Treponema pallidum* immobilisation test. The ESR was 44. It was established that the primary exposure to the disease was probably some four months previously. The contact was traced and both were given   intensive antisyphilitic treatment over a period of two months. The scleral inflammation disappeared within a week and has never recurred.

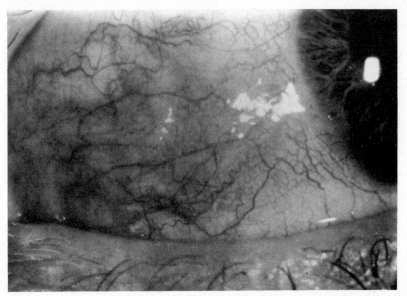

Figure 8.5.   Nodular scleritis, the presenting feature of secondary syphilis, in a young woman.

The cerebrospinal fluid remained normal in this patient but must always be checked because they may require special treatment. Four of the seven patients in whom scleritis was the presenting feature of syphilis had an increase in cells and protein and the Lange curve showed a first or mid-zone rise. All of our patients have responded to nonspecific anti-inflammatory therapy, suggesting that scleral inflammation is not necessarily caused by the organism.

The spirochaete, *Treponema pallidum*, invades all tissues and the sclera is not exempt; the scourge of the late fifteenth century which swept Europe after the siege of Naples led directly to the abandonment once and for all of the theory of humors, and its replacement by the theory of transmission of disease by contagion. It was then realised that syphilis was spread by direct contact, usually sexual, but in the case of the outer eye, by hand or mouth (Fracastoro, 1530).

Between two and four weeks after infection the primary chancre appears on the site of inoculation together with an enlargement of the local lymph glands. The secondary lesions, which usually appear six to eight weeks later,

consist of a generalised non-irritant skin rash and mucous membrane involvement. These manifestations are followed at a much longer interval, often four
or five years, by the final stage in which the deeper structures are involved
by generalised granulomas in the form of gummas. The histological reaction
in every stage of the disease is a lymphocytic and plasma cell granuloma
with endarteritis obliterans of the medium and small vessels of the body wherever
found.

Primary syphilis

MacKenzie (1854) described a primary chancre which involved the sclera.
Figure 8.6 shows a sketch taken from the fly-leaf of his annotated copy

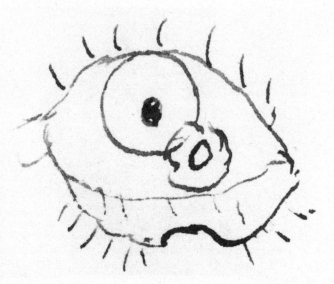

Figure 8.6. Sketch from the annotated copy of MacKenzie's *A Practical Treatise in Diseases of
the Eye* (1854) of a primary chancre involving both lid and sclera.

of *A Practical Treatise in Diseases of the Eye*, with the comment in his
handwriting. Although primary diseases of the conjunctiva are relatively
common and they always involve the episclera, the sclera is able to resist
the infection at this stage. According to Duke Elder and Leigh (1965) most
people who develop this lesion are innocently infected, but they quote the
story of the Russian who removed foreign bodies from the eye with his tongue
and left behind 34 chancres!

The commonest site of these ulcers, which are straight-edged with a sloughing
grey base, is adjacent to the lower lid, where MacKenzie has drawn it. The
surrounding inflammation of the conjunctiva and episclera is intense. The pre-
auricular and submaxillary lymph glands become very swollen, hard and tender.

Secondary syphilis

Although involvement of the episclera and sclera is rare in the primary disease, it is common in the secondary stage and is termed syphilitic scleroconjunctivitis, first described by Gunn in 1894 and characterised by Elschnig in 1897. At the same time as, or slightly after the skin rash appears (Figure 8.7) a severe

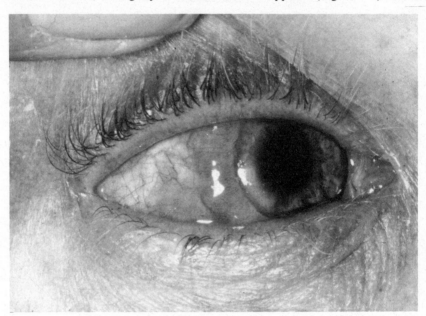

Figure 8.7.   Limbal episcleritis with conjunctival chemosis in secondary syphilis. This lesion is very similar to that seen in Reiter's disease.

simple episcleritis and conjunctivitis occur. The appearance is unusual because most of the inflammatory changes occur at the limbus in the region of the limbal arcade and the inflammation lessens towards the equator although the conjunctiva is chemosed. It is difficult to see the scleral vessels but the sclera is not swollen. The limbal swelling may be so great as to overlap the corneal margin which may also become infiltrated. Biopsy reveals a massive round cell infiltration, neovascularisation and endarteritis (Elschnig, 1897; Trantas, 1911). The only patient we have seen with this condition responded extremely rapidly to treatment with penicillin without any additional local medication.

Tertiary syphilis

Patients seen in this stage of the disease present with a scleritis indistinguishable by its clinical appearance from that due to any other cause. Almost all the patients have an anterior diffuse scleritis of insidious onset, but we have seen it in nodular disease and it has been described as a cause of posterior scleritis (Simon, 1919). Evans' (1905) histological specimen also showed the lesion to be posterior, involving the rectus muscle and showed a typical endarteritis obliterans of the ciliary vessels. Deodati, Bec and Labro (1971) have confirmed this by angiography in a patient with syphilitic scleritis.

Even though endarteritis obliterans is diagnostic of the syphilitic lesion, it is not always present in those in whom syphilis should be the cause of the scleritis. Although such a patient may have a true gumma, they may also be free of other symptoms of syphilis (Bhaduri and Basu, 1956).

Case study. While serving near Armentières with the British Expeditionary Force in 1915, Mr R.T. acquired a chancre of the penis which was treated with neosalvarsan. In 1920 he was hospitalised with a gastrointestinal complaint, neurasthenia and chronic conjunctivitis possibly of syphilitic origin. He therefore had another course of antisyphilitic treatment and remained well until 1933 when he developed other systemic symptoms. He was given yet another course of antiluetic treatment which gave him severe jaundice. Having lost all faith in doctors, he was not seen again until 1947 by which time he was having difficulty doing his job working on a lathe. He was found to be hypertensive (220/130) and to have arteriosclerosis and neurological syphilis (GPI). He refused the treatment offered and was not seen for a further two years, by which time his speech had become slurred.

Lumbar puncture revealed a mid-zone rise in the Lange curve of 123432100. He was therefore treated with 20 000 units of penicillin intrathecally, but the disease progressed over the next five years and he developed weakness of the legs and difficulty in walking.

In 1954, 39 years after his original infection, he suddenly developed a bilateral, entirely symptomless necrotising scleritis with very little surrounding inflammation (Figure 8.8). It was exactly like that seen with long-standing rheumatoid arthritis, of which there was no clinical and serological evidence.

Treatment, including a further course of penicillin, was not effective. However, the sclera, although thin, did not perforate before his death four years later. Pathologically the eye showed a typical necrotising scleritis involving only the anterior segment with thinning and infiltration of both sclera and cornea. The cellular infiltrate was exactly as seen with any necrotising scleritis. There was no evidence of endarteritis in the anterior ciliary vessels or the vessels in the granuloma. The posterior segment was entirely normal.

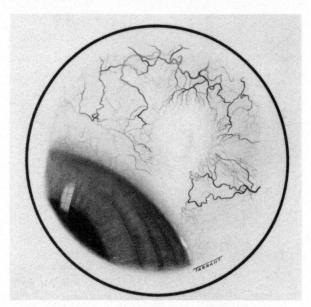

Figure 8.8. Necrotising scleritis in a patient with tertiary syphilis. The sclera became very thin before his death four years later.

Congenital syphilis

The commonest ocular manifestation of this condition is interstitial keratitis, which forms one of the three cardinal signs, the others being 'peg top' teeth and deafness (Figure 8.9, a, b, c).

In later life these patients can develop scleritis which is very resistant to treatment by anti-inflammatory agents or by further antisyphilitic treatment. The scleritis in these patients is always of the diffuse anterior or posterior variety with long duration and mild severity.

Case study. Mrs L.B., aged 47, was known to have congenital syphilis, diagnosed at the age of six when she developed a mild interstitial keratitis. The treatment given at that time

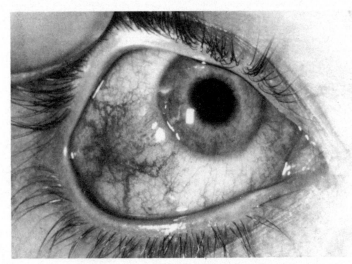

Figure 8.9(a). Nodule adjacent to the sclera in a patient with congenital syphilis. She also had a mild posterior scleritis.

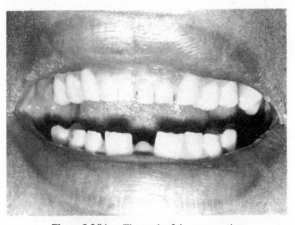

Figure 8.9(b). The teeth of the same patient.

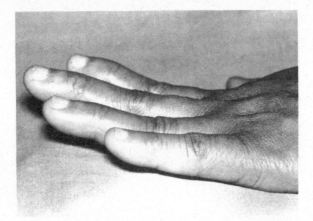

Figure 8.9(c).   The short little finger of the same patient.

is not known but the eyes were not grossly affected until the age of 40 when the vision rapidly deteriorated and the eyes became protruding and painful. The cornea became opaque and the upper half of the sclera of both eyes became red and congested.

For religious reasons she did not seek treatment for three years and by the time she was first seen she had no perception of light in either eye, one of which was very painful and was excised.

Macroscopic examination showed a staphyloma involving the sclera and cornea. Microscopically the corneal stroma was heavily vascularised and infiltrated with focal areas of chronic inflammatory cells and many plasma cells. The sclera adjacent to the staphyloma showed large areas of necrosis with dense infiltration of the plasma cells and some epithelioid proliferation but no specific changes which could be related to the vessels themselves.

It is known that progressive vascular changes occur in patients with congenital syphilis: the fact that both the sclera and the cornea were affected probably led to the eventual destruction of this eyeball.

There is a group of patients who develop interstitial keratitis which when inactive looks exactly like that seen in congenital syphilis, but whose serological tests are all negative and they have no history of contact. Many of these patients have an associated scleritis which may or not be combined with the uveitis and deafness of Cogan's syndrome.

VIRAL INFECTIONS

The conjunctiva is never involved in leprosy and the episclera and sclera commonly so; the reverse is the case in viral infections. Whereas practically all the viral and rickettsial organisms will cause a conjunctivitis and keratitis, the sclera and episclera only very rarely become involved. It seems probable that the viruses are present in the sclera during the stage of viraemia and an increase in the cellular content of the sclera is seen if there is concomitant keratitis or uveitis, but there are few lesions which could be ascribed to viruses.

Herpes Simplex

Herpes simplex regularly affects the corneal epithelium, sometimes the conjunctival epithelium, and very rarely the conjunctival stroma or episclera. Cases of episcleritis occurring in the course of herpes simplex have beeen recorded by Panzardi (1947), Saba (1947), and Sanna (1950), but this is probably unusual (Figure 8.10).

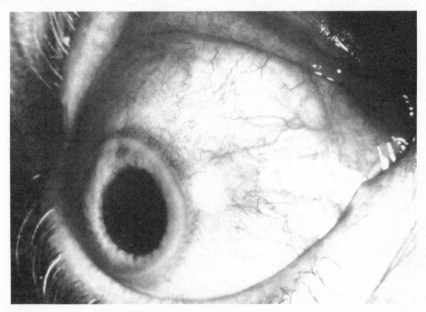

Figure 8.10. A conjunctival/episcleral lesion from which herpes simplex virus was isolated.

Herpes Zoster

Scleral and episcleral complications of herpes zoster occur in six per cent of patients with herpes zoster ophthalmicus (Marsh, 1975, personal communication), and need careful treatment if they are not to become the most severe of the patient's handicaps. It is also the exception to prove the rule that episcleritis does not progress to a scleritis, although it is probable that this is the result of two different reactions to the same stimulus.

The manifestations of herpes zoster ophthalmicus are due to infection with, or reactivation of latent varicella virus lying within the trigeminal ganglion (Garland, 1943; Hope-Simpson, 1965).

The virus replicates in response to an unknown trigger factor and migrates down the radicles of the trigeminal nerve, eventually reaching the skin, and, in 50 per cent of patients, the eye, particularly if the nasociliary branch of the nerve is involved.

The patient, who is generally elderly, complains of sudden onset of pain in the upper part of the face, is usually ill with a moderate fever and is often nauseated. Direct enquiry may elicit a history of contact with chicken pox (varicella) some 14 days before. After three or four days, the same side of the face becomes flushed and very shortly afterwards blisters filled with clear fluid appear on the skin. Later these turn yellow and scab and the surrounding soft tissues become oedematous (Figures 8.11 and 8.12); the eyelid swelling spreads to the other side, closing both eyes and worrying the patient a great deal. Over the next three to four weeks the scabs separate, leaving deeply pitted scars in the skin, and frequently a distressing severe neuralgia develops which in the elderly patients may last the rest of their lives. The area which has been affected with herpes zoster always has altered sensation and may be extremely sensitive to even slight changes of temperature and draughts of cold air.

If the nasociliary branch is involved the vesicles appear on the side of the tip of the nose, in which case the eye is almost always involved (Hutchinson, 1886).

At the time the vesicles are just showing, particularly if there are any on the lid margin, the conjunctiva flushes and becomes oedematous. In a few patients a definite simple or nodular episcleritis occurs with marked infiltration of the episcleral tissues. The episcleral inflammation may occur together

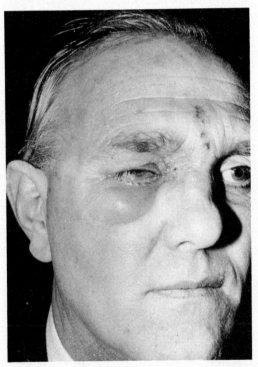

Figure 8.11. Herpes zoster ophthalmicus. The vesicles involve the inner canthus and episclera and, although small, also reach the hairline. The swelling of the periorbital tissues has not yet involved both sides.
Courtesy of R. Marsh, London.

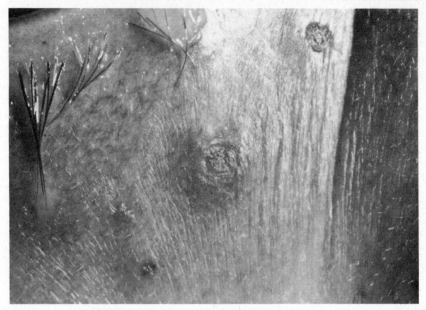

Figure 8.12. Vesicles of herpes zoster. The lesion below the eyelashes on the left of the figure still contains fluid but this is getting thick and yellow. The other vesicles have burst and scarring is drawing up the edge of the lesion on the right.

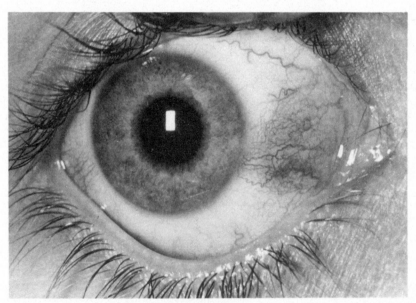

Figure 8.13. Episcleritis which persisted for three months after the vesicles had scarred. There is another lesion at 7 o'clock.

with corneal and conjunctival involvement or be entirely separate from it (Figure 8.13). If the conjunctiva is involved there is mucopurulent discharge; the membrane itself is swollen and chemosed and stains lightly with Bengal rose. The cornea is commonly affected, the first lesion being an epithelial one which is raised and close to the limbus and often develops into a fine dendritic pattern. The lesions rarely last longer than a few days and parallel the episcleral inflammation which starts at the same time and lasts for the same period.

After about ten days, at which time the skin lesions are beginning to crust, some patients will suddenly develop either a nodular episcleritis or, less commonly, a nodular scleritis, and rarely a diffuse anterior scleritis of great severity (Arducci and Cappelli, 1968). At the same time stromal infiltrates appear in the cornea just below Bowman's membrane, adjacent to visible large corneal nerves. A sectorial iris atrophy sometimes develops in the same segment as the corneal opacities. Both the stromal keratitis and the nodular episcleritis disperse spontaneously in the majority of patients, but in those with scleritis the condition persists. In these patients recurrences are the rule; the recurrences not necessarily occurring at the same site as the previous inflammation. Some of the patients with the stromal keratitis also have a persistence of the condition but the keratitis and the scleritis are not necessarily associated.

The majority of patients with the early episcleritis recover completely and have no residual changes; in about 20 per cent, however, the episcleritis clears leaving a white eye and then two months to several years later the patient suddenly develops a severe necrotising or nodular scleritis (Figure 8.14). This

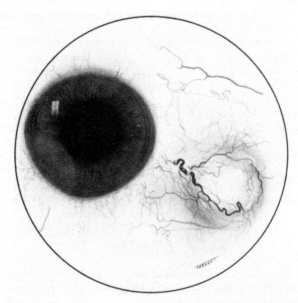

Figure 8.14. Nine months later. The same patient as Figure 8.13. A nodular scleritis has developed at the site of the original lesion. The cornea shows diffuse stromal infiltrate adjacent to the site of the lesion at 7 o'clock.

is often accompanied by a uveitis and a disciform keratitis which consists either of deep stromal opacities (sometimes with immune rings around them) which progress to a sclerosing keratitis, or epithelial dendritic lesions which leave a persistent stromal haze. There may also be an iritis accompanying this inflammatory change and the intraocular pressure may rise. This type of necrotising scleritis is extremely resistant to treatment and may give rise to a punched-out area in the sclera, a very thin atrophic scar, or very occasionally perforation (Levy and Lobstein, 1952) or staphyloma formation (Arducci and Cappelli, 1968). Fortunately, however, the necrotising process does not extend and always remains localised to the site of the original patch of episcleritis. This type of scleritis and keratitis sometimes becomes manifest when local steroids are withdrawn following healing of the corneal disc and is very liable to recur at intervals over many years. Corneal sensation is always reduced in the affected area and some of the corneal changes which may then arise may be attendant on this.

There appear then to be three separate patterns as a consequence of episcleral and scleral involvement in herpes zoster with some overlap between them. In some patients in the early vesicular stage an episcleritis occurs which clears spontaneously and is presumably due to viral infiltration of the tissue. In others who have had no previous episcleral involvement a transient episcleritis or occasionally scleritis develops between 10 days and a fortnight after the start of the disease. This has been shown histologically to be accompanied by a vasculitis of the episcleral and scleral vessels and is probably therefore an immune response, either to degenerate nerve fibre products, or persisting virus, although corneal buttons examined at this stage are always free of virus particles. Finally, in the late recovery stage, some patients develop a relapsing necrotising or nodular scleritis at the site which has previously been involved by an episcleritis early in the course of the condition. This presumably results from an immunologically induced granulomatous change occurring in tissue previously sensitised by the virus. All of these stages have equivalent changes in the cornea. If the late nodular scleritis is neglected, perforation or anterior staphylomata can occur (Adelung, 1951; Levy and Lobstein, 1952).

Treatment of the early episcleritis should be with idoxuridine (IDU) and local steroids on the assumption that this is caused by the virus. The treatment of those who develop episcleritis after ten days should be with local steroids and if there is a scleritis oxyphenbutazone should be given as well. The late variety may require intermittent treatment with systemic anti-inflammatory agents and occasionally systemic steroids. If the topical steroids are withdrawn too quickly, the episcleritis will recur and it may be necessary to continue them, but slowly reduce the dosage over at least two months.

Mumps

Transient scleritis and episcleritis have been described by Berg (1927), Rieger (1935), North (1953) and Swan and Penn (1962). The course and nature of the inflammation seem to be the same as that seen in herpes zoster, but the inflammation is transient and does not appear to have a recurrent nature.

Q Fever

Perdriel et al (1961) described transient episcleritis as a complication of Q fever. This is an acute febrile illness caused by *Rickettsia burneti* and characterised by sudden onset and interstitial pneumonitis.

Infectious Mononucleosis

During an epidemic of infectious mononucleosis (glandular fever) in a university population, 103 patients had eye changes. One of these patients had a scleritis and peripheral choroiditis and developed a temporary axial myopia (Jones, Howie and Wilson, 1952).

CHLAMYDIAL INFECTION

Scleritis has been produced by intracorneal injection of chlamydia by Jones, Al-Hussaini and Dunlop (1966) and it is possible that some cases of nonspecific scleritis are due to this cause, but so far we have been unable to find any evidence of chlamydial infection from conjunctival culture or scrapings over the superficial episcleral nodules.

HISTOPLASMOSIS

Histoplasmosis is caused by infection by the gram-positive fungus *Histoplasma capsulatum* which has a yeast-like and mycelial phase. Infection can be fatal following widespread dissemination of the organism, or benign in which case the organism can rarely, if ever, be isolated from the tissues, its causeative role being implied by skin testing and the appearance of the clinical lesions. Although the disease is found throughout the world it is common in certain areas such as the Mississippi valley in the United States. Systemically the disease manifests itself by lesions of the reticuloendothelial system, the lungs, liver, spleen, lymph nodes and bone marrow and may mimic Hodgkin's disease. The patients are anergic to tuberculin (Duke Elder and Leigh, 1966).

Scleritis has never been described in human histoplasmosis; however, in eyes examined from dogs who had been given systemic histoplasmosis, scleritis developed in half the animals (Salfelder, Schwarz and Akbarian, 1965). The scleritis in these animals accompanied a uveitis or a choroiditis. The lesions, which were sometimes necrotic, consisted of circumscribed granulomatous foci of histiocytes and lymphocytes with occasional leucocytes and plasma cells. The organisms were not found in the lesions.

This nonspecific granulomatous change is typical of that found in scleritis from other causes and it does not seem improbable that in areas where histoplasmosis is common it could be a potent initiating cause. We have not seen scleritis result from histoplasmosis but then histoplasmosis is rare in England.

In North America histoplasmosis is a common cause of anterior uveitis (Woods and Wahlen, 1960) and also gives rise to small discrete peripheral choroidoretinal lesions which are often accompanied by a cystic, central, haemorrhagic lesion at the macula. These lesions are very similar to those found in the experimental disease so that in areas in which histoplasmosis is common a histoplasma skin test should be undertaken in patients who develop scleritis.

TOXOPLASMOSIS

Toxoplasmosis occurs everywhere in the world and not uncommonly causes choroiditis and granulomatous uveitis (Wilder, 1952). It is therefore surprising that it has been proved to cause scleritis only once (Tokuda, Okamura and Kamano, 1970). Histological sections from patients whose eyes have been removed with the granulomas of toxoplasmosis show only a chronic inflammatory reaction in the sclera but no granuloma affecting the collagen fibres. Tokuda's patient was a 45-year-old female who first developed a severe, diffuse anterior 'brawny' scleritis in both eyes. This was followed by a uveitis which was so severe in one eye that it became an endophthalmitis. Because it became phthisical the eye was removed and histopathological study suggested a reticulum sarcoma but the crescentic *Toxoplasmona gondii* organisms and cysts were found in the specimen. The aqueous humor was aspirated from the opposite eye and cysts were detected in the aspirate by fluorescent antibody techniques.

Diagnosis of toxoplasmosis depends on serological tests of which the dye test is the most commonly used. Antibodies in the patient's serum inhibit the uptake of methylene blue by the parasites, the end-point of the test being when 50 per cent fail to do so. Many healthy adults have a low titre to the dye test and it is generally accepted that titres of less than 1:16 under 10 years, less than 1:32 under 20 years, and less than 1:64 in the adult should only be regarded as significant if the titre is rising. For technical reasons we have not performed toxoplasmosis dye tests on our patients as a routine but we have recently found high titres in a few patients. It may be that scleritis due to acquired toxoplasmosis is more common than was previously thought. It is unlikely that congenital toxoplasmosis is significant in the production of scleral disease.

RHINOSPORIDIOSIS

Rhinosporidiosis is a chronic granulomatous infection caused by the fungus *Rhinosporidium seeberi*, occurring mainly in South-East Asia, South America and rarely in Africa and Europe. Most recorded cases are from South India and Ceylon. The most common age incidence is 20 to 30 years; however, no age is exempt and infections in a four-year-old child and 90-year-old man have been reported. The organism which becomes implanted in the nasal or ocular mucosa through small abrasions is transmitted from infected cattle and is endemic in certain agricultural communities where cattle and humans bathe in the same stagnant pool of water.

The main sites of infection are the nose, nasopharynx, conjunctiva, lacrimal sac and larynx. When the lacrimal sac is infected it presents as a boggy swelling feeling like a bag of worms due to polypoid masses. Similar lesions are found on the conjunctiva and look like a strawberry or a minute pair of lungs attached by a trachea to the conjunctiva (Suseela and Subramaniam, 1976).

Among other sites, granulomas occur in the sclera (Lamba, Shukla and Ganapathy, 1970), the scleral granuloma presenting either as a chronic necrotising nodular scleritis which eventually causes ectasia as the necrotic area separates, or as solitary lesions as large as 1.5 cm in diameter. All cases show a mulberry-like mass on one edge of the lesion, which if biopsied can be found to contain the fungus. The visual acuity is unaffected and as the disease tends to run a benign course, treatment, which can only be surgical, is not usually necessary. Complete excision of the lesion and replacement with grafted cornea on sclera give excellent results.

METABOLIC DISEASES IN WHICH THE SCLERA IS INVOLVED

Gout

Classical gout is generally thought to be easy to diagnose: the patient, who is usually male, wakes in the early hours of the morning with severe pain in the big toe. In fact, the picture is not always quite so simple; only three attacks in four affect this joint and one attack in ten affects more than one joint. The inflammation results from the deposition of uric acid crystals into the joint. Similar symptoms can be produced by the other known type of crystal synovitis (pyrophosphate arthropathy) which results from the deposition of calcium pyrophosphate dihydrate crystals. This condition, sometimes termed pseudogout, is in most cases quite the classic disease; the knee is most commonly involved, the big toe rarely affected, and never the eye. The diagnosis of both these conditions can only be made with certainty by identifying the characteristic crystals in the joint fluid.

Gout classically occurs in postpubertal males and postmenopausal females as an acute inflammatory process affecting the first metatarsophalangeal joint, which settles in a couple of weeks. However, almost any joint can be affected. Acute synovitis after trauma or an operation should lead one to suspect gout. Usually the clinical diagnosis is obvious with severe pain, swelling and redness with overlying dry skin and accompanying gross tenderness. Further acute attacks can occur leading to the development of tophi in and around the joints which can cause destructive changes. Deposition of urates in the kidneys can cause renal impairment and renal stones.

During an acute attack the joint is hot and so exquisitely tender that the patient often cannot even bear the weight of the bedclothes. 'I feel as if I am walking on my eyeballs' was how Sidney Smith (1771–1845) described an attack. If left untreated, the pain will remain very severe for several days and then slowly subside. As this occurs, the outer layers of the skin often peel from the area that was most severely inflamed.

In clinical practice, gout is usually divided into primary gout, in which no obvious immediate cause can be found, and secondary gout, in which there is a pathological increase in uric acid production or decrease in its excretion. As the main source of uric acid is the cell nucleus, any condition in which there is increased cell destruction may lead to overproduction of uric acid, e.g. leukaemia, and the treatment of malignant conditions by cytotoxic agents which kill rapidly dividing cells (Watts, 1966).

More commonly, secondary gout is caused by decreased excretion of uric acid in the urine as a result of a general failure of the excretory mechanism in the kidney. A cause of increasing importance is the blocking of uric acid excretion by drugs; the use of thiazide diuretics is a common example (Klemperer and Bauer, 1944; Yu and Gutman, 1959).

Not all patients with high plasma uric acid levels develop gout, but the chances of doing so increase as the plasma uric acid level rises. Asymptomatic hyperuricaemia merits treatment if the serum uric acid values are consistently above 9.0 to 9.5 mg/100 ml, because gouty arthritis is very likely to occur in such patients (Hall et al, 1967). They are also exposed to the risk of developing chronic hyperuricaemic nephropathy (Talbott and Terplan, 1960).

The chances of suffering from gout increase as the plasma uric acid level rises. This was clearly shown by a population study in which the prevalence of gout was related to the level of serum uric acid:

Serum uric acid (mg/100 ml)	6–7	7–8	8–9	9+
Incidence of gout	2.5%	15%	40%	80%

The plasma uric acid concentration depends mainly on the sex, age and genetic constitution of the subject (Mikkelsen, Dodge and Valkenburg, 1965). There is also a racial factor. Polynesian men have a high incidence of hyperuricaemia and there is a high incidence of gout. Contrary to popular belief, dietary factors are relatively unimportant. The numerical values for uric acid levels are also influenced by the analytical method used (Dodge and Mikkelsen, 1970) and therefore the normal range for individual laboratories must be ascertained.

The presence of crystals in the joint is usually but not always associated with acute synovitis, although crystals also can be present without producing symptoms. It seems that the uptake of crystals by polymorphonuclear leucocytes causes the joint inflammation, and if the polymorphs are diminished there is a reduced inflammatory response (Phelps and McCarty, 1972). When crystals are phagocytosed they enter an endocytic vacuole (phagosome). Fusion of lysosomes occurs, and these contain hydrolytic and digestive enzymes. Interaction occurs between the crystals and the phospholipid of the lysosomal membrane, possibly due to the weak acidic groups on the surface of the crystal forming hydrogen bonds (Nash, Allison and Harington, 1966; Weissmann and Rita, 1972); disruption of the membrane, and release of lysosomal enzymes and the crystal follows. Phagocytosis of urates leads to increased production of lactic acid which causes further precipitation of crystals (Goldfinger, Howell and Seegmiller, 1965).

Crystal ingestion stimulates the production of a chemotactic factor producing further recruitment of leucocytes (Phelps, 1972). Hageman factor is activated and leads to a series of further reactions releasing chemical mediators of inflammation, including kinins (Goldfinger, Melmon and Webster, 1964).

Colchicine in vitro has been shown to stabilise the lysosomal membrane, block the release of chemotactic factor (Allison, 1973) and hinder the assembly of intracellular microtubules involved in lysosomal release (Malawista and Bensch, 1967).

The presence of monosodium urate in the external structures of the eye precipitates the inflammation in the same way as it does in the joint. This may presumably produce a simple hyperaemic conjunctivitis or, more frequently, conjunctivoepiscleritis which was originally described by Jonathan Hutchinson in 1886 as the 'gouty hot eye' (Figure 8.15).

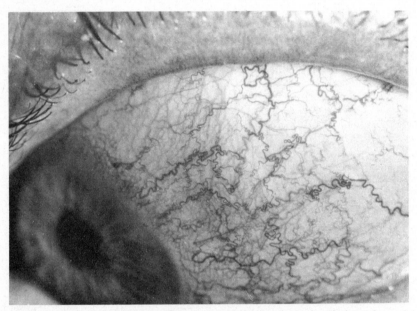

Figure 8.15.   Conjunctivoepiscleritis of acute gout. Notice that the conjunctival vessels are almost as congested as the deeper episcleral ones.

The onset, as with all manifestations of acute gout, is sudden, the eyes feel uncomfortable, pricking, sore, and there is some difficulty in moving them, particularly in the morning. Attacks, which may be precipitated by cold, excessive heat and sometimes indiscretions of diet or psychological upsets, usually last for about ten days before gradually fading away. It seems to be characteristic that if the patient recognises he is about to develop an attack and treats himself, then the attack may be aborted, but if he allows the eye to become even slightly inflamed, the inflammation will persist for ten days whatever is done. On occasion aggregations of urate crystals can be seen in the episcleral tissue of both conjunctiva and episclera. The combination of conjunctivitis and episcleritis, which can be extremely severe, is extremely unusual and if seen is almost certainly gout even though there are no joint symptoms.

The sclera is rarely involved in acute gout, but when it is the attacks are very much more painful than when the episclera is involved alone or with the conjunctiva. The attacks may be accompanied by a uveitis, and if the intraocular pressure rises the attack may be mistaken for a closed angle glaucoma.

It is extremely difficult when consulting the old literature to decide what conditions are due to gout and what are not because almost any eye symptoms and signs which could not readily be explained were put down to it. Our experience is that, discounting the acute gouty conjunctivitis and conjunctivo-episcleritis, clinical gout has been found to be present in seven per cent of the patients with episcleritis and two per cent of those with scleritis.

Uric acid may become deposited in the joint, causing erosion of bone. In contrast to rheumatoid arthritis, these erosions give the appearance of punched-out holes in normal bone. A more obvious appearance of uric acid deposition is the formation of tophi. These are yellowish nodules which tend to occur especially over cartilage, particularly in the ear (Figure 8.16). Before modern treatment was available, they would tend to ulcerate, the uric acid being extruded from them.

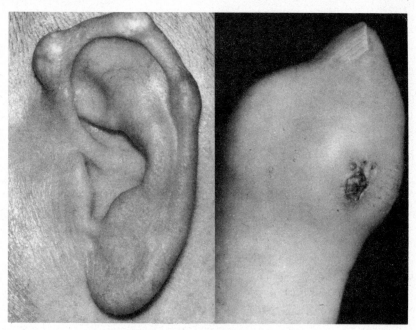

Figure 8.16.   Tophaceous gout of the ear and finger tip.
Courtesy of Alan Murley, Cambridge.

Tophi have been described in the sclera, but this is extremely unusual. In Figure 8.16 the patient, who had chronic tophaceous gout, presented with a nodular scleritis, which did not differ from that which would be seen in scleritis of any other cause. McWilliam (1952) and Heinz (1971) have however described hard, chalk-like masses of uric acid crystals symmetrically in the bulbar conjunctiva which looked like a pinguecula.

Wood (1936) described a patient who also had tophaceous gout in whom the crystals could be seen in the episclera and had widespread intraocular inflammation. Heinz (1971) has reviewed 63 patients with gout and found eight to have the signs of an ocular tophus, conjunctivitis, episcleritis, subconjunctival deposits and two had crystalline deposits in the lens. He also found 25 per cent had the fundus changes of an associated systemic hypertension.

Cystine Storage Disease (Lignac–Fanconi Syndrome, Cystinosis)

In this unusual and fatal condition there is an inability to secrete cystine and other amino acids, as a result of which cystine crystals are deposited in every tissue of the body, including the eye. The crystals, which can be detected in and under the child's episcleral tissue, can be seen easily by using the polarised beam on the pantoscope, even when they are invisible on the slit-lamp microscope. The changes in the cornea are diagnostic, occupying the whole thickness of the cornea. The deposition of crystals becomes more and more intense as the condition itself progresses, but never seems to cause any inflammatory reaction within the sclera itself.

The renal tubular defects may be due to reduction in available thiol groups (due to the presence of cystine) which are necessary for enzyme function. Administration of penicillamine, which increases the available thiol groups, has been shown to lead to improvement. The tubular lesion, which resembles that in the adult Fanconi syndrome, i.e. leads to mixed proximal and tubular defects, is always present in early life, usually a few months after birth, when polyuria, thirst, weakness and signs of rickets appear. The patients who are mentally retarded die early.

Alkaptonuria (Ochronosis)

This autosomal recessive disorder is characterised by dark pigmentation of skin, sclera and cartilage by arthritis, and is caused by absence of the enzyme homogentisic acid oxidase which converts homogentisic acid to malylacetoacetic acid during the degradation of tyrosine. The urine and tissues contain an excess of homogentisic acid and its precursors (Zannoni, Seegmiller and LaDu, 1962). Alkaptonuria is one of the conditions which Sir Archibald Garrod included in his now famous concept of inborn errors of metabolism (Garrod, 1908).

The urine turns a dark colour on oxidation. The clinical manifestations, known as ochronosis, similarly depend on its deposition in connective tissue, especially sclera and cartilage. Thus the ears become discoloured, developing a slate-blue appearance, and both sweat and cerumen are also coloured. Pigmentation occurs of the skin of the axillae and groin and over the nose (Martin et al, 1955). The urinary discolouration is distinguished from that of porphyria, bile pigments, melanoma, intravascular haemolysis and drug-induced discolouration by the high homogentisic acid content. Although the urine becomes brown at an early age, the other manifestations do not usually become apparent until middle-age and the disease is compatible with longevity.

The interpalpebral region of the sclera and the episclera is particularly pigmented. The areas can be mistaken for scleral hyaline plaques, being adjacent to the recti muscles and about the same size in both eyes. However, the plaques appear at a very much younger age. The pigmentation of the centre of the area is dark brown merging gently through yellow-brown, into the normal sclera. The area of pigmentation is always said to be triangular in shape, but this is by no means always so because Allen, O'Malley and Straatsma (1961) have reported cases in which the pigmentation involved the whole sclera.

Histological appearance of the sclera shows the collagen fibres to be swollen and the elastin fibres in particular disrupted with loss of the stromal cells (Ashton, Kirker and Lavery, 1964). The pigment is extracellular and all the scleral stroma and even the dural optic nerve sheath show pigmentation. Even though there may be large patches of intense pigment deposition, there is little, if any, inflammatory reaction to the pigment. A similar change in the eye has been noticed in factory workers as a toxic reaction to prolonged exposure to phenol derivatives, particularly hydroquinone (Anderson, 1947).

The locomotor manifestations are usually confined to the spine, giving rise to backache and stiffness and leading to complete spinal rigidity. Radiologically, the intravertebral discs are narrowed and the discs themselves calcified. Secondary degenerative changes with osteophyte formation subsequently develop (Martin et al, 1955). Occasionally a peripheral arthropathy develops; the features are essentially those of degenerative joint disease caused by a deposition of the pigment.

The Porphyrias

This series of conditions is associated with abnormal porphyrin metabolism. Porphyrins and their precursors are produced in excess, can be measured in the blood, urine and faeces and have a wide range of symptoms and signs involving almost every system in the body.

Porphyrin is a by-product of haem synthesis and hence of haemoglobin, myoglobin and the cytochromes. The steps in the pathway are shown in Figure 8.17. It will be seen that haem synthesis takes place by the Series III isomers and that Series I isomers are, if anything, by-products. Almost every cell in the body is capable of forming porphyrins, but the major sites of production are the liver and the bone marrow, and abnormal production of porphyrins is virtually restricted to these sites. Delta aminolaevulic acid (ALA) synthetase activity is known to be increased in every form of porphyria (Granick and Urata, 1963) and there is evidence that the different biochemical patterns characteristic of each of the porphyrias are related to anomalies of other enzymes at later stages in the pathway.

Classification of the porphyrias (Table 8.1) is based on the major site of abnormal porphyrin production, which may be liver or bone marrow, the hepatic porphyrias being more common (Schmid, Schwartz and Watson, 1954).

In England one person in 50 000 has some form of porphyria and 80 per cent of these are either acute, intermittent or cutaneous hepatic porphyria.

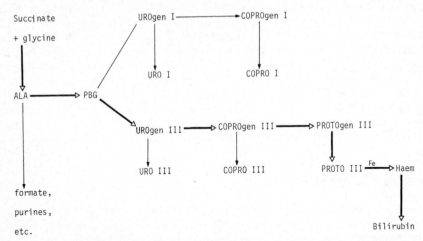

Figure 8.17. Biosynthesis of haem. ALA = aminolaevulic acid; PBG = porphobilinogen; UROgen = uroporhyrinogen;   COPROgen = coproporphyrinogen;   PROTOgen = protopor-phyrinogen.

Table 8.1. *Classification of the porphyrias*

Hepatic porphyrias
1. Acute intermittent porphyria
2. Cutaneous hepatic porphyria
     (a) Hereditary type — porphyria cutanea tarda
     (b) Possibly genetically predisposed — alcoholism
     (c) Acquired — hexachlorobenzene-induced
3. Variegate porphyria — mixed porphyria
4. Hereditary coproporphyria

Erythropoietic porphyrias
1. Congenital (erythropoietic) porphyria
2. Erythropoietic protoporphyria

In South Africa, cutaneous hepatic porphyria has a high prevalence amongst the Bantu, while porphyria variegata has been found in about 9000 of the white population (Dean, 1969).

Acute intermittent porphyria

This is the most severe of the hepatic porphyrias; it occurs in acute attacks, followed in most cases by complete remission. It is inherited as an autosomal dominant character but in one-third of reported cases there is no family history.

Gastrointestinal symptoms are common, most patients presenting with colicky central abdominal pain (Goldberg, 1959). Involvement of the central nervous system may lead to cranial nerve palsies and optic atrophy but these patients *do not* develop any changes in the sclera.

This diagnosis should be suspected if a patient who is also found to have hypertension, tachycardia or some neuropsychiatric disorder presents with abdominal pain. This suspicion is increased if there is a family history and if the urine turns dark on standing, or if the symptoms are aggravated by taking certain drugs, particularly barbiturates. Sulphonamides, methyldopa, chlorpropamide and anticonvulsants are also known to aggravate porphyria.

The diagnosis is confirmed by testing the urine for porphobilinogen and by chemical tests of porphyrin abnormalities in the blood. Treatment involves management of the various presenting features and prophylaxis is important. No specific therapy is available which will reverse the biochemical abnormalities.

Cutaneous hepatic porphyria

The main clinical findings appear in the skin and are related to the photo-sensitising property of porphyrins. Hepatocellular disease is common. A small proportion of cases appear to be inherited as an autosomal dominant (Holti et al, 1958). Symptoms may also be precipitated by taking a number of drugs, including alcohol.

The most striking and consistent clinical feature of this condition is a bullous dermatosis and hyperpigmentation on exposure to sunlight. The skin may be fragile and pruritus is often troublesome.

Histological examination of the skin shows gross hyaline swelling in the walls of the capillaries at the periphery of the bullae. Studies have shown that light of 400μm wavelength is absorbed by the porphyrin molecule and causes these skin lesions (Rimington et al, 1967).

Porphyria variegata

This form of porphyria gets its name because it combines the various clinical features of acute intermittent and cutaneous hepatic porphyrias. It is inherited as an autosomal dominant trait. A number of large family trees have been compiled and the longest is that of a South African family which can be traced back to a Dutch settler who arrived at the Cape of Good Hope in 1688 (Dean and Barnes, 1955).

Like acute intermittent porphyria, porphyria variegata attacks young adults but is very rare in childhood. Systemic attacks are nearly always precipitated by a drug.

Patients are liable to develop in the second or third decade conjunctival changes similar to benign mucous membrane pemphigoid except that they extend on to the lids and lead to scarring and symblepharon.

Douglas (1972) described three female patients. Two of these had presented many years before with similar facies, the skin of the areas exposed to sun being covered with an increased amount of downy hair and deeply pigmented. There was severe scarring of the lids, nose, mouth, circumoral area and ears. The feet and hands were also severely scarred and superficially the digits resembled those of a patient with scleroderma. The skin was smooth but not excessively taut. The x-ray showed destruction of the terminal phalanges of one of the patients, a finding also described in scleroderma.

They both had rose-coloured teeth due to deposits of type I porphyrins. Areas containing concentrations of type I porphyrins fluoresced with this rose colouration when exposed to ultraviolet light; this can be demonstrated by exposing the patients' teeth to a Wood's light. This rose discolouration was also seen in bone. Three of the four eyes of these two patients perforated spontaneously, but prior to that they were reported as having yellow-brown thickening of the episclera/conjunctiva in the palpebral area which extended on to the limbus. These areas looked like 'milk curds' in ultraviolet light. The eyes were otherwise normal.

His final patient spontaneously perforated one eye and was found to have a scleral excavation without surrounding inflammation (scleromalacia perforans), exposing the choroid in the other. He was treated by an autogenous scleral overlay graft with good results.

Histological studies show that the superficial lamellae of the sclera are affected more than the deep lamellae. The superficial lamellae sequestrate, leaving the lamina fusca, whilst the deep lamellae show hyaline change or calcium deposition and perhaps elastin degeneration.

If the area of collagen destruction is close to the limbus, the cornea can also become involved, the cornea becoming infiltrated. It may even be destroyed or a leucoma may form (Garrod, 1936; Castex and Lopez-Garcia, 1970). Aguarde et al (1969) described lid vesicles, ciliary changes, conjunctival bullous keratoconjunctivitis and scleritis, together with abnormal fundus pigmentation, although the scleral collagen is preferentially attacked in this condition, giving rise to the typical changes of scleromalacia perforans (Barnes and Boshoff, 1952; Miani, 1958; Aguarde et al, 1969). Similar changes can be found in the joints.

GENETIC AND METABOLIC DISORDERS OF CONNECTIVE TISSUE

These are uncommon disorders and whilst metabolic abnormalities are known in a number of instances, and almost certainly exist within the group as a whole, diagnosis of these disorders rests on clinically recognisable features.

Genetic disorders can affect connective tissue in various ways:

1. There may be a defect in the synthesis of components such as collagen. Such defects are suspected of being the cause of Marfan's syndrome and osteogenesis imperfecta, and may result from an abnormal amino acid sequence in the protein chains.
2. There may be a deficiency of a synthesising enzyme as, for example, in homocystinuria.
3. There may be a disturbance of the normal breakdown of connective tissue. This is seen in the mucopolysaccharidoses where the common denominator is storage of mucopolysaccharides and glycolipids due to deficiency of lysosomal hydrolases.

Marfan's Syndrome

The most conspicuous feature of Marfan's syndrome is the generalised over-growth of long bones, resulting in tallness, long slender fingers and toes (arachnodactyly) (Figure 8.18) and a long head. The span will exceed the height and the heel to pubis distance exceeds that from crown to pubis. Sternal deformity, excurvature and scoliosis are common. The skeletal muscles are hypoplastic, there is deficiency of cutaneous fat which emphasises the ungainly appearance, and there is joint laxity (McKusick, 1955a).

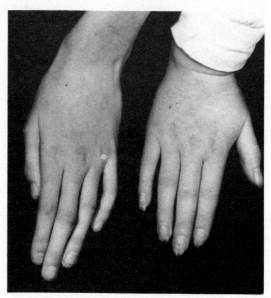

Figure 8.18.   The long thin hand and fingers of a patient with Marfan's syndrome compared to a normal adult of the same age to the right.

This condition is inherited as an autosomal dominant although mutations occur. Cardiac lesions occur in some 36 per cent (McKusick, 1955b), the prognosis depending largely on whether aortic involvement occurs. Aortic dilatation—by far the gravest complication—leads in a proportion of cases to aneurysm formation and rupture. The 50 per cent risk of inheriting the disease for each child of an affected person proves unacceptable for many couples and all should be made aware of the genetic risk.

The diagnosis is clinical and the differential diagnosis is principally from homocystinuria (Brenton et al, 1972) and from constitutional tall structure.

Ocular abnormalities

Ectopia lentis occurs in over 95 per cent of patients with the syndrome. Dislocation of the lens is usually partial, bilateral or symmetrical. The direction of displacement is usually upwards (Figure 8.19) but when subluxation occurs

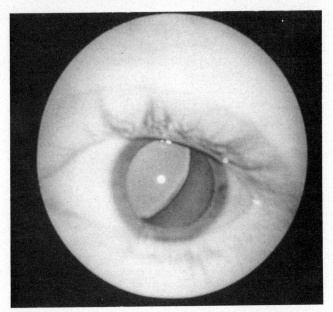

Figure 8.19. Dislocation of the lens in the same patient.

it can be either forwards into the anterior chamber or backwards into the vitreous in which case secondary glaucoma usually supervenes. Unfortunately, the glaucoma is extremely difficult to control and may eventually destroy vision. The scleral collagen, like the aorta is unable to resist intraluminal pressure and will, if the intraocular pressure is even slightly above normal, allow the globe to expand, producing a staphyloma at its weakest part, the limbus. Surgery on the eye for glaucoma and scleral repair should be avoided if at all possible as results are poor.

Homocystinuria

This condition is an inborn error of metabolism inherited as an autosomal recessive characteristic in which homocystine accumulates in the blood and urine. It was discovered in 1962 by Carson and Neill but several years passed before it was realised that a considerable number of patients thought to have Marfan's syndrome in fact had homocystinuria (Schimke et al, 1965). The similarity is sufficient for a urine test for homocystine to be worthwhile in any suspected Marfan patient.

Complications include mental retardation and a thrombotic tendency which may cause infarction of an organ. When the lens dislocates, it does so downwards, and the scleral collagen appears to be stronger, thicker and more resistant to raised intraocular pressure than in Marfan's syndrome.

In most cases of homocystinuria the underlying metabolic defect is absence of the enzyme cystathionine synthetase (Mudd et al, 1964). The cyanide-nitro-prusside test on urine acts as a simple screening procedure for the detection of homocystinuria, a reddish colour developing if the test is positive. Since the test is also positive in cystinuria, the diagnosis must be confirmed by chromatography.

Osteogenesis Imperfecta

The cardinal manifestations of this condition are blue sclerae, brittle bones and deafness. The classic appearance is typified by Toulouse Lautrec (see McKusick, 1972). The basic pathology is of mesodermal hypoplasia, which manifests itself mostly in the bony tissue but also produces thinning of the sclera so that the choroid is readily visible through the scleral coat. Ruedemann (1953) and de Leonibus and Gemolotto (1954) showed that not only were the sclera and cornea thin but there was also a gross deduction in the number of collagen fibrils present, a persistence of precollagenous reticulin and an increase in the procollagen content of the tissue. The epithelium, endothelium and elastic tissue appear normal in consistency. Eichholtz and Muller (1972) have examined the sclera by electron microscopy and have confirmed Ruedemann's findings but have also noted deposits between the scleral lamellae (possibly chondroitin sulphate) and vacuoles in the endoplasmic reticulum. They consider that these point to a disturbance of the fibroblasts and help account for the increased transparency. Whatever the underlying cause, the results of the thin sclera and cornea are the same: the thin sclera and cornea can normally withstand the normal intraocular pressure, but occasionally both the sclera and cornea may become ectatic. Three main types of this disease occur: osteogenesis imperfecta (Vrolik's type), osteopsathyrosis (Lobstein's type) and the tardive type (Spurway's disease). If blue sclera occurs in any of these types the histological appearance is the same.

The systemic manifestations of the condition include hypermobility of the joints, and the musculature is poorly developed. Fractures are multiple and distressing, occurring with the minimum of trauma as early as intrauterine life and at any time thereafter. The fractures themselves unite, but somewhat abnormally with excessive deposition of fibrous tissue. However, it must be emphasised that while some individuals have multiple fractures dating from birth, others go through life without a fracture. The deafness in due in part to otosclerosis and in part to nerve involvement and occurs in 30 per cent of patients.

The prognosis depends on the type and severity of the disease. Vrolik's type is fatal in infancy but for the other types, even in severely crippled cases, the expectation of life is generally good, there may be improvement at puberty, and the tardive type may reproduce. The inheritance is autosomal dominant in the majority of cases and genetic counselling is of great importance.

Other Causes of Blue Sclerotics

Recently patients have been described who have developed blue sclera, kera-toglobus and brittle corneas which can sometimes perforate spontaneously.

These patients are without any or with only a few other systemic signs, which consist of hyper-extensible joints and pes cavus (Babel and Houber, 1969; Gregoratos, Bartosocas and Papas, 1971; Lamba, Shukla and Ganapathy, 1971). All seem to be inherited as an autosomal or sex-linked recessive, but whether they represent an incomplete form of osteogenesis inperfecta or Type VI Ehlers–Danlos syndrome is uncertain. Blue sclerotics have also been described in iron deficiency (Hall, 1971; Pope and Agnoletto, 1971).

Pseudoxanthoma Elasticum

This is a rare form of atrophy which appears in early life. It is characterised by the appearance of small yellow striae on the neck, axillae and abdomen, and sometimes on the elbows and knees, and also gastrointestinal bleeding and retinal changes.

Pathologically the streaks consist of a degeneration of elastic tissue which may also involve the aorta and peripheral blood vessels. Angioid streaks occur in the eye caused by splits in Bruch's membrane, which, if they pass close to the macula, will severely affect vision. Scleral dehiscences very similar to those in Figure 9.3 can also occur. There may also be a more widespread retinal degeneration. The sclera does not become inflamed in this condition but of 180 patients studied by Pope (1971), thin blue sclera were commonly found and occurred in 32 to 62 per cent of the probands, depending on the type of pseudoxanthoma elasticum. Between three and 20 per cent of these patients also described similar scleral changes in their relatives.

The diagnosis, once thought of, is not difficult to make by observation of the facial appearance, the redundant folds of loose skin, the striae and the fundal appearances.

Ehlers–Danlos Syndrome

Hypermobile joints, fragile and elastic skin and a tendency to bleed are the main signs of this disorder. Beighton (1970) classified the Ehlers–Danlos syndrome into five varieties, to which a sixth and a seventh have since been added: Type VI by Pinelli et al (1972) and Lichtenstein et al (1972) and Type VII by McKusick (1972).

Table 8.2. *Classification of the Ehlers–Danlos syndrome*

Type	Common name	Mode of inheritance	Basic defect
I	Gravis type	AD	?
II	Mitis type	AD	?
III	Benign hypermobile type	AD	?
IV	Ecchymotic or vascular type	AD	?
V	X-linked type	X-linked	Lysyl oxidase deficiency
VI	Ocular type	AR	Lysyl hydroxylase deficiency
VII		AR	Procollagen peptidase deficiency

AD = autosomal dominant.
AR = autosomal recessive.

The sixth type is characterised by ocular symptoms out of proportion to the systemic findings and these consist of microcornea or megalocornea, extreme thinning of the cornea and sclera, keratoconus, dislocated lenses, cataracts and retinal detachments. The extreme thinning of the sclera gives it a pale blue tinge which is very striking and occurs in seven per cent of the patients. Spontaneous rupture of the cornea and sclera occurs in many of these patients; McKusick (1972) described it as fragilitas oculi and related it to Marfan's syndrome and, as in this syndrome, surgery should be avoided if possible because suturing, which is always difficult, may be impossible because of the fragility of the tissues. Many eyes have to be enucleated because of failed surgery.

Lysyl hydroxylase converts lysine to hydroxylysine. Aldehydes are formed which subsequently cross-link spontaneously. If there is interference at any one of these steps, the connective tissue is weakened, because of the absence of cross-linking.

Table 8.3.   *Disorders associated with cross-linking of collagen*

Cause	Enzyme defect	Syndrome
	Peptidyl lysine and hydroxylysine	1. Ehlers–Danlos syndrome Type VI (lysyl hydroxylase deficiency). 2. Aneurysm-prone mice. 3. Menke's kinky hair syndrome. 4. Ehlers–Danlos syndrome Type V.
1. Lathyrogens 2. Copper deficiency	Lysyl oxidase	
	Peptidyl allysine and hydroxylysine	
3. D-penicillamine 4. Homocysteine	Cross links	5. Ehlers–Danlos syndrome Type VII (procollagen peptidase deficiency).

From Maumenee (1974).

In Type V and Type VII Ehlers–Danlos syndrome, deficient cross-linking is the outstanding feature. In Type V there is reduced lysyl oxidase activity (Leachman et al, 1974) and in Type VII there is absence of procollagen peptidase, leading to excess procollagen in the extracellular space and impaired cross-linking.

In patients with Menke's kinky hair syndrome—a hereditary copper deficiency resulting in poor cross-linking—ocular symptoms are absent (Danks et al, 1972). It might, therefore, be suggested that there is only defective ocular tissue in Type VI Ehlers–Danlos syndrome, the ocular collagen being affected by lysyl hydroxylase deficiency, but not by procollagen peptidase deficiency.

Scleral Icterus

'All looks yellow to the jaundic'd eye' (Alexander Pope, 1688–1744).

The yellow discolouration of the conjunctiva and sclera which accompanies hepatic or haemolytic jaundice must be practically the oldest recognised physical sign in medicine. Bilirubin derived from the breakdown of haem is conjugated in the liver with glucuronic acid by the microsomal enzyme glucuronyl transferase. This renders it soluble and not tightly bound to plasma albumin, so that it can be excreted in the urine. If jaundice is due to an excessive breakdown of haemoglobin then there will be an excessive amount of unconjugated bilirubin in the blood, and if due to biliary obstruction there will be considerably more of the conjugated form.

Clinical discolouration of the sclera does not occur before the level of bilirubin in the blood rises above 1.5 mg/100 ml plasma (Thompson, 1973) and its appearance and disappearance lags behind the rise and fall in plasma level because the bilirubin binds strongly to the elastin fibres of the sclera. Because it is in the soluble form, jaundice caused by an increase in conjugated bilirubin in the plasma becomes clinically apparent at a lower plasma level than that caused by free bilirubin (Knell, 1973). It is because of this and because the conjunctival staining comes and disappears before the scleral staining that the depth of the jaundice cannot be estimated as accurately by looking at the eye as by analysing the blood.

Unilateral icterus has been described following choroidal haemorrhage which occurred during or following intraocular manipulations in surgery for retinal detachment (Tolentino and Brockhurst, 1963). In this case the scleral staining is caused by haemolysis of the extravasated blood, haemoglobin being released and broken down to bilirubin (Figure 8.17). The bilirubin diffuses into the sclera in its unconjugated form and is taken up weakly by the elastin and to a less extent by the collagen fibres of the sclera. Choroidal haemorrhage is difficult to distinguish from choroidal tumours. If icterus is present haemorrhage is the most likely diagnosis.

The discolouration of the sclera produced by icterus needs to be distinguished from that seen in natural pigmentation, the porphyrias and alkaptonuria. The prolonged use of local eye preparations, particularly proteinated silver preparations, mercurials and iodides, causes discolouration and pigmentation of the conjunctiva, episclera and occasionally also the sclera but the colour of staining is very different from the deep yellow of jaundice.

REFERENCES

Adelung, J. C. (1951) Skleralstaphylom nach Herpes zoster ophthalmicus. *Klinische Monatsblatter für Augenheilkunde*, **118**, 620–629.

Agnoletto, A. (1971) Blue sclerotics in iron deficiency. *Lancet*, **ii**, 1160.

Aguarde, J. P., Mascaro, J. M., Galy-Mascaro, C. & Capedevila, J. M. (1969) Some little known cutaneous and ocular manifestations of porphyria. *Annales de Dermatologie et de Syphiligraphie*, **96**, 265–270.

Allen, R. A., O'Malley, C. & Straatsma, B. R. (1961) Ocular findings in hereditary ochronosis. *Archives of Ophthalmology*, **65**, 657–658.

Allison, A. C. (1973) *Ciba Foundation Symposium on Locomotion of Tissue Cells* (Ed.) Fitzsimons, D., p. 109. Amsterdam: Elsevier.

Anderson, B. (1947) Corneal and conjunctival pigmentation among workers engaged in manufacture of hydroquinine. *Archives of Ophthalmology*, **38**, 812–826.

Andreani, D. G. (1954) Tuberculoma of the sclera. *Giornale Italiano di Oftalmologia*, **7**, 506–515.

Arducci, F. & Cappelli, I. (1968) Scleral staphyloma after scleritis caused by herpes zoster. *Annali di Ottalmologia*, **94**, 187–192.

Ashton, N., Kirker, J. G. & Lavery, F. S. (1964) Ocular findings in a case of hereditary ochronosis. *British Journal of Ophthalmology*, **48**, 405–415.

Babel, J. & Houber, J. (1969) Keratoconus and blue sclerae in a congenital anomaly of connective tissue. *Journal de Génétique Humaine*, **17**, 241–246.

Barnes, H. D. & Boshoff, P. H. (1952) Ocular lesions in patients with porphyria. *Archives of Ophthalmology*, **48**, 567–580.

Barros, J. M. de (1939) *Aspectos Clinicos do Comprolimento Ocular da Lepra*. Sao Paulo: Companhia Melhoramentos.

Bauer, W. & Klemperer, P. (1944) Medical progress: treatment of gout. *New England Journal of Medicine*, **231**, 681–685.

Beighton, P. (1970) *The Ehlers–Danlos Syndrome*. London: Heinemann.

Bell, G. H. (1914) Report of a case of tuberculosis of the sclera of probable primary origin. *Transactions of the American Ophthalmological Society*, **13**, 787–795.

Berg, F. (1927) Scleritis pericornealis nach Parotitis epidemica. *Berichte uber die Versammlungen der deutschen ophthalmologischen Gesellschaft*, **46**, 368–372.

Bhaduri, B. N. & Basu, S. K. (1956) Scleral gumma. *British Journal of Ophthalmology*, **40**, 504–505.

Borthen, L. & Lie, H. P. (1899) *Die Lepra des Auges*, p. 182. Leipzig: Engelmann.

Brenton, D. P., Dow, C. J., James, J. I. et al (1972) Homocystinuria and Marfan's syndrome. *Journal of Bone and Joint Surgery*, **54**, 277–298.

Brini, A., Quéré, M. & Achard, M. (1953) Sclerite nodulaire nécrosante (presence de bacille de Koch). *Bulletin des Sociétés d'Ophtalmologie de France*, **7**, 822–825.

Carson, N. A. & Neill, D. W. (1962) Metabolic abnormalities detected in a survey of mentally backward individuals in Northern Ireland. *Archives of Disease in Childhood*, **37**, 505–513.

Castex, M. R. & Lopez-Garcia, A. (1970) Clinical aspects of porphyria. *Boletin de la Academia Nacional de Medicina de Buenos Aires*, **70**, 265–279.

Colrat, A. (1930) Vaso dilatation épisclérale et conjunctival consécutive aux oreillions. *Archives d'Ophtalmologie*, **47**, 839–840.

Courtis, B. (1928) *Tuberculosis Experimental del Ojo*. Thesis, Universidad Nacional de Buenos Aires.

Danks, D. M., Campbell, P. E. & Stevens, B. J. (1972) Menkes' kinky hair syndrome. An inherited defect in copper absorption with widespread effects. *Pediatrics*, **50**, 188–201.

Das Gupta, B. K. & Usman, M. (1949) Bilateral symmetrical tuberculous ulcers of bulbar conjuntivae treated with streptomycin. *British Journal of Ophthalmology*, **33**, 501–505.

Dean, G. (1969) The porphyrias. *British Medical Bulletin*, **25**, 48–51.

Dean, G. & Barnes, H. D. (1955) Inheritance of porphyria. *British Medical Journal*, **ii**, 89–94.

Dejean, C. (1953) La scléro-kératite tuberculeuse atypique experimentale. *Bulletin et Memoires de la Société Française d'Ophtalmologie*, **66**, 316–320.

Deodati, F., Bec, P. & Labro, J-B. (1971) Syphilitic scleritis; clinical and angiographic study. *Bulletin des Sociétés d'Ophtalmologie de France*, **71**, 63–65.

Dodge, H. J. & Mikkelsen, W. M. (1970) Observations on the distribution of serum uric acid levels in participants of the Tecumseh, Michigan Community Health Studies. A comparison of results of one method used at two different times and of two methods used simultaneously. *Journal of Chronic Disease*, **23**, 161–172.

Douglas, W. H. (1972) Congenital porphyria: general and ocular manifestations. *Transactions of the Ophthalmological Societies of the United Kingdom*, **92**, 541–553.

Duke Elder, W. S. & Leigh, A. G. (1965) *System of Ophthalmology,* Vol. 8, (a) p. 1029, (b) p. 845, (c) p. 237. London: Kimpton.

Eichholtz, W. & Muller, D. (1972) Electron microscopy of cornea and sclera in osteogenesis imperfecta. *Klinische Monatsblatter für Augenheilkunde,* **161,** 646–653.

Ellis, O. H. & Holtz, M. J. (1953) Scleromalacia perforans. *California Medicine,* **78,** 60–63.

Elschnig, A. (1897) Syphilitische Infiltration der conjunctiva bulbi. *Klinische Monatsblatter für Augenheilkunde,* **35,** 155–159.

Evans, J. J. (1905) Diffuse gummatous infiltration of scleral and episcleral tissues. *Transactions of the Ophthalmological Societies of the United Kingdom,* **25,** 188.

Finnoff, W. C. (1931) Tuberculosis in etiology of acute iritis. *American Journal of Ophthalmology,* **14,** 127–132.

Fracastoro, G. (1530) *Syphilis Sive Morbus Gallicus.*

Garland, J. (1943) Varicella following exposure to herpes zoster. *New England Journal of Medicine,* **228,** 336–337.

Garrod, A. (1908) Croonian lectures on inborn errors of metabolism. *Lancet,* **ii,** 73.

Garrod, A. (1936) Congenital porphyrinuria. *Quarterly Journal of Medicine,* **5,** 473–480.

Goldberg, A. (1959) Acute intermittent porphyria. *Quarterly Journal of Medicine,* **28,** 183–209.

Goldfinger, S. E., Howell, R. R. & Seegmiller, J. (1965) Suppression of metabolic accompaniments of phagocytosis by colchicine. *Arthritis and Rheumatism,* **8,** 1112–1122.

Goldfinger, S., Melmon, K. L. & Webster, M. E. (1964) The presence of kinin-peptide in inflammatory synovial effusions. *Arthritis and Rheumatism,* **7,** 311.

Granick, S. & Urata, G. (1963) Increase in activity of α-aminolevulinic acid synthetase in liver mitochondria induced by feeding of 3,5-dicarbethoxy-1,4-dihydrocollidine. *Journal of Biological Chemistry,* **238,** 821–827.

Gregoratos, N. D., Bartosocas, C. S. & Papas, K. (1971) Blue sclera with keratoglobus and brittle cornea. *British Journal of Ophthalmology,* **55,** 424–426.

Gunn, D. (1894) Syphilitic subconjunctival infiltration. *Transactions of the Ophthalmological Societies of the United Kingdom,* **14,** 68.

Hall, A. P., Barry, P. E., Dawber, T. R. & MacNamara, P. M. (1967) Epidemiology of gout and hyperuricemia. *American Journal of Medicine,* **42,** 27–37.

Hall, G. H. (1971) Blue sclerotics in iron deficiency. *Lancet,* **ii,** 1377.

Heinz, K. (1971) Ocular findings in cases of gout and hyperuricemia. *Wiener klinische Wochenschrift,* **83,** 42–44.

Hibi, H. & Shiozawa, E. (1965) Ocular symptoms of erythema nodosum leprosum. *Journal of Clinical Ophthalmology* (Tokyo), **9,** 779–782.

Holti, G., Rimington, C., Tate, B. C. & Thomas, G. (1958) An investigation of porphyria cutanea tarda. *Quarterly Journal of Medicine,* **27,** 1–17.

Hope-Simpson, R. E. (1965) The nature of Herpes zoster: a long term study and a new hypothesis. *Proceedings of the Royal Society of Medicine,* **58,** 9–20.

Hutchinson, J. (1886) Hot eye in association with gout. *British Medical Journal,* **i,** 1018.

James, D. G., Anderson, R., Langley, D. & Ainslie, D. (1964) Ocular sarcoidosis. *British Journal of Ophthalmology,* **48,** 461–470.

Jones, B. R., Al-Hussaini, K. M. & Dunlop, E. C. (1966) Infection by tric agent and other members of the Bedsonia group, with a note on Reiter's disease. *Transactions of the Ophthalmological Societies of the United Kingdom,* **86,** 291–312.

Jones, B. R., Howie, J. B. & Wilson, R. P. (1952) Ocular aspects of an epidemic of infectious mononucleosis. *Proceedings of the University of Otago Medical School,* **30,** 1–2.

Jones, D. B., Visvesvera, G. S. & Robinson, N. M. (1975) Acanthamoeba polyphaga keratitis and acanthamoeba uveitis associated with fatal meningoencephalitis. *Transactions of the Ophthalmological Societies of the United Kingdom,* **95,** 221–231.

Knell, A. (1973) In *Diseases of the Liver, Gall Bladder and Pancreas* (Ed.) Williams, R. pp. 521–526. London: Medicine Education International.

Krantz, W. (1950) Tuberculous manifestations affecting the skin and eye. *Dermatologische Wochenschrift,* **121,** 447.

344   *The Sclera and Systemic Disorders*

Kuriakose, E. T. (1963) Oculosporidiosis rhinosporidiosis of the eye. *British Journal of Ophthalmology*, **47**, 346–349.

Kuriakose, E. T. (1964) Oculosporidiosis. Clinical manifestation and treatment. *Proceedings of the All-India Ophthalmological Society*, **21**, 151–158.

Lagrange, H. (1933) Diagnosis of iridociliary tuberculosis. *British Journal of Ophthalmology*, **17**, 679–685.

Lamba, P. A., Shukla, K. N. & Ganapathy, N. (1970) Rhinosporidium granuloma of conjunctiva with scleral ectasia. *British Journal of Ophthalmology*, **54**, 565–568.

Lamba, P. A., Shukla, K. N. & Ganapathy, N. (1971) Blue sclera with keratoglobus. *Oriental Archives of Ophthalmology*, **9**, 123–126.

Leachman, R. D., Angelini, P., Di Ferrante, N. & Donnelly, V. (1974) Lysyl oxidase deficiency in Ehlers–Danlos syndrome type V. In *Birth Defects Original Article Series* (Ed.) Bergsma. California: Torrence.

Leonibus, F. de & Gemolotto, G. (1954) Rilievi istologici su di un caso di sclera blu. *Bolletino di Oculistica*, **33**, 789–795.

Lévy, R. & Lobstein, A. (1952) Une complication rare du zona ophtalmique; l'atrophie sclérale avec perforation. *Bulletin des Sociétés d'Ophtalmologie de France*, **3**, 256–258.

Lichtenstein, J. R., Martin, G. R., Kohn, L. D. & Byers, P. H. (1972) Defect in conversion of procollagen to collagen in a form of Ehlers–Danlos syndrome. *Science*, **182**, 298–300.

MacKenzie, W. (1854) *A Practical Treatise in Diseases of the Eye*, 4th edition. London: Longman.

Maitre-Jan, A. (1907) *Traite des Maladies de l'oeil et des Remedes pour leur Guerijon*. Paris: Laurent d'houry.

Malawista, S. E. & Bensch, K. G. (1967) Human polymorphonuclear leukocytes: demonstration of microtubules and effect of colchicine. *Science*, **156**, 521–522.

Martin, W. J., Underdahl, L. O., Mathieson, D. R. & Pugh, D. G. (1955) Alkaptonuria: report of 12 cases. *Annals of Internal Medicine*, **42**, 1052–64.

Maumenee, I. H. (1974) Hereditary connective tissue diseases involving the eye. *Transactions of the Ophthalmological Societies of the United Kingdom*, **94**, 753–761.

McKusick, V. A. (1955a) Cardiovascular aspects of Marfan's syndrome: heritable disorder of connective tissue. *Circulation*, **11**, 321–342.

McKusick, V. A. (1955b) Heritable disorders of connective tissue: Marfan's syndrome. *Journal of Chronic Disease*, **2**, 609–644.

McKusick, V. A. (1972) *Heritable Disorders of Connective Tissue*, 4th edition, (a) p. 407, (b) p. 317. St. Louis: Mosby.

McWilliams, J. R. (1952) Ocular findings in gout; a report of a case of conjunctival tophi. *American Journal of Ophthalmology*, **35**, 1778–1783.

Miani, P. (1958) Ocular manifestations in congenital porphyria. *Giornale Italiano di Oftalmologica*, **11**, 381–400.

Mikkelsen, W. M., Dodge, H. J. & Valkenburg, H. (1965) The distribution of serum uric acid values in population unselected as to gout or hyperuricaemia: Tecumseh, Michigan 1959–1960. *American Journal of Medicine*, **39**, 242–251.

Mudd, S. H., Finkelstein, J. D., Irreverre, F. & Laster, L. (1964) Homocystinuria: an enzymatic defect. *Science*, **143**, 1443–1445.

Nagington, J., Watson, P. G., Playfair, T. J. et al (1974) Amoebic infection of the eye. *Lancet*, **ii**, 1537–1540.

Nash, T., Allison, A. C. & Harington, J. S. (1966) Physicochemical properties of silica in relation to its toxicity. *Nature*, **210**, 259–261.

Naumann, G., Gass, J. D. & Font, R. L. (1968) Histopathology of herpes zoster ophthalmicus. *American Journal of Ophthalmology*, **65**, 533–541.

North, D. P. (1953) Ocular complications of mumps. *British Journal of Ophthalmology*, **37**, 99–100.

Panzardi, D. (1947) Contributo alla conoscenza delle lesioni erpetiche oculari: su di un particolare caso di compromissiono della conjunctiva, cornea ed episclera da virus erpetico. *Bollettino d'Oculistica*, **26**, 465–470.

Parducci, F. & Carpelli, L. (1968) Su di un caso di stafiloma sclerale consequente a sclerite da herpes zoster. *Annali di Ottalmologica*, **94**, 187–192.

Paufique, L., Audibert, J. & Paupert-Ravault, M. (1961) Necrosing nodular scleritis associated with skin lesions; probably tuberculous in nature. *Bulletin des Sociétés d'Ophtalmologie de France*, **58**, 473–474.

Perdriel, G., Michel, A., Guyard, M. & Hoel, J. (1961) The ocular manifestations of Q fever. *Annales d'Oculistique*, **194**, 957–970.

Phelps, P. (1972) quoted by McCarthy, D. J. in *Phagocytic Mechanisms in Health and Disease* (Ed.) Williams, R. C. & Fudenberg, H. H. p. 107. New York, London: Intercontinental Medical Book Corporation.

Phelps, P. & McCarthy, D. J. (1966) Crystal induced inflammation in canine joints. III Importance of polymorphonuclear leukocytes. *Journal of Experimental Medicine*, **124**, 115–126.

Phillips, S., Williams, M. L. & Maiden, S. D. (1950) Chronic miliary tuberculosis. *American Review of Tuberculosis*, **62**, 549–554.

Pinnell, S. R., Krane, S. M., Kenzora, J. E. et al (1972) A hereditable disorder of connective tissue: hydroxylysine-deficient collagen disease. *New England Journal of Medicine*, **286**, 1013–1020.

Pope, F. M. (1971) Blue sclerotics in iron deficiency. *Lancet*, **ii**, 1160.

Rao, P. N. & Ramalingan, T. T. (1969) Rhinosporidiosis manifesting as unusual scleral staphyloma. *Journal of the All-India Ophthalmological Society*, **17**, 59.

Rieger, M. (1935) Uber subconjunctivitis epibulbaris metastatica bei Parotitis epidemica. *Archiv für Ophthalmologie*, **133**, 505–507.

Rimington, C., Magnus, I. A., Ryan, E. A. & Cripps, D. J. (1967) Porphyria and photo-sensitivity. *Quarterly Journal of Medicine*, **36**, 29–57.

Ruedemann, A. D. (1953) Osteogenesis imperfecta congenita and blue sclerotics. *Archives of Ophthalmology*, **49**, 6–16.

Saba, V. (1947) Sullo episcleriti erpetishe: contributo clinico. *Annali di Ottalmologia e Clinica Oculistica*, **73**, 168–170.

Salfelder, K., Schwarz, J. & Akbarian, M. (1965) Experimental histoplasmosis in dogs. *American Journal of Ophthalmology*, **59**, 290–299.

Sanna, M. (1950) Episclerite erpetica. *Bollettino d'Oculistica*, **29**, 173–177.

Sarda, R. P., Mehrotra, A. S. & Adnani, K. (1969) Nodular episcleritis (a proved case of tubercular origin). *Indian Journal of Ocular Pathology*, **3**, 24–26.

Satyendran, O. M., Row, N. V., Phatak, B. H. & Sarma, S. R. (1965) Rhinosporidiosis of the eye and adnexa. *Oriental Archives of Ophthalmology*, **3**, 332–335.

Saxena, R. C. (1963) Ocular involvement in leprosy. *Journal of the All-India Ophthalmological Society*, **11**, 13–16.

Schimke, R. N., McKusick, V. A., Huang, T. & Pollack, A. D. (1965) Homocystinuria: studies of 20 families with 38 affected members. *Journal of the American Medical Association*, **193**, 711–719.

Schmidt, R., Schwartz, S. & Watson, C. J. (1954) Porphyrin content of bone marrow and liver in various forms of porphyria. *Archives of Internal Medicine*, **93**, 167–190.

Simon, H. (1919) *Ein Fall von Scleritis Posterior*. Dissertation, University of Heidelberg.

Sorsby, A. (1963) *Modern Ophthalmology*, Vol. 2 p. 123. London: Butterworth.

Suseela, V. & Subramaniam, K. S. (1976) *Rhinosporidiosis and the Eyes*. Unpublished.

Swan, K. C. (1951) Some contemporary concepts of scleral disease. *Archives of Ophthalmology*, **45**, 630–644.

Swan, K. C. & Penn, R. F. (1962) Scleritis following mumps. Report of a case. *American Journal of Ophthalmology*, **53**, 366–368.

Talbott, J. H. & Terplan, K. L. (1960) The kidney in gout. *Medicine*, **39**, 405–467.

Thompson, R. (1973) In *Diseases of the Liver, Gall Bladder and Pancreas* (Ed.) Williams, R. pp. 528–533. London: Medicine Education International.

Tokuda, H., Okamura, R. & Kamano, H. (1970) A case of brawny scleritis caused by toxoplasma gondii. *Rinsho Ganka*, **24**, 565–571.

Tolentino, F. I. & Brockhurst, R. J. (1963) Unilateral scleral icterus due to choroidal haemorrhage. *Archives of Ophthalmology*, **70**, 358–360.

Trantas, M. (1911) Bourrelet périkératique syphilitique. *Archives d'Ophtalmologie*, **31**, 320–325.

Verhoeff, F. H. (1907) Tuberculous scleritis, a commonly unrecognised form of tuberculosis. *Boston Medical and Surgical Journal*, **156**, 317–321.

Walker, C. (1966) Conglomerate tuberculosis of the iris with scleral perforation. *Transactions of the Ophthalmological Societies of the United Kingdom*, **86**, 169–175.

Watts, R. W. (1966) Allopurinol in the therapy of neoplasia and blood diseases. Metabolic aspects. *Annals of the Rheumatic Diseases*, **25**, 657–659.

Weissmann, G. & Rita, G. A. (1972) Molecular basis of gouty inflammation: interaction of monosodium urate crystals with lysosomes and liposomes. *Nature, New Biology*, **240**, 167–172.

Wood, D. J. (1936) Inflammatory disease in the eye caused by gout. *British Journal of Ophthalmology*, **20**, 510–519.

Woods, A. C. & Wahlen, H. E. (1960) The probable role of benign histoplasmosis in the etiology of granulomatous uveitis. *American Journal of Ophthalmology*, **49**, 205–220.

Yu, T. F. & Gutman, A. B. (1959) A study of the paradoxical effects of salicylate in low intermediate and high dosage on the renal mechanisms for excretion of urate in man. *Journal of Clinical Investigation*, **38**, 1298.

Zannoni, V. G., Seegmiller, J. E. & LaDu, B. N. (1962) Nature of the defect in alcaptonuria. *Nature*, **193**, 952–953.

CHAPTER NINE

Other Affections of the Sclera

'*Have you not a moist eye? a dry hand? a yellow cheek? a white beard?
a decreasing leg? an increasing belly? is not your voice broken? your
wind short? your chin double? your wit single? and every part about
you blasted with antiquity? and will you yet call yourself young?*'
Lord Chief Justice, *Henry IV*, part 2, I ii (Shakespeare).

AGE CHANGES

As all artists know, the sclera and its coats change with age both in colour and
consistency. In the infant the white of the eye appears almost transparent,
like best quality bone china, and as childhood advances it becomes a denser
white, the thickness of the episclera and Tenon's capsule giving it a shimmering,
glistening look. From the age of 20 onwards, the sclera becomes increasingly
yellow and by the mid-forties irregularly so. As the stroma of the conjunctiva
breaks down and the episclera thins, the eye loses its lustre and takes on
a yellow, blotchy appearance. These colour changes are much more marked
in the perilimbal regions than at the equator which retains its youthful appearance because of the persistence of thick fascia. These changes with age, which
go hand in hand with the loss of subcutaneous tissue and elasticity of the
lid, enable one to judge the age of anyone from the appearances of the eyes
alone. In the infant the collagen is in a very immature form with different
bonding structure from that found in the adult. This immature form continues
until the age of three by which time the eye has reached 90 per cent of
its adult size of 24 mm. Whether the mucopolysaccharide structure is also
changed at the end of that period of rapid growth is as yet unknown, but
it probably is. In congenital glaucoma the scleral fibres are stretched and
attenuated, partly because of the immature collagen structure which allows
stretching of each bundle to occur, but also because the cement substances
cannot resist the consistently high intraocular pressure. After the age of five,
the collagen becomes almost mature and no further growth occurs after the
age of 13.

In early childhood the sclera is slightly thicker anteriorly than posteriorly;
in later childhood and adolescence it is slightly thicker posteriorly than

347

anteriorly. As age advances, it becomes generally thinner and less hydrated (Figure 9.1). There is an increase in the thickness of the collagen fibres if not an increase in the amount of collagen itself and a decrease in the ground substance, although the proportion of mucopolysaccharides may increase, particularly in certain zones, reducing the hydration and increasing the transparency in a patchy manner. Vannas and Teir (1960) noted a zonal concentration of proteoglycan in the anterior sclera and perpendicular tubular structures in the sclera and felt that these structures become more prominent with age. The sclera and the collagen become almost acellular and the collagen itself changes with increasing age; clumps of curly fusiform collagen are found at first irregularly

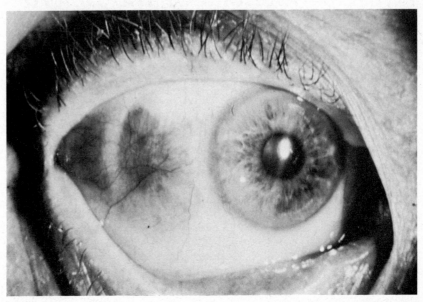

Figure 9.1. Increased transparency in the region of the lateral rectus muscle in an otherwise perfectly healthy 50-year-old patient. This patch, which had been present for at least ten years, has remained unaltered over four years and may be an age change or scleral ectasia.

and sparsely scattered but later they are found throughout the sclera. The number of elastic fibres also decreases. These changes with age have a direct application to the practice of tonography and Schiøtz tonometry (Friedenwald, 1937), the readings of intraocular pressure being of little value in the very young. After the age of 50 when the middle layers of the sclera become firm and hard, there is a very marked rise in the scleral rigidity which has to be compensated for in any calculations.

The colour changes in the sclera are due to an increase in lipid deposition among the scleral fibres and this becomes particularly obvious in old scars. In certain areas the sclera may well become transparent due to calcium deposition; where the calcium concentration is very high, the sclera can become totally transparent, as in the scleral hyaline plaques.

Scleral Hyaline Plaques

These scleral plaques have excited a considerable amount of interest (Norn, 1974) because superficially they appear to be of an inflammatory nature and have been mistaken for scleromalacia perforans (Graves, 1937; Norn, 1974). In fact they are of no pathological significance whatever and require no treatment. The plaques, which are common and symptomless, occur in patients over the age of 50 in the interpalpebral region close to the insertion of the recti muscles. The appearance is of an area of sclera about 2 mm in diameter, the centre of which appears to be slightly facetted, surrounded by a dense yellow ring (Figure 9.2). The sclera at the centre of the spot is translucent

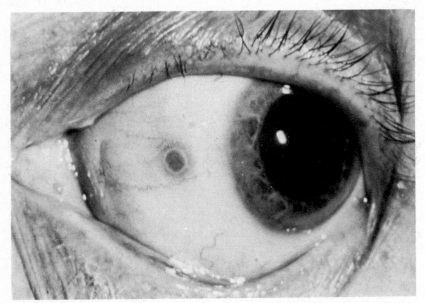

Figure 9.2.   Scleral hyaline plaque; a senile change of no pathological significance.

and can be transilluminated by shining the light through the pupil. The thickness of the sclera is reduced there from 0.6 to 0.3 mm (Culler, 1939). There is no surrounding inflammation nor any sign that there ever has been any. When examined in a pathological specimen the plaques can be shelled out and are hard and seed-like. Although clinically the episclera and conjunctiva can be seen over the lesion, histologically the episclera is thin, atrophic and often avascular. The centre of the plaque is entirely acellular, containing large masses of hyaline material. Opinions vary as to whether the central appearance is caused by calcification or by hyalinisation. Cogan, Hurlbut and Kuwabara (1958), using various staining methods and x-ray diffraction, found that it contains calcium sulphate and is therefore unique in animal tissue. The collagen in the area immediately adjacent to the plaque is swollen, fragmented and contains very few nuclei; the layers of calcium may lie between the fibres but this finding is not universal.

The cause of these lesions is not known, but they are probably caused by a degeneration of the collagen of the sclera which makes it structurally weak. The plaque thus appears at the site of maximal tension of the muscle, the increased transparency being partly due to the loss of mucopolysaccharide ground substance which accompanies the degeneration of the collagen fibrils.

Scleral hyaline plaques have to be distinguished from scleromalacia perforans and from the hyaline degeneration which occurs universally in old age, particularly in those tissues which have been inflamed. This type of hyaline degeneration can also be calcareous and of such severity that it leads to bony deposits in the sclera. It is always found in old age underlying a pinguecula.

Amyloid Degeneration

Although clinically unrecognisable, small deposits with many of the features of amyloid can be found when eyes are examined histologically. Their incidence increases with age, and it may be that these deposits will ultimately be shown to be an invariable accompaniment of ageing (Wright et al, 1969).

Amyloid is commonly found in the tissues of patients suffering from long-standing connective tissue disease of all types and is discussed in Chapter 6.

Coats (1915) first described a syphilitic patient who, following an injury to the eye, developed amyloidosis of the conjunctiva which became hypertrophic. The amyloid tissue eventually invaded the sclera throughout its full depth. We have seen two patients, one a young man similar to Coats' patient, who had no systemic disease and who for no apparent reason developed conjunctival and scleral changes in one eye. Another patient who had long-standing rheumatoid arthritis and diffuse anterior scleritis developed hypertrophic nodules under the conjunctiva which stained with Congo red, the specific stain for amyloid.

Calcareous Degeneration

If we live long enough, this type of change will undoubtedly occur in us all. Deposits of calcium between the scleral fibres are universal and were first noticed by Pagenstecher (1860). The calcareous change is much more marked in eyes which have previously been inflamed and occurs more often from the equator backwards. Pagenstecher found that when the lime salts were extracted, the scleral fibres which remained were perfectly normal, but we have repeated this and have found that although the gross appearance of the fibres is normal, there are areas of patchy necrosis, and the nuclei are infrequent and often completely absent in the areas where the calcium has been deposited.

In patients with metastatic calcification due to hypervitaminosis D, hypercalcaemia (particularly when it is due to renal disease), sarcoidosis and hyperparathyroidism, calcium becomes deposited in the interpalpebral region in both episclera and sclera and can be leached out when the patient receives the appropriate systemic treatment. Local chelating agents are not effective in removing the deposits. The calcium can be seen as fine white deposits under the episclera and between the scleral fibres. The deposits are much more common near the limbus than the equator and they appear to be slightly irritative because the overlying conjunctiva and the episcleral blood vessels are often congested.

Cartilaginous deposition common in birds and reptiles only occurs in degenerative or malformed human eyes, probably due to metaplasia of the collagen matrix.

SCLERAL ECTASIA

Ectasia of the sclera occurs when the scleral coat becomes stretched for any reason (if the uvea is involved the stretching is then termed a staphyloma).

Congenital Anomalies as a Cause of Scleral Ectasia

Ectasia can result from failure of the optic vesicle to close. Colobomas of the uveal tract and retina are relatively common. Similar changes in the sclera are rare, presumably because if the distal end of the embryonic fissure fails to close, the eye becomes microphthalmic or fails to develop at all. Occasionally, however, the sclera fuses and develops but leaves a large ectatic area inferiorly from the disc. This ectatic area is of course always accompanied by a coloboma of the uveal tract. The most common anomaly of this type is when the proximal end of the fissure fails to close and then the defect in the optic nerve and adjacent retina and choroid occurs. The retinal vessels pass upwards into normal retina from the upper end of the defect. If the very far end of the optic vesicle fails to close then a coloboma of the optic nerve alone occurs and this is usually incompatible with reasonable vision. Ectasia of the anterior sclera is much less usual (Fuchs, 1924), but congenital weakness has been said to occur in sclera near to the attachments of the extra-ocular muscles (Vail, 1948; Klemanska, 1954) because of an insufficient number of fibres or stretching of those which are present (Figure 9.1).

In peripapillary ectasia the mesoderm around the papilla fails to form normally (Donaldson et al, 1969). The whole of the area around the true disc bulges outwards giving rise to the appearance of an enormous but normal disc with normal central vessels down the bottom of a deep pit. The vessels pass out of the true disc over bare sclera or atrophic choroid, then into normal retina over the sharp margins of the ectatic sclera.

Scleral ectasia has been known to occur close to the macula and not affect the rest of the sclera. Kraupa (1914) and Lisch (1949) reported a bilateral case who retained normal vision in spite of the fact that the defect involved both maculae.

Gruenwald (1944) has suggested that the pigment epithelium might exert an influence on the formation of the sclera. Although its absence does not completely prevent the formation of the sclera, the base of the coloboma is nevertheless thin. In addition, if there is a generalised defect of pigment epithelium, the sclera under it will be thin and abnormal. If this theory is correct then abnormalities of the pigment epithelium could account for the posterior staphylomas found with retinal detachment and degenerative myopia.

Very occasionally the whole of the sclera can expand. Virgilio, Williams and Klintworth (1976) have entered the *Guinness Book of Records* with an eye measuring 40 × 40 × 37 mm taken from a young man whose eye expanded after developing uveitis and secondary glaucoma at the age of 18. They found that the thin collagen fibres of the inner portion of the sclera were not present. Whether this loss is due to all the fibres being taken up by the enlarged globe, or to a defect in the formation of the innermost collagen fibrils because of a congenital defect, or because of the intercurrent uveitis is not clear.

Corneoscleral Cysts

These cysts, which appear spontaneously at the limbus at any early age from five months to 20 years were first described by Mackenzie in 1854. They are epithelial-lined and are thought to be pouchings of Schlemm's canal (Custodis, 1932) or perhaps a diverticulum of the anterior chamber itself (Friede, 1920). The cysts appear in the region of the limbus, usually remaining very small but occasionally increasing to 3 or 4 mm in size such that they cause symptoms. As the cyst expands, it splits the scleral lamella and later the cornea. The cysts themselves, which contain a clear watery fluid, can be removed or punctured without difficulty if they cause symptoms, but may well be left in situ. Although they cause much alarm and despondency when they are first seen, they are without any pathological significance and the cause of their appearance is totally unknown; it may well represent a defect in the scleral coats adjacent to the perforating anterior ciliary vessels. Some may be akin to epibulbar dermoid cyst and be caused by islands of epithelial cells. Very similar cysts, one of enormous size, have been described following trauma to the eye (Garzino, 1953; Borello, 1960).

Acquired Ectasia

Areas of ectatic sclera are not uncommonly seen at surgery in patients with retinal detachments; whether the thin sclera has any part in the development of the detachment is still uncertain (Dufour, Seddick and Gailloud, 1969). They are commonly radially arranged, passing backwards from the equator like spokes of a wheel and although the anterior end of one of these spokes may be related to a retinal break this is not universally found (Figure 9.3). Many of these patients are myopic but not all and there does not seem to be any direct association between scleral ectasia and progressive or degenerative myopia. The vascular supply of the episclera is poor near to the equator so that the nutrition of both the sclera and the overlying retina is in part dependent on the integrity of the choriocapillaris. Reduction in the blood supply to the choriocapillaris could lead to retinal damage and to a reduction in the number and nutrition of scleral fibres, which being weakened pouch outwards or disappear. In areas where the choroid appears to be normal, the retina seems to function normally. Ectatic sclera is always bridged by choroid and retina, and connective tissue derived from Tenon's capsule fills the gaps (Vail, 1948; Watzke, 1963).

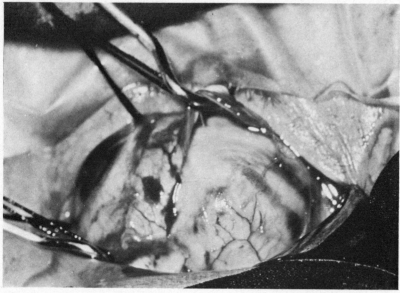

Figure 9.3. Scleral ectasia in a myopic patient with a retinal detachment. The ectatic areas pass backwards, like the spokes of a wheel, from the equator.
Courtesy of J. D. Scott, Cambridge.

Spontaneous Intercalary Scleral Perforation

This curious and unusual form of scleral ectasia can easily be mistaken for scleromalacia perforans. Perforation of the sclera occurs at the limbus without any surrounding inflammation or any other evidence of systemic disease, probably due to some collagen defect in the anterior scleral sulcus at the site of a large perforating vessel (Figure 9.4). The patient, who is usually between 20 and 40, has no pain or any other complaints except perhaps blurring of vision due to a slightly changed refraction. Sometimes the blurring is of acute onset as the limbus gives way. On examination of the eye, a small neat hole can be seen punched through the sclera adjacent to the limbus covered with oedematous conjunctiva and which looks exactly like an Elliot trephine operation done just a little too far posteriorly. The intraocular pressure is low when the perforation occurs but rises rapidly to near normal. The pupil may be drawn up into the wound but this does not always happen. No other abnormality can be found in the eye. Once the perforation has occurred, the appearance remains unaltered and although there is no tendency for the aperture to fill in, the hole is not large enough to require surgical closure. Any patients who present in this way but have systemic disease such as rheumatoid arthritis, like the patients described by Eber (1939) and Mitter (1948), should probably be regarded as a true necrotising scleritis without inflammation (scleromalacia perforans).

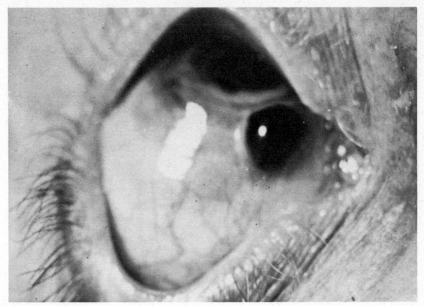

Figure 9.4. Spontaneous intercalary perforation in a 34-year-old male who had no pain or discomfort, only noticing a very slight alteration in visual acuity. The defect was repaired with a scleral patch.

Scleral Staphyloma

Ectatic sclera which has become attached to the underlying uvea is referred to as a staphyloma—a phrase coined by Scarpa (1801) from the Greek word *staphylos* (a bunch of grapes). Staphylomas occur because of severe pathological change induced in the sclera either by scleral or underlying uveal inflammation. A long-standing chronic rise in intraocular pressure, particularly in young or chronically inflamed eyes, also causes scleral expansion. If the inflammation is behind the equator, fusion of the uvea to the sclera occurs with loss of the choriocapillaris. Nutritional changes in the sclera follow, leading to loss of scleral fibres which, if severe enough, allow the underlying uvea and retina to prolapse outwards. An equatorial staphyloma forms in this way at the site of the vortex veins or close to the equator, presumably because the fibres here are less closely arranged than elsewhere and more easily spread by the inflammatory process.

More commonly recognised are staphylomas which occur anterior to the equator, calary (over the ciliary body) and intercalary (between the ciliary body and the limbus). The reason for their occurrence is far less obvious: for some reason they rarely occur after inflammatory changes in the sclera itself and then only if the intraocular pressure is very high. Certainly the pressure has to be constantly around 40 mm Hg before the uvea is forced into an inflammatory scleral defect. Calary and intercalary staphylomas are more usually found in eyes where there has been chronic anterior uveitis

(Figure 9.5), massive anterior synechiae with secondary glaucoma, or following perforation of a globe in which a large area of iris has become adherent to the sclera. When this occurs, nutrition of both the underlying iris and the sclera is disturbed, the scleral fibres become attenuated and thin, the inner fibres fragmenting first (Fuchs, 1893; Mattice, 1913; Vail, 1948; Watzke, 1963). The peripheral retina, choroid or iris adheres to this inner surface. The retina at the site of the staphyloma is always degenerate and cystic and sometimes a large cyst may form within the retina itself, the outer side of which is adherent to the staphyloma. Retinal tears may occur at this site, particularly after minor trauma (Young, 1955; Catford, 1963).

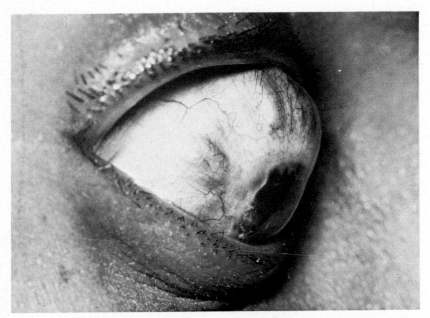

Figure 9.5.   A large intercalary staphyloma in a patient with diffuse anterior scleritis complicated by uveitis and glaucoma which was inadequately controlled.

Clinically, anterior staphylomas appear as areas of gradually increasing transparency or thinning of the sclera. The process begins in multiple small areas, or even over the whole of the anterior segment of the globe. Each thin area, which is easily detectable by transillumination, gradually increases in size. Some exceptionally firm strands of sclera may however bridge the large thin area so that it becomes divided, giving the bunch-of-grapes appearance which Scarpa described in 1801. The ectatic areas can be so large as to prevent the lids from shutting over the eye but in spite of this spontaneous perforation is extremely rare.

Treatment is difficult, partly because by the time the staphylomas have occurred, severe intraocular damage has also taken place. Glaucoma procedures such as trabeculectomy or Krasnov's iridocyclo retraction in an area of moderately normal sclera will sometimes prevent the extension of the staphyloma. Other procedures used have included iridectomy but the eyes must not be touched in the region of the staphyloma or the eye will split open from a perforation in either direction, like tearing a rotten sheet. Smith in 1931 described the use of broad iridectomy which he felt prevented extension of the staphyloma for 28 years. Payrau and Remky in 1961 reported five successful cases of overlay scleral graft but it is most important to cover these grafts with a large conjunctival flap, if possible including episcleral tissue and suturing the flap into cornea as near normal sclera as possible using mattress sutures. The chances of rupturing an eyeball in this situation are very high indeed, so that simple procedures such as that used by Stallard (see Chapter 10) in which the sclera is infolded or excised, are preferable. If major surgery is contemplated in those cases where the eye otherwise is normal, then an anterior segment graft such as that used by de Jaeger, Ooms and Bernolet (1956) should be performed if the sclera is so thin that a complete scleral overlay cannot be undertaken (page 425). It is rarely justifiable to operate on an eye where the major disability is the abnormal shape of the eyeball itself.

Posterior staphylomas, in which the posterior part of the sclera possibly including the disc bulge outwards, were first described by Antonio Scarpa in 1801. He described two cases, the first of which was almost certainly due to degenerative myopia. The second, although similar, experienced very severe pain; it is difficult to understand why she had this unless the cause of the staphyloma was either an inflammatory scleral disease or a long-standing closed angle glaucoma.

Scleral straps or supporting fascial slings have been advocated for the treatment of posterior staphylomas, but there is no convincing evidence that they have either prevented an increase in the extension of the staphyloma or improved the vision.

Degenerative Myopia

In degenerative myopia, as opposed to simple myopia, the axial length of the globe is enlarged, the major expansion being at the posterior pole. Changes in the choroid and retina occur concurrently in the same region, leading to macular changes and loss of central vision. Using the indirect ophthalmoscope, the sharp well-defined edge of the posterior scleral out-pouching, i.e. the posterior staphyloma, can easily be seen. It develops first temporal to, but eventually includes the disc and those areas adjacent to it. Degenerative myopia is often genetically determined and is the commonest cause of registration for blindness in the United Kingdom (Sorsby, 1956).

The myopia may be present from birth and if unilateral leads to intractable amblyopia unless treated with contact lenses in infancy. More commonly the child becomes myopic between the ages of 5 and 12 with a further rapid increase during adolescence as a result of the increase in the axial length of the globe which occurs at puberty. Unlike simple myopia, degenerative myopia continues to increase throughout life, sometimes unilaterally, often reaching between 20 and 30 dioptres by middle life. In the early stages the disc and surrounding fundus look normal, but very soon a temporal crescent of exposed choroid and sclera develops. Concomitant with the out-pouching of the posterior sclera, degenerative changes appear in the choroid. These are generally seen on the temporal side of the disc and at first consist of pigment migration and a concomitant loss of the related retinal elements. Eventually there is a total loss of choroidal and retinal tissue which allows first the underlying choroidal vessels and then the underlying sclera to be seen. The retinal vessels become straight and thin as the retina degenerates. When the macula becomes involved in the degenerative process the vision deteriorates rapidly and although some patients can re-educate other parts of the retina to give them useful, if poor, vision, eventually all central vision goes.

Throughout the course of the condition the disc looks its normal pink colour until or unless the patient develops glaucoma, the onset of which is insidious. Glaucoma is common in degenerative myopia and difficult to diagnose because of the bizarre field changes and the abnormal scleral rigidity. Blach and Jay (1965) feel that when investigating glaucoma in these patients, apart from the use of applanation tonometry which is obligatory, the field of vision should be checked with the patient wearing corneal contact lenses.

The glaucomatous disc in degenerative myopia may show the classical glaucomatous cup, but often, because of the straightening and flattening of the cribriform plate and attenuation of the precribriform tissue, it assumes simply a sloping or concentric outline, so that the disc is flat rather than cupped. Stretching of the sclera adjacent to an optic disc in glaucomatous myopes was noted by Polatti in 1906 and Hotta in 1904. The glaucomatous disc appears orange/grey rather than white because of the contrast with bare sclera (Blach and Jay, 1965).

The macroscopic appearances of 'an eye taken from the body of a woman 40 years old for another purpose' were described by Scarpa (1801).

'This eye was of an oval figure and upon the whole larger than one found on the opposite side. On the posterior hemisphere of this eye and on the external side of the entrance of the optic nerve or on the part corresponding to the temple of that side, the sclerotica was elevated in the form of an oblong tumour, of the size of a small nut; and as the cornea was sound and pellucid and the humours still preserved their transparency, on looking through the pupil, there appeared within it, towards the bottom, an unusual brightness, produced by the light penetrating that part of the sclerotica which had become thin and transparent where it was occupied by the staphyloma. When the eye was opened I found the vitreous humour entirely disorganised and converted into limpid water, and the crystalline lens rather yellowish, but not opaque. When the posterior hemisphere of the eye was immersed in spirit of wine, with a few drops of nitrous acid to it, in order to give the retina consistence and opacity, I could perceive distinctly that there was a deficiency of the nervous expansion of the retina within the cavity of the staphyloma; that the choroid coat was very thin and discoloured at this part and wanted its usual vascular plexus, and that the sclerotica, particularly at the apex of the staphyloma, was rendered so thin as scarcely to equal the thickness of writing paper'.

Heine in 1899 measured the thickness of various portions of myopic sclera and found that in the anterior half of the eye the sclera was normal, but posterior to the equator the sclera, instead of increasing in thickness as in normal eyes, became very much thinner particularly temporal to the disc.

Histologically, Blach (1963) found that the episcleral vascular network was normal, but the choroidal circulation was generally thinned and the choriocapillaris completely absent in the atrophic areas over the staphyloma.

Curtin and Teng (1958) found that the meridional bundles of sclera showed thinning, some loss of fibrous striations and bundle birefringency. The cross bundles showed separation, splaying and diminution in size. The sclera itself showed amorphous acellular patches in places. Blach (1963) confirmed these findings and found that there were fewer scleral lamellae more loosely arranged, with some patches where the scleral fibres themselves lost their normal consistency. It appears that in staphylomas here as elsewhere the inner lamellae were most affected. The scleral fibres did not fuse as closely as normal with the outer layers of the optic nerve, leaving a large intervaginal space. All of these findings are consistent with a concept of gradual stretching of the fibres.

The posterior sclera is the last to develop, not being completely formed until after the fifth month of fetal life, and continues to thicken until the age of 14 (Sondermann, 1950; von Ammon, 1858). Sondermann suggested that the sclera in this region may fail to thicken, that is to say the collagen and ground substance may fail to mature normally, and, as a result of this, the normal intraocular pressure may well expand the globe to form a staphyloma.

This is probably not the whole story because the choroidal changes can occur even if there is no increase in the myopia; Goldsmith (personal communication, 1971) has observed one such case for 30 years. The sclera may be thin in the region of a choroidal coloboma and there is some evidence that pigment epithelium of the retina is abnormal. As it has been suggested by Gruenwald (1944) that this influences the growth of the sclera, Blach (1963) suggests the schema in Figure 9.6 as the possible sequence of events in the development of degenerative myopia. The evidence is still inconclusive but this explanation would appear to satisfy the observed physical signs. The retinal and choroidal changes are secondary and caused by excessive stretching of the limited amount of retina and choroid.

Buphthalmos

This condition, caused by the high intraocular pressure of congenital glaucoma, results in the uniform stretching of the sclera before the collagen fibres have matured. This leads to the very large 'ox eye' which affects the whole sclera, increasing the diameter of the cornea to as much as 15 mm. The very thin anterior sclera, normally relatively transparent in the small infant, is even more transparent and the underlying uveal structures can sometimes be seen in detail through it; this gives a grey/blue hue to the sclera. The thinning becomes less obvious posteriorly and the sclera around the disc is of normal thickness. Relief of the glaucoma prevents further stretching of the sclera, but once it has become stretched it never returns to normal, probably because after the sclera has become organised, no further normal scleral fibres can be laid down. The lamina cribrosa is thin and stretched backwards but appears otherwise normal in this condition.

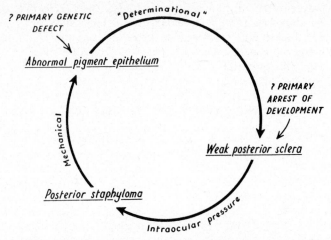

Figure 9.6. The possible aetiology of degenerative myopia.
Courtesy of R. K. Blach.

Buphthalmos can sometimes be mistaken for a congenital anterior staphyloma.

Congenital Anterior Staphyloma

This condition is either the result of an intrauterine infection (Parsons, 1904; Coats, 1910) or a developmental abnormality of the anterior chamber cleavage syndrome type, in which the cornea and sometimes the iris fail to form. The lens may also be absent or become adherent to the cornea (Peters, 1906; Delmarcelle and Pivont, 1957).

The cornea is opaque and the whole anterior segment bulges forwards so that the eye becomes flask-shaped. Although the sclera may be very thin all over, it is usually of normal thickness in front of the muscle insertions and very thin behind them. The sclera behind the equator is normal. These changes contrast markedly with scleralisation of the cornea.

Scleralisation of the Cornea

In this condition, which is not progressive, the peripheral cornea appears to be continuous with the cornea, so that there is only a small central aperture of clear corneal tissue. Very rarely the whole cornea can become opaque (Goldstein and Cogan, 1962). Sclerocornea may be associated with other mesodermal abnormalities not only in the eye but elsewhere (Friedman et al, 1975).

Crespi (1947) described a bilateral segmental scleralisation of the cornea which he attributed to a disturbance of the anterior end of the embryonic cleft, akin to a coloboma. As buphthalmos and the anterior chamber cleavage syndrome are not uncommon, with or without aniridia, it is probable that sclerocornea is the result of a developmental defect of the eye at its earliest stage. None of the cases examined histologically has had a normal or even complete Descemet's membrane, and in most Bowman's membrane was absent, the corneal collagen anteriorly looking like sclera.

INFECTIONS OF THE SCLERA

Infection of the sclera itself is very rare because the blood supply is sparse and the collagen fibres are tightly bound within the fibrous tunic. One of the reasons why so little interest has been shown in the sclera in the past is because pus and tumours do not penetrate the scleral coat readily, giving it an unjustified reputation for inertness. Although polymorphs can migrate freely through the sclera in response to an antigenic stimulus, it is common experience that the products of intraocular suppuration remain confined to the inside of the eye until it can contain no more. The evisceration operation is based on the fact that an intraocular abscess can be removed knowing that the suppuration is most unlikely to have spread outside the sclera. Very occasionally infections can be seen to track through the intrascleral vascular channels, and focal abcesses can remain even after evisceration, necessitating further surgery for their treatment (Votočková, 1957). If the globe ruptures in a panophthalmitis it does so at its weakest point—the corneoscleral junction —and phthisis bulbi inevitably follows.

von Arlt's statements made in 1856 cannot be challenged: 'Specifically diagnosable infection of the sclera which has not spread from an adjacent focus of infection is an extreme rarity, and usually follows injury or a retained intrascleral foreign body'. We have seen two of these cases, one of which was similar to that described by von Graefe in 1857 and was the result of a stitch abscess following squint surgery from an entirely scleral buried catgut suture. This patient had been told to expect some inflammation following squint surgery and had therefore not troubled until the eye became extremely red, painful and proptosed. There was a large abscess over the lateral rectus which was still covered by conjunctiva. Cultures obtained when the abscess was opened surgically grew *Staphylococcus pyogenes aureus*. The abscess was curetted leaving only a very thin scleral lamella over the uveal tract. During the next four months, the defect filled in with scar tissue and the patient now has a slightly transparent area at the site of the abscess, but no other detectable defect. Our second patient gave a history of having jabbed his eye on a stake whilst tying up his chrysanthemums, and developed an intrascleral abscess from a piece of bamboo. The suppuration cleared up following its removal (Figure 9.7).

Infection of scleral plombs placed on the outside of the eye during retinal detachment surgery is commonplace, almost ten per cent having to be removed for this reason. Scleral abscesses from this cause are rare (Lincoff, McLean and Nano, 1965) but do nevertheless occur. It is important to treat them adequately when first seen because continuing infection can act as a sensitising stimulus to induce a severe intractable granulomatous necrotising scleritis (page 173).

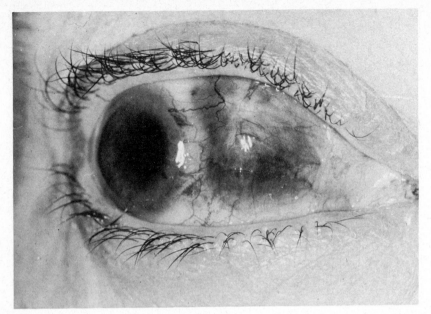

Figure 9.7. Extremely thin sclera following a scleral abscess which resulted from a buried piece of bamboo.

Scleral abscesses caused by pyogenic metastases from furunculosis and other pyogenic infections elsewhere used to be fairly common but, since the introduction of antibiotics have become a rarity. That they do occur from time to time cannot be doubted because blood cultures have confirmed that the abscess contained the same organism as that in the circulation (Figure 9.8) (Thiel, 1929). Recent reports have cited the nasal sinuses (Düring, 1952), a parotitis (Paez-Allende, 1958), the bladder (Otto and Hild, 1957) and puerperal infection (Shindo, 1969) as the sources of the infection, so there is no doubt that they can arise from a generalised septicaemia. Brand (1952), following a review of the literature, suggested that there are three recognisable types:

1. Simplex, in which a circumscribed abscess confined to episcleral tissue is formed.
2. Necrotica, in which the abscess involves scleral tissue and causes scleral necrosis.
3. Progrediens, in which multiple abscesses form in the region of the ciliary veins from abscesses in the sclera, iris and the rest of the uveal tract.

Before the antibiotic era the low resistance of the patient allowed these abscesses to advance very rapidly, particularly if they were posterior to the equator where they commonly led to perforation and loss of the eye (Natanson, 1908). Nowadays intensive systemic and subconjunctival antibiotics, removal of infected scleral plombs, and occasional recourse to incising the abscess lead to a rapid cure.

Duke Elder and Leigh (1965) quoted the case of a doctor who had surface

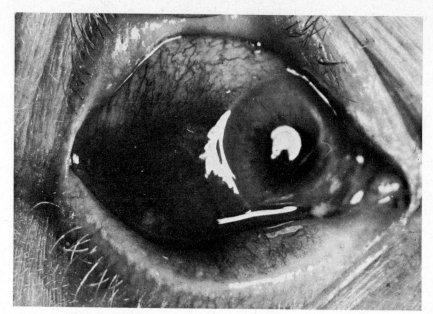

Figure 9.8. Scleral abscess from pyogenic metastatic furunculosis.

diathermy for retinal detachment. He had furunculosis and developed a scleral abscess at the site of the diathermy; the globe perforated and although a little vitreous was lost, the inflammation anchored the retina in place, his visual acuity remained at 6/6 and the sclera healed over the surface.

All infective lesions of the sclera present in a similar way, i.e. the sudden appearance of a localised tender swelling at the site of the underlying abscess and extreme congestion of the overlying episclera. Over a period of 24 to 48 hours it becomes more and more obvious with swelling of the sclera and a yellow/white central opacity. The progression of the lesion from here onwards depends on the nature of the organisms; some take many months to progress to their full extent. The eye and face become extremely painful, presumably due to the stretching and destruction of the nerve endings, and the sclera gradually disintegrates, eventually forming a staphyloma unless the abscess is treated. Usually the inflammation involves the underlying ciliary body or choroid giving rise to a marked uveitis and exudate into the anterior or posterior chambers. If the inflammation is posterior then the abscess causes proptosis and all the appearances of a posterior scleritis (Dubois-Poulsen, François and Tibi, 1950).

The commonest organism found in these abscesses is *Staphylococcus aureus* (Friedman and Henkind, 1974), but Streptococci (Bonnet and Bonnet, 1950), Pneumococci (Hudson, 1933; Coriglione, 1961), and *Pseudomonas pyocyanea* (Jain and Gupta, 1969) have all been implicated (Figure 9.8). Fungus infections follow a similar but much slower course and have been described from time to time: aspergillosis (Köllner, 1906), sporotrichosis (Chaillous, 1912), rhino-sporidiosis (see Chapter 8) and other unidentified mycotic lesions (Podedworney and Suie, 1964). Diagnosis is by culture of the organism and fungal infections must be looked for in all discharging or suspicious abscesses of the episclera and sclera.

Acanthamoeba

Acanthamoebae are ubiquitous in the air, soil and water throughout the world and require some change in host resistance before they can seriously infect the human host. As their food is bacteria they thrive in abscesses, but because they readily encyst in a hostile environment they are extremely difficult to treat.

Infections with *Acanthamoeba polyphaga* and *Acanthamoeba castellanii* can however occur in the cornea without any obvious predisposing cause and may even metastasise from the bloodstream following an initial pharyngeal infection (Nagington et al, 1974; Jones et al, 1975). If the organism enters the central nervous system the disease is fatal.

In Jones' first case, probably produced by directly injecting the organism into the cornea after scratching it with straw or washing it with infected water, the disease ran a protracted course of corneal ulceration which involved the adjacent sclera (Figure 9.9) with multiple scleral nodules. The patient was eventually treated with keratoplasty and retained the eye. The scleral nodules responded to treatment with polymyxin, natamycin, fluorocytosine, gentamicin and prednisolone. Scleral biopsy revealed inflammation with lymphocytes, plasma cells, Russell bodies but was negative for *Amoeba*.

Cestode Infection

Hunter, Pye and Schwartz Guedder (1960) described the affection of the sclera with *Diphyllobothrium latum*. A poultice had been applied to the eye using animal flesh and tapeworms had migrated into the conjunctival sac and thus involved the episclera, orbit and lids.

FOREIGN BODY GRANULOMAS

Although a foreign body embedded in the episclera usually gives rise to a scleral abscess it can, if it is not very toxic or is sterile, produce a granulomatous reaction which looks very much like a nodular scleritis. The inflammation in these lesions is confined to the nodule itself, not affecting the surrounding episclera very much, and is unresponsive to anti-inflammatory therapy. The foreign body can usually be seen after careful inspection on the slit-lamp after the conjunctival congestion has been cleared with 1/1000 adrenaline.

Commonly caterpillar hairs or vegetable matter cause these granulomas as part of the condition known as ophthalmia nodosa. All of these foreign bodies have spines like arrow-heads which carry the foreign body further and further into the tissue. As it progresses it excites a typical chronic granulomatous reaction which may or may not be successful in extruding the hair

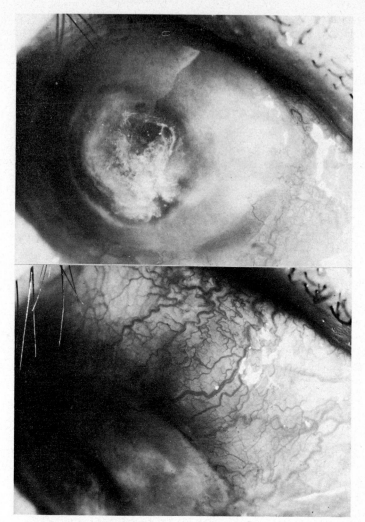

Figure 9.9.   Acanthamoeba of cornea and sclera; a partially treated corneal abscess caused by
Acanthamoeba polyphaga. The lower figure shows a scleral nodule.
Courtesy of D. Jones, Houston, Texas.

or fibre. If a large number of hairs are able to enter the eye, the granulomatous
uveitis caused can be so severe as to lead to the loss of the eye. The scleral
nodules containing the hairs are easily excised and this should be done (Figure
9.10), but individual hairs, provided they are not causing a severe reaction,
should be left alone because they are small, friable and difficult to remove, the
damage caused in the attempt being more than that caused by the foreign body.

The caterpillars which carry these hairs are the pine processionary (*Thaumatopoea pityocampa*)—the scourge of the pine forests of Southern Europe and
the Middle East, and the fox moth (*Euproctia chryssorrhoea*) common in

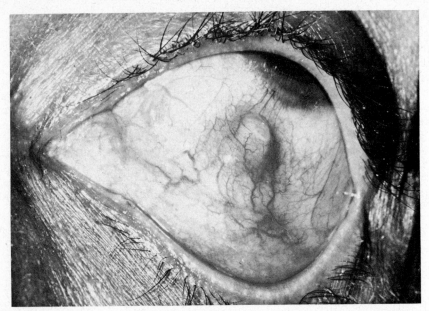

Figure 9.10. Ophthalmia nodosa. Scleral nodule caused by the hairs of the caterpillar *Thaumatopoea pityocampa* (pine processionary) in a man who was employed to remove the nests from the pine trees because they were known to cause skin irritation.

Table 9.1. *Caterpillars known to cause urticaria and ophthalmia nodosa*

British Isles	Other countries
Caterpillars causing urticaria	
Arctia caja (garden tiger moth)	46 species from the
Orgyn antigua (vapourer moth)	following families of
Euproctia similis (goldtail moth)	Lepidoptera:
Euproctia chrysorrhoea (browntail moth)	Lasiocampidae
Lasiocampa quercus (oak eggar)	Thaumatopoeidae
Macrothylacia rubi (fox moth)	Arctiidae
Caterpillars causing ophthalmia nodosa	*Thaumatopoea pityocampa*
Macrothylacia rubi (fox moth)	(pine processionary)
Arctia caja (tiger moth; caterpillar named 'wooly bear')	*Thaumatopoea jordana*
	Isia isabella
	Dendrolimus pini

orchards in England. Although the hairs of an individual caterpillar can cause the lesions, particularly when used as a missile by children, they are usually rubbed into the eye after touching the nests which contain many millions of hairs. A similar scleral lesion has been found to be due to mite mouth parts

(Friedman and Henkind, 1974). The vegetable matter commonly responsible includes the hairs of everlasting flowers (*Helichrysum*), ears of barley and the needles of burdock. Eyelashes, a chalazion bursting through the lid under the conjunctiva, oyster shells, sea urchin spines, pieces of stone or even a contact lens have all been known to cause granulomas. A chronic granuloma of the sclera can follow surgery, either because of talc in the wound or from failure to remove a suture. Episcleral and conjunctival granulomas from this cause are common, but silk or catgut sutures which appear to be completely buried can also do this. Diagnosis is rarely difficult because of the previous history of surgery. A true persistent granulomatous necrotising scleritis has followed cataract extraction on several occasions. This is of late onset and starts at the site of the surgical incision. The reason why this occurs is unknown but it may be that buried sutures have provided the continuing stimulus which has encouraged perpetuation of the inflammatory reaction.

TUMOURS OF THE SCLERA

Tumours of the sclera are exceptionally rare, but episcleral tumours are not uncommon. They may be derived from the episcleral tissues themselves, from the vascular or nervous tissue which pass through the episclera, from extension of the lesions of conjunctiva or inner eye or be a manifestation of a systemic neoplastic process. Neoplastic changes need to be considered here because they can sometimes be mistaken for inflammatory lesions of the episclera and sclera.

Epibulbar Dermoids

Epibulbar dermoids are common and when they occur at the limbus rarely cause any difficulty in diagnosis. However, when a limbal dermoid is confined to the sclera, episclera and conjunctiva, it can cause confusion. The commonest site for the entirely conjunctivoscleral dermoid is the same as that which also involves the cornea, i.e. the lower temporal quadrant. The conjunctiva and episclera are raised and the whole mass is fixed and vascularised, so it looks like a grey rough lump with a pink flush. Careful examination will almost always detect the fine hairs on the surface of the lump which confirms the diagnosis.

Dermoids, which may be solid or cystic, are formed from inclusions of epidermal and connective tissues at sites of closure of the fetal clefts. Histologically they consist of dense collagenous connective tissue covered by stratified epithelium which produces keratin and usually contains hair follicles and the shafts of sebaceous glands. If there is a disproportionate amount of fat in the dermoid then they become dermolipomas; their appearance is similar but yellower and histologically they contain very few epithelial structures.

All forms of dermoids may continue to grow from birth, having a burst of activity at puberty, but fortunately do not usually require treating unless unsightly. They are difficult to remove if the sclera is involved; the defective tissue has to be replaced by a graft because the dermoid may be so deep as to be impossible to remove without rupturing the globe (Miller, 1925).

All the mesoblastic tumours and some epithelial tumours which involve the conjunctiva also affect the episclera and sometimes penetrate the sclera. Although some have characteristic physical signs which help in the diagnosis, most require biopsy to be certain of their cause. Rather than describe all these tumours in detail, we will concentrate on those which are known to give difficulty in differential diagnosis or treatment, summarised in the Table 9.2.

Table 9.2.   *Tumours of the conjunctiva, episclera and sclera*

Tumours of conjunctiva
   Epithelial tumours:
      (A) Surface epithelium
         1. Benign keratoacanthoma
         2. Benign but potentially precancerous
            (a) Dyskeratoses, e.g. epithelial plaques, intraepithelial epithelioma
            (b) Papilloma
         3. Malignant epithelioma
      (B) Glandular tumours
         Benign adenoma: papillary cystadenoma, oncocytoma
         Malignant: pleomorphic adenoma

Tumours of episclera and conjunctiva
   1. Mesoblastic tumours
      (A) Inflammatory hyperplasias: granuloma, plasmoma
      (B) Connective tissue tumours
         1. Benign: fibroma, myxoma, osteoma
         2. Malignant: sarcoma
   2. The reticuloses: lymphoma, lymphosarcoma, mycosis fungoides
   3. Vascular tumours
      1. Benign: haemangioma, lymphangioma
      2. Malignant: angiosarcoma, Kaposi sarcoma
   4. Pigmented tumours
      1. Benign: naevus, epithelial, subepithelial
      2. Malignant: malignant melanoma
   5. Peripheral nerve tumours
      1. Benign: neurofibroma, neurilemmoma
      2. Malignant: malignant melanoma

Tumours of the sclera
   True primary tumours of the sclera are unknown

Modified from Duke Elder (1964).

Epithelial Tumours

The epithelial tumours rarely cause difficulty in diagnosis particularly in the early stages because the mass itself is confined to the superficial tissue which is readily mobile. Although intraepithelial epitheliomas tend to be limbal and not to invade deeply, this is not always the case (Pichion and Trigonidis, 1965); Bowen's disease indeed can metastasise without any evidence of local infiltration. Some papillomas and epitheliomas which arise away from the limbus may be difficult to diagnose in the early stage, particularly if they start in the fornix and are tethered to the deeper tissues. The vascularised mass, which can be well circumscribed before it forms its fronds, can look very like a granuloma. The malignant nature of an epithelioma soon becomes apparent, but we have seen a patient who had been treated as a nodular episcleritis for many months and was referred not because of the conjunctival involvement which was not very obvious, but because the cornea in the same area was becoming cloudy. Close inspection of the conjunctiva in this patient revealed a change in colour, loss of lustre and a diffuse thickening extending over the whole temporal half, the downward extension apparently being localised to one small area. The surrounding reactive hyperaemia and inflammatory cell exudate gave it the appearance of an inflammatory nodule.

Intraocular spread of surface epitheliomas can occur with columns of cells penetrating the sclera via the vascular channels and the episclera and Tenon's capsule by a posterior direct extension of tumour cells. Dejean et al (1958) described a patient with 'Brai' disease in which there are multiple skin epitheliomas and papillomas. An exactly similar lesion occurred at the limbus and progressed by penetration of the limbus by long tubes of cells.

Treatment depends on the site and extent of the growth and can therefore vary from β radiation to local or very extensive excisions of the lesions. Enucleation or evisceration as a primary treatment is virtually never justified.

Mesoblastic Tumours

Nodular fasciitis

Nodular fasciitis is a benign nodular proliferation of fibroblasts and vascular tissues involving the superficial fascia anywhere in the body, including Tenon's capsule. In the eye, the tumour usually presents as a painless vascularised pinkish lump attached to the underlying sclera and may increase rapidly in size. The nodules can also affect the eyelid, periorbital tissue or present as a limbal tumour. Both the appearance of the lesion and the speed of its increase in size suggest a malignant tumour, particularly a lymphoma or sarcoma, but excision of the tumour reveals its true nature which is of proliferating fibroblasts. Treatment is simply by excision, which is necessary in any case for the diagnosis of all tumours in this region. The wounds heal well without recurrence.

Fibromas

Fibromas of the episclera alone are not attached to the underlying sclera and, because they are heavily vascularised, tumours appear very like papillomas except that they have a smooth surface. Fibromas occur on any part of the episclera but are usually anterior around the limbus, firm, fixed and of variable size, consisting of densely packed fibroblasts intermingled with inflammatory cells. The histological diagnosis will vary with the amount of the different connective tissue elements which are in excess. The tumour may be classified as a myxoma if there is a great deal of ground substance, a fibroma or elastoma if only fibrous elements are present, and a myxofibroma if it contains a mixture of each.

The old literature contains many descriptions of fibromas of the sclera, but none of them seems to fit with the diagnosis of a true fibroma. Schöbl (1889) describes a two-year-old child whose whole sclera was so hypertrophic that it was thought that he had a glioma. The thickening however was of innumerable round cells. Similarly, Gayet's patient (1888) could have had a posterior scleritis of inflammatory origin. Saemisch's (1872) case in a ten-year-old child seems also to have been a necrotising anterior and posterior scleritis.

Epibulbar osteomas and choriostomas

This rare tumour was first described by von Graefe (1863) and Critchett (1882) in the earliest editions of ophthalmology journals—these contain many oddities. It is a chromophytic teratoblastoma (Duke Elder, 1964), i.e. an aberration of one germinal layer only and probably not, as has been suggested by Kreibig and Nehm (1969) and Mullaney Coffey and Fenton (1971), atavistic —a throwback to the bony and cartilaginous lamellae of birds and fishes. The osteoma consists of a hard pellet of bone lying freely mobile within the episcleral tissue. The conjunctiva surrounds the bony ossicle which is never found within the sclera itself. These tumours may grow very large; Bengisu, Tahsinoglu and Toker (1973) reported a case of an eight-year-old boy who had a plexiform neurofibroma. After the eye was excised he was found to have a cartilaginous choriostoma in the episclera, suggesting that the two conditions are related. However, it would seem that the combination of the two conditions could have occurred by chance as the lesions were separate and there was no direct continuation with the neurofibroma. Calcified scleral nodules have been described in hypervitaminosis D (Gartner and Rubner, 1955) and in carcinoma of the kidney (Timm, 1964) and need to be distinguished from true osteomas.

Neurofibromas

Although a rare occurrence as a part of von Recklinghausen's disease, neurofibromas can occur as hard immobile masses in the episclera and superficial sclera (Nitsch, 1929; Dabezies and Penner, 1961). Histologically it is extremely difficult to decide the nature of these solitary neurofibromas (Kuwabara and Sakanoue, 1965), and they must be distinguished from the lesions of tuberose sclerosis (Luo, 1940) and intrascleral nerve loops of Axenfeld (1902). In plexiform neurofibromatosis the tumour can extend from the orbit to involve the episclera, looking like a bag of worms (Verhoeff, 1903).

Sarcomas

To verify that sarcomas arise de novo in the sclera is also difficult; a 35-year-old male patient of Hirschberg (1868) was reported to have a sarcoma entirely within the deep episclera and sclera. All the other cases quoted in the literature, summarised by Lagrange (1901), Betetto and Amidei (1954) and Erbakan (1961), are either descriptions of granulomas, invasive tumours of the ciliary body and choroid, leukaemic infiltrates or lymphosarcoma passing outwards from the eye, or epitheliomas passing inwards. It must be concluded that if true tumours of the sclera occur they must be an extreme rarity. Secondary deposition in the episclera from elsewhere does sometimes occur, however.

Reticuloses

The 'reticuloses' is the generic term given to tumours arising from the reticulo-endothelial system. These are commonly present as epibulbar, usually episcleral tumours. They are classified according to cell type so they can only be diagnosed by biopsy of the scleral/episcleral nodule. If they contain primitive lymphocytes, as when they present in acute leukaemia, they are lymphoblastic lymphomas. If the lymphocytes are more mature, as in the chronic leukaemias, they are lymphocytic lymphomas. If they are composed mainly of histiocytic cells or bizarre forms of these—the Reed–Sternberg cell—the mass is presumed to be part of Hodgkin's disease. Sarcomas can develop from each type.

Most of these tumours start as small, red or pinkish nodules within the episclera (Figure 9.11). Others develop as pink or yellowish fleshy masses which rapidly spread over one segment of the globe. The nodules, which are always sharply demarcated, do not excite an inflammatory response and may extend into or arise from an orbital mass. Whilst the eye lesions can be solitary, some other physical signs of systemic involvement can usually be found and should always be looked for. Full haematological investigations are essential.

Lymphosarcomas present in a similar way with similar looking tumours except that they increase in size with alarming rapidity and with evidence of systemic spread.

Treatment of all small lesions is by excisional biopsy; this is easy and most satisfactory because of the thin avascular nature of the tumour. Thereafter treatment is with local irradiation supplemented by systemic antimetabolites.

Vascular Tumours

Angiomas

Angiomas are classified according to the type of vessels involved in the mass; plexiform (with normal vessel form), capillary (small vessels only), venous (veins only), cavernous (cystic spaces), and lymphangioma (lymph vessels only). All of these types involve the episcleral vessels but very few present a difficulty in diagnosis.

Cavernous haemangiomas

The commonest variety is a cavernous haemangioma which presents as a mass of vessels, dark red in colour and sometimes associated with a gross

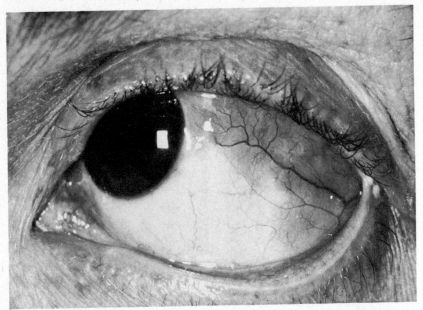

Figure 9.11. The lower edge of a conjunctival episcleral lymphoma. It gradually increased in size over a period of three months and responded to low dosage radiotherapy.

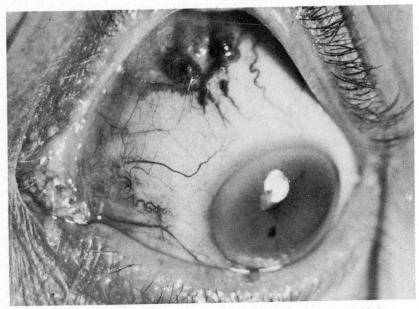

Figure 9.12. Cavernous haemangioma as a forward extension of an orbital lesion.

overgrowth of the conjunctiva. The mass and overlying conjunctiva are freely mobile on the underlying sclera and can be partially emptied on pressure. They are always present at birth, grow in early life and start to sclerose spontaneously from the age of six onwards; they may bleed spontaneously and severely. Whilst the lesion can be localised to the conjunctiva it is more usually a peripheral manifestation of an orbital cavernous haemangioma (Figure 9.12). As most tumours will improve with age, removal can be left till late childhood unless they are cosmetically intolerable or keratinisation of the overlying conjunctiva occurs. At some stage excision will be required. This is a very satisfactory form of treatment in the majority but occasionally persistent chemosis of the conjunctiva occurs. Thermocoagulation as a first procedure in patients who already have conjunctival changes seems to prevent the persistent conjunctival oedema.

Capillary haemangiomas

Although less common than nodular episcleritis, this small, circumscribed and congested lesion can easily be mistaken for it (Figure 9.13). It has, of course, a very different history, being present for many years and not altering in size. Because of its small size it does not often need to be removed. It may be the only peripheral manifestation of the Sturge–Weber syndrome, which usually presents as a naevus flammeus of the face, mucous membranes, choroid and, most important, of the meninges which can give rise to epilepsy and mental retardation. Takahashi (1966) described two patients in whom the sole physical signs were extensive telangiectasia of the episcleral and conjunctival capillaries and large microaneurysms at the limbus.

Other forms of angioma are rare. Redslob (1926) and Knobloch (1951) described racemose angioma which involved not only the episcleral vessels but the whole underlying network. These lesions must be viewed with suspicion; the case illustrated in Figure 9.14 appeared to be due to an angioma but careful examination revealed that the vessels were arising from an underlying melanoma. The genuine deep racemose angiomas do not require treatment.

Telangiectatic granulomas

The exact nature of this lesion is uncertain, but its appearance is dramatic and it is quite painless. A bright red spot appears in the subconjunctival tissues which increases rapidly in size and eventually bursts through the conjunctiva until it becomes a pedunculated mass. Removal requires a wide conjunctival opening and the large vessels feeding the base of the lesion are cauterised as the peduncle is approached. The base is then cauterised and tied if possible (sutures usually cut through). Cautery and excision of the base must be done cautiously otherwise profuse bleeding occurs which is difficult to stop. After removal, histology reveals that it contains multiple vascular channels and chronic granulation tissue. Thus it is possible that it represents an unusual reaction to infection in an already existing angioma.

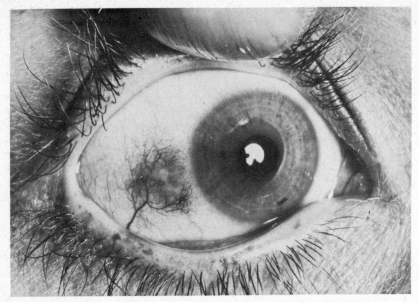

Figure 9.13. Capillary haemangioma of the episclera confirmed by biopsy.

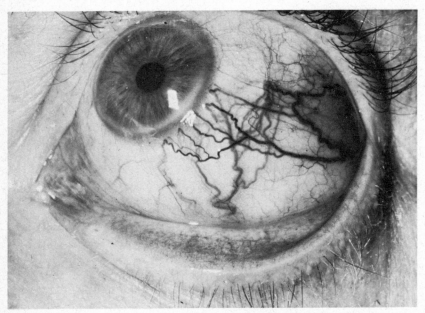

Figure 9.14. Large vascular channels were thought at first to be due to a haemangioma but were later found to be due to an underlying malignant melanoma.

Lymphangiomas

Whilst isolated lymph vessel obstruction which gives rise to transparent tube-like excrescences under the conjunctiva is common, true lymphangiomas are rare. Jones (1961) says that 19 per cent of epibulbar lesions are lymphangiomas, which are more common than realised because many are diagnosed as cavernous haemangiomas. Like these tumours they are present from birth and can present as a red fleshy mass because bleeding occurs into them. Most commonly, however, they present as a white, transparent or fleshy mass at the limbus or on the bulbar conjunctiva which may extend back into the orbit. The surrounding conjunctiva may be congested. Treatment is not usually necessary but simply injecting saline into the tubules may disperse the small lesions. Larger lesions need to be excised.

Pigmented Tumours

The pigmented tumours which involve the subconjunctival tissues are not only common but also cause much confusion in diagnosis, particularly if the amount of pigment they contain is small. Correct diagnosis is important; neoplastic pigmented lesions must be differentiated from simple scleral pigmentation which can occur in all races (Figures 3.1 and 9.16). Deeply pigmented lesions often overlie the nerve loops of Axenfeld (see Chapter 2) (Figure 9.17).

The naevus, although it contains melanocyte naevus cells, need not be pigmented. In affected individuals this common lesion (30 per cent of epibulbar lesions) is always present at birth but may not be noticed until middle childhood, by which time it has reached an appreciable size (Figure 9.18). Like its counter-part in the skin, it can suddenly and rapidly increase in size at puberty with the change from junctional to compound state and can even become malignant. The lesions are usually darkly pigmented, flat and close to the limbus, but every variation between this and the non-pigmented, diffuse, fleshy tumour exists. Many lesions look like a nodular episcleritis or angiomas. The pigmentation varies at puberty and in pregnancy. Most lesions have somewhat larger than normal episcleral vessels running to them and one of the first signs of a change from the benign to malignant state is a great increase in this vascularity without any obvious increase in size. The lesions then become more pigmented and start to expand outwards, upwards and downwards becoming fixed to the sclera. Viewing in ultraviolet light helps to assess this change as the naevus and melanoma cells fluoresce (Duke Elder, 1964). Diagnosis is rarely in doubt once a malignant melanoma has occurred in the deep episcleral tissues (Figure 9.19), nor is there any difficulty with the intraepithelial conjunctival melanomas.

Treatment is usually difficult. If the diagnosis of a naevus is certain then it should be photographed and followed at regular intervals. If the growth is abnormal, then local excision is acceptable if only to obtain a definite diagnosis. Excision must be performed with great care and precision because cells remaining after excision of a true naevus can become malignant. If malignancy is confirmed the whole gamut of surgical and radiotherapeutic armamentarium must be ranged against it.

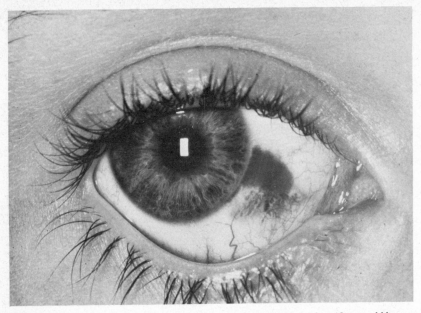

Figure 9.15. Spontaneous haemorrhage from a small haemangioma in a 12-year-old boy.

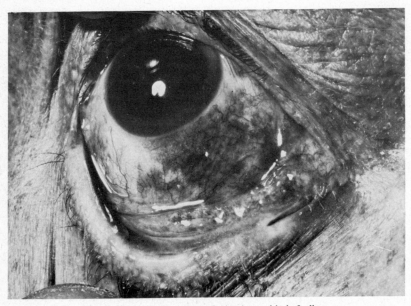

Figure 9.16. Scleral pigmentation in an elderly Indian.

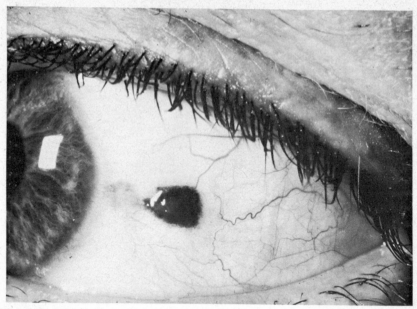

Figure 9.17. Deeply pigmented naevus. This was extremely tender and may have been overlying a nerve loop of Axenfeld.

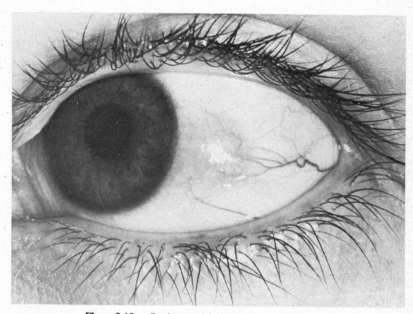

Figure 9.18. Conjunctival /episcleral naevus in a child.

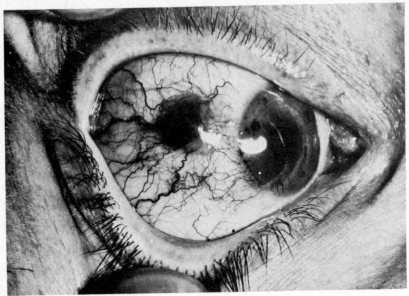

Figure 9.19. Densely pigmented malignant melanoma in a young white child.

Secondary Tumours

Although secondary epithelial tumours can involve episcleral or scleral tissue by direct extension, the secondary tumours which arise in the episcleral tissue are sarcomas or secondary pigmented tumours. An angiosarcoma (Kaposi sarcoma) often presents as a mass in the episclera and conjunctiva looking initially like a lymphoma which grows rapidly in size, becoming much more pink in colour. This lesion appears at the same time as multiple similar tumours elsewhere, or together with lymphomatous disease elsewhere (Sacks, 1956). Garrett (1957) described an episcleral secondary from a seminoma. He also discussed cases said to have come from the breast, thyroid, lung, uterus, prostate and pancreas. We have seen one secondary from a breast carcinoma which responded rapidly to local irradiation.

Diagnosis and treatment is by excision.

REFERENCES

Axenfeld, T. (1902) Uber intrasklerale Nervenschleifen. *Sitzungsberichte der Ophthalmologischen Gessellschaft in Wein*, **1903**, 134–137.

Bengisu, U., Tahsinoglu, M. & Toker, G. (1973) Neurofibromatosis associated with cartilaginous choristoma of the episclera. *Annales d'Oculistique*, **206**, 401–403.

Betteto, G. & Amidei, B. (1954) Fibrous sarcoma of the sclera. *Annali di Ottalmologia*, **80**, 495–510.

Blach, R. K. (1963) *The Nature of Degenerative Myopia.* MD thesis, University of Cambridge.

Blach, R. K. & Jay, B. (1965) Glaucomatous disc in degenerative myopia. *Transactions of the Ophthalmological Societies of the United Kingdom*, **85**, 161–168.

Bonnet, P. & Bonnet, J. L. (1950) Sclérite furonculiforme au cours d'un septicémie à staphylocoques. *Bulletin des Sociétés d'Ophtalmologie de France*, **3**, 104–106.

Bonuik, M. & Zimmerman, L. E. (1961) Necrosis of uvea, sclera and retina following operation for retinal detachment. *Archives of Ophthalmology*, **66**, 318–326.

Bonuik, M. & Zimmerman, L. E. (1962) Episcleral osseous choristoma. *American Journal of Ophthalmology*, **53**, 290–296.

Borello, C. (1960) A scleral cyst of traumatic origin. *Rassegna Italiana d'Ottalmologia*, **29**, 89–102.

Brand, I. (1952) Uber die Episkleritis metastatica furunculiformis. *Klinische Monatsblätter für Augenheilkunde*, **120**, 393–396.

Calhoun, F. P. (1924) A dermoid tumour of corneoconjunctiva associated with scleral ectasia. *American Journal of Ophthalmology*, **7**, 669–670.

Catford, G. V. (1963) Distension retinal detachment. *British Journal of Ophthalmology*, **47**, 266–270.

Chaillous, J. (1912) Sporotrichose gommeuse disseminée, gomme intra-oculaire, perforation de la sclérotique. *Annales d'Oculistique*, **148**, 321–328.

Coats, G. (1910) Congenital anterior staphyloma. *Ophthalmoscope*, **8**, 248–257.

Coats, G. (1915) Hyperplasia, with colloid and amyloid degeneration, of the episcleral and circumdural fibrous tissue. *Transactions of the Ophthalmological Societies of the United Kingdom*, **35**, 257–274.

Cogan, D. G., Hurlbut, C. S. & Kuwabara, T. (1958) Crystalline calcium sulphate (gypsum) in scleral plaques of a human eye. *Journal of Histochemistry and Cytochemistry*, **6**, 142–145.

Coriglione, G. (1961) A case of bilateral episcleritis in atypical primary pneumopathy. *Rivista Italiana del Tracoma e di Patologie Oculare Virale ad Esotica*, **13**, 102–116.

Crespi, G. (1947) Coloboma de la cornea. *Archivos de la Sociedad Oftalmologica Hispano-Americano*, **7**, 577–586.

Critchett, A. (1882) A case of bony tumour of the conjunctiva. *Transactions of the Ophthalmological Societies of the United Kingdom*, **2**, 254.

Culler, A. M. (1939) Pathology of scleral plaques. *British Journal of Ophthalmology*, **23**, 44–50.

Curtin, B. J. & Teng, C. C. (1958) Scleral changes in pathological myopia. *Transactions of the American Academy of Ophthalmology and Otolaryngology*, **62**, 777–790.

Custodis, E. (1932) Uber skleral cysten. *Albrecht v. Graefes Archiv für Ophthalmologie*, **128**, 112–118.

Dabezies, O. H. & Penner, R. (1961) Neurofibroma and neurilemona of the bulbar conjunctiva. *Archives of Ophthalmology*, **66**, 73–75.

de Jaeger, A., Ooms, P. & Bernolet, J. (1956) Giant intercalary staphyloma. *Bulletin de la Société Belge d'Ophtalmologie*, **114**, 613–616.

Dejean, C., Boudet, C., Paycha, M. & Jaulmes, C. (1958) Sclerocorneal limbus tumour due to 'Brai' disease. *Montpelier Medicine*, **53**, 726–728.

Delmarcelle, Y. & Pivont, A. (1957) Staphylôme cornéen à heredité dominant. *Bulletin de la Société Belge d'Ophtalmologie*, **117**, 560–568.

Donaldson, D. D., Bennett, N., Anderson, D. R. et al (1969) Peripapillary staphyloma. *Archives of Ophthalmology*, **82**, 704.

Dubois-Poulsen, A., François, P. & Tibi, J. (1950) Pseudo-tumeur orbitaire par abcès episclérale postérieur enkysté. *Bulletin des Sociétés d'Ophtalmologie de France*, **6**, 480–484.

Dufour, R., Seddik, N. & Gailloud, C. (1969) Retinal detachment and scleral thinning. *Bulletin et Memoires de la Société Francaise d'Ophtalmologie*, **82**, 208–209.

Duke Elder, S. (1964) *System of Ophthalmology*, Vol. 3, p. 825. London: Kimpton.

Duke Elder, S. & Leigh, A. S. (1965) *System of Ophthalmology*, Vol. 8: (a) p. 1027, (b) p. 1213. London: Kimpton.

Düring, E-G. (1952) Ulceration of the sclera. *Deutsche Gesundheitswesen*, **7**, 1159–1162.

Eber, C. T. (1939) Fistula at limbus (scleromalacia perforans). *American Journal of Ophthalmology*, **17**, 921–923.

Erbakan, S. (1961) Intraocular lymphosarcoma. *American Journal of Ophthalmology*, **52**, 412–413.

Feigenbaum, A. (1936) Typical and atypical episcleritis metastatica furunculiformis and their relation to rheumatic episcleritis and to erythema nodosum. *Folia Ophthalmologica Orientalia*, **2**, 27–37.

Ferry, A. P. & Sherman, S. E. (1974) Nodular fasciitis of the conjunctiva apparently originating in the fascia bulbi. *American Journal of Ophthalmology*, **78**, 514–517.

Friede, R. (1920) Ein Fall von Kongenitaler Skleralzyste mit Stauungspapille. *Klinische Monatsblätter für Augenheilkunde*, **64**, 666–671.

Friedenwald, J. S. (1937) Contribution to the theory and practice of tonometry. *American Journal of Ophthalmology*, **20**, 985–1024.

Friedman, A. H. & Henkind, P. (1974) Unusual causes of episcleritis. *Transactions of the American Academy of Ophthalmology and Otolaryngology*, **78**, 890–895.

Friedman, A. H., Weingeist, S., Brackup, A. et al (1975) Sclerocornea and defective mesodermal migration. *British Journal of Ophthalmology*, **59**, 683–687.

Fuchs, E. (1893) *Liehrbuch der Augenheilkunde*. Leipzig: Deuticke.

Fuchs, E. (1924) *Textbook of Ophthalmology* (Ed.) Duane, A. 8th edition. Philadelphia: Lippincott.

Garrett, M. (1959) Ocular metastasis from seminoma. *British Journal of Ophthalmology*, **43**, 759–761.

Gartner, S. & Rubner, K. (1955) Calcified scleral nodules in hypervitaminosis D. *American Journal of Ophthalmology*, **39**, 658–663.

Garzino, A. (1953) Post-traumatic cyst of the sclera of remarkable size. *Rassegna Italiana d'Ottalmologia*, **22**, 308–317.

Gayet, A. (1888) Deux tumeurs symetriques des globes oculaire. *Archives d'Ophtalmologie*, **8**, 18–28.

Goldstein, J. E. & Cogan, D. G. (1962) Sclerocornea and associated congenital anomalies. *Archives of Ophthalmology*, **67**, 761–768.

Graves, B. (1937) Bilateral mesial superficial deficiency of the sclera. *British Journal of Ophthalmology*, **21**, 534–539.

Gruenwald, P. (1944) Studies on developmental pathology, II: Sporadic unilateral microphthalmia and associated malformation in chick embryos. *American Journal of Anatomy*, **74**, 217–257.

Heine, L. (1899) Beitrage zur Anatomie des myopischen Auges. *Archiv für Augenheilkunde*, **38**, 277.

Hirschberg, J. (1868) Casuistiche Mittheilungen uber Geschwulste der orbita und des bulbus. *Klinische Monatsblätter für Augenheilkunde*, **6**, 153–178.

Hotta, G. (1904) Ueber die pathologische-anatomischen Veränderungen hochgradig myopischer Augen durch Glaukom. *Klinische Monatsblätter für Augenheilkunde*, **42**, 84–94.

Hudson, A. C. (1923) Two cases of primary band shaped opacity of both corneae. *Proceedings of the Royal Society of Medicine*, **16**, 31–33.

Hunter, G. W., Pye, W. W. & Schwartz Guedder, J. C. (1960) Diphyllobothrium latex. In *Manual of Tropical Medicine*. Philadelphia: W. B. Saunders.

Jain, I. S. & Gupta, S. D. (1969) Multiple scleral abscesses due to pseudomonas pyocyaneus. *Oriental Archives of Ophthalmology*, **7**, 325–326.

Jehanin, H. (1966) A case of mycosis of the sclera cured by surgery. *Bulletin des Sociétés d'Ophtalmologie de France*, **66**, 117–119.

Jones, D. B., Visvesvara, G. S. & Robinson, N. M. (1975) Acanthamoeba polyphaga keratitis and acanthamoeba uveitis associated with fatal meningoencephalitis. *Transactions of the Ophthalmological Societies of the United Kingdom*, **95**, 221–231.

Jones, I. (1961) Lymphangiomas of the ocular adnexa. *American Journal of Ophthalmology*, **51**, 481–509.

Klemanska, K. (1954) Scleral staphyloma and retinal detachment. *Klinika Oczna*, **24**, 143–145.

Knell, A. (1973) In *Diseases of the Liver, Gallbladder and Pancreas in Medicine* (Ed.) Williams, R. pp. 521–528. London: Medical Education International.

Knobloch, R. (1951) Scleral and corneal haemangioma. *Československa Oftalmologie*, **7**, 336–337.

Köllner, H. (1906) Schimmelpilzerkrankung der Sklera. *Zeitschrifte für Augenheilkunde*, **16**, 441–447.

Kraupa, E. (1944) Ueber 'zirkumskripte grübenförmige Ektasie' am Augengrunde. *Zeitschrifte für Augenheilkunde*, **31**, 149–152.

Kreibig, W. & Nehm, O. (1969) The episcleral bone lamella. *Klinische Monatsblätter für Augenheilkunde*, **155**, 707–712.

Kuwabara, Y. & Sakanoue, M. (1965) An unusual case of scleral tumour. *Rinsho Ganka*, **19**, 191–192.

Lagrange, H. (1901) *Traité des Tumeurs de l'Oeil.* Paris: Stenheil.

Lincoff, H. A., McLean, J. M. & Nano, H. (1965) Scleral abscess, I. A complication of retinal detachment buckling procedures. II. The experimental production in animals. *Archives of Ophthalmology*, **74**, 641–648, 665–668.

Lisch, K. (1949) Uber hinter Skleraktase. *Berichte der Deutsche Ophthalmologischen Gesellschaft*, **55**, 402–404.

Luo, T. H. (1940) Conjunctival lesions in tuberous sclerosis. *American Journal of Ophthalmology*, **23**, 1029–1034.

MacKenzie, W. (1854) *A Practical Treatise on Diseases of the Eye*, 4th edition. London: Longman.

Masselon, J. (1894) De la sclerectasie nasale dans la myopie. *Annales d'Oculistique*, **112**, 20–29.

Mattice, A. F. (1913) On the pathogenesis of scleral staphyloma. *Archives of Ophthalmology*, **42**, 612–617.

Miller, T. (1925) Congenital dermoid cyst of cornea in conjunction with dermolipoma. *American Journal of Ophthalmology*, **7**, 703–704.

Mitter, S. N. (1948) Scleral degenerations—a case of sclero :alacia perforans. *British Journal of Ophthalmology*, **32**, 899–904.

Mullaney, J., Coffey, V. P. & Fenton, M. (1971) Atavistic ocular ossicle. *British Journal of Ophthalmology*, **55**, 243–247.

Nagington, J., Watson, P. G., Playfair, J. et al (1974) Amoebic infection of the eye. *Lancet*, **ii**, 1537–1540.

Natanson, A. N. (1908) Zur Kasuistik der subkonjunktivalen Abszesse. *Klinische Monatsblätter für Augenheilkunde*, **46**, 528–530.

Nitsch, M. (1929) Neurofibromatose des Auges. *Zeitschrift für Augenheilkunde*, **69**, 117–143.

Norn, M. S. (1974) Scleral plaques. I. Incidence and morphology. II. Follow up, cause. *Acta Ophthalmologica*, **52**, 96–106, 512–520.

Otto, J. & Hild, E. (1957) Metastatic episcleritic abscesses. *Klinische Monatsblätter für Augenheilkunde*, **131**, 541–543.

Paez-Allende, F. (1958) Diffuse episcleritis caused by parotitis. *Archivos e Memorias de la Sociedad Oftalmologia del Litoral*, **11**, 88–91.

Pagenstecher, A. (1860) Beitrage zur pathologischen Anatomie des Auges. *Albrecht v. Graefes Archiv für Ophthalmologie*, **7**, 92–118.

Parsons, J. H. (1904) Congenital anterior staphyloma. *Transactions of the Ophthalmological Societies of the United Kingdom*, **24**, 47–63.

Payrau, P. & Remky, H. (1961) Scleroplasty with stored sclera. *Klinische Monatsblätter für Augenheilkunde*, **138**, 797–804.

Peters, A. (1906) Uber angeborene Defektbildung der Descemetschen Membran. *Klinische Monatsblätter für Augenheilkunde*, **44**, 27–40.

Pichion, A. & Trigonidis, G. (1965) Presentation of a case of intraepithelial carcinoma in situ. *Archeia Ophthalmologiks Hetaireias Boreiou Hellados*, **14**, 63–64.

Podedworney, W. & Suie, T. (1964) Mycotic infection of the sclera. *American Journal of Ophthalmology*, **58**, 494.

Polatti, A. (1906) Kavernose (lakunare) Sehnervenatrophie und Dehiscenz der Sklera bei hochgradiger Myopie. *Klinische Monatsblätter für Augenheilkunde*, **44**, 14–27.

Redslob, E. (1926) Anéurisme cirsoide de la conjunctive bulbaire. *Bulletin et Memoires de la Société Française d'Ophtalmologie*, **39**, 91–95.

Sacks, I. (1956) Kaposi's disease manifesting in the eye. *British Journal of Ophthalmology*, **40**, 574.

Saemisch, T. (1872) Fibrom der Sklera. *Archiv für Augenheilkunde*, **2**, 115–121.

Scarpa, A. (1801) *Saggio di Osservazione e d'Esperienze sulla principale Malattie degli Occhi.* Pavia: Presso Baldassare Comino.

Schöbl, J. (1889) Über hyperplastiche Entzündungen der Augenhaüte. *Archiv für Augenheilkunde*, **20**, 98–122.

Shindo, S. (1969) Case of metastatic suppurative scleritis. *Rinsho Ganka*, **23**, 403–405.

Smith, J. (1931) Total ectasia of the sclera. *Archives of Ophthalmology*, **5**, 990.

Sondermann, R. (1950) Die Bedeutung der Vererbung für die Entwicklung der Myopie. *Albrecht v. Graefes Archiv für Ophthalmologie*, **151**, 200–208.

Sorsby, A. (1956) *Blindness in England, 1951–1954.* London: Her Majesty's Stationery Office.

Takahashi, H. (1966) Two cases of simple scleral haemangioma. *Folia Ophthalmologica Japonica*, **17**, 671–675.

Thiel, R. (1929) Gutartige Staphylokokken-Metastasen im Bereich der vorderen Ziliagefässe. *Klinische Monatsblätter für Augenheilkunde*, **82**, 78–84.

Thompson, R. (1973) In *Diseases of the Liver, Gallbladder and Pancreas in Medicine* (Ed.) Williams, R. pp. 523–533. London: Medical Education International.

Timm, G. (1964) Calcium deposits in the sclera in primary carcinoma of the kidney. *Ophthalmologica*, **148**, 252–262.

Vail, D. (1948) Scleral staphyloma and retinal detachment. *Transactions of the American Ophthalmological Society*, **46**, 58–72.

van der Hoeve, J. & de Kleijn, A. (1917) Blue sclerotics, fragility of bones and disorders of audition. *Nederlandsch Tijdschrift voor Geneeskunde*, **1**, 1003–1010.

Vannas, S. & Teir, H. (1960) Observations on structures and age changes in the human sclera. *Acta Ophthalmologica*, **38**, 268–279.

Verhoeff, F. H. (1903) Discussion on Snell, S.: Plexiform neuroma. *Transactions of the Ophthalmological Societies of the United Kingdom*, **23**, 176–177.

Virgilio, L. A., Williams, R. J. & Klintworth, G. K. (1976) An unusually large human eye with abnormal scleral collagen. *Archives of Ophthalmology*, **94**, 101–105.

von Ammon, A. (1858) Die Entwicklungsgesichte des menschlichen Auges. *Albrecht v. Graefes Archiv für Ophthalmologie*, **4**, 1–8.

von Arlt, . . (1856) *Die Krankheiten des Auges.* Prague: Credner.

von Graefe, A. (1857) Kleinere Mittheilungen Verschwarung der sclera nach einer Schieloperation. *Albrecht v. Graefes Archiv für Ophthalmologie*, **3**, 409–411.

von Graefe, A. (1863) Tumor im submucosen Gewebe der lid eine dehaut von eigenthumlicher Beschassenheit. *Klinische Monatsblätter für Augenheilkunde*, **1**, 23.

Votočková, J. (1957) Scleromalacia following evisceration of the eye. *Československá Oftalmologie*, **13**, 294–297.

Watson, P. G. & Sevel, D. (1966) Ophthalmia nodosa. *British Journal of Ophthalmology*, **50**, 209–217.

Watzke, R. C. (1963) Scleral staphylomas and retinal detachment. *Archives of Ophthalmology*, **70**, 796–804.

Wright, J. R., Calkins, E., Breen, W. J. et al (1969) Relationship of amyloid to ageing. *Medicine*, **48**, 39–60.

Young, C. A. (1955) Equatorial scleral staphyloma. Surgical treatment in a case with retinal detachment. *American Journal of Ophthalmology*, **40**, 12–14.

CHAPTER TEN

Treatment of Scleral Disease

'Irritations of the eyes, which are caused by smoke, overheating, dust or similar injury, are easy to heal; the patient being advised first of all to avoid the irritating causes; .. next, to bathe the eyes, in the beginning with lukewarm water, later with cold, also to avoid bright light. For the disease ceases without the use of any kind of medicine, if only a proper way of living be adopted'. Tetrabiblon (Aetios, c.535 AD).

It will have become obvious that episcleritis is a benign condition which, by nature of its recurrences, is of considerable nuisance to the patient but does not constitute any menace to the patient himself or his eyesight. Scleritis on the other hand may be the result of or portend serious systemic disease and may destroy the eye.

The effective management of patients with these conditions depends on their being diagnosed early and accurately, and the ability to deal swiftly and decisively with any underlying systemic disease. Investigations to eliminate serious disease can be kept to a minimum in episcleritis, but need to be more extensive in patients with diffuse and nodular scleritis and exhaustive in patients with necrotising scleral disease.

In the past many patients have been overtreated for benign conditions and undertreated for serious eye disease which has progressed so that they have eventually lost vision or the eye (Fraunfelder and Watson, 1976). Ophthalmologists have failed to understand the nature of the underlying systemic disease which has sometimes been left untreated and physicians have failed to recognise the eye disease or the need for particular methods of management required for the eye complications of systemic disease. No effective treatment is free of side-effects; in fact, it could be said that unless a drug has side-effects it is ineffective, but fear of these should not deter the doctor from giving that treatment which will cure a disease or suppress its effects sufficiently to prevent it causing permanent harm to the patient. This inevitably leads to a conflict of interests between ophthalmologist and physician or rheumatologist who must therefore work together in the care of the patient. A clear understanding and appreciation of the needs of each speciality involved is bound to lead to the best treatment of the patient.

Problems do not arise when the scleritis is associated with an underlying condition for which there is a specific treatment, but rather when the underlying condition cannot be cured but can only be kept from advancing rapidly or be symptomatically improved by suppressing inflammation. Unfortunately, the drugs which achieve effective suppression systematically are often ineffective in controlling the eye complications.

Although there are exceptions, the activity of the associated eye complications tends to mirror the activity of the underlying connective tissue disorder. For instance, Jayson and Jones (1971) demonstrated a significant association between scleritis and rheumatoid nodules, arteritis, pericarditis, pleurisy and the systemic complications of rheumatoid arthritis as a whole. They also found that exacerbations of scleritis often coincided with the activity of the underlying joint inflammation and that the patients with eye complications often required the more 'powerful' drugs which are usually reserved for patients with the most agressive disease.

DRUGS AVAILABLE FOR THE TREATMENT OF GRANULOMATOUS SCLERAL DISEASE

The antirheumatic and anti-inflammatory agents now available are legion, but surprisingly only a few are effective in the active treatment of scleral disease. Although inhibition of the inflammation can be shown to prevent the advance of scleral disease, there is no definite evidence that a decrease in inflammation reduces joint damage. Drugs can be classified as:

1. Simple analgesics, e.g. paracetamol.
2. Analgesics with major anti-inflammatory properties, e.g. aspirin, phenylbutazone.
3. Analgesics with anti-inflammatory properties, e.g. propionic acid derivatives.
4. Pure anti-inflammatory drugs, e.g. corticosteroids.
5. Compounds with more specific action in rheumatoid arthritis, e.g. gold, penicillamine.
6. Compounds with a more specific action in other diseases, e.g. allopurinol in gout.

Many patients with chronic recurrent disease often request a new or more effective drug. Time spent in general discussion about the disease and its implications will often reveal the patient's real needs.

The increasing number of drugs available requires increasing vigilance, particularly with regard to changes in drug metabolism, drug interaction and errors in dosage and consumption.

Simple Analgesics

Simple analgesics include paracetamol, dihydrocodeine (DF 118), dextropropoxyphene (Depronal SA, Doloxene) and pentazocine (Fortral). These drugs have no anti-inflammatory activity and should not normally be used alone for treating an inflammatory arthropathy. They can be useful in alleviating pain in degenerative joint disease and as a supplement to an anti-inflammatory agent in rheumatoid arthritis.

Phenacetin-containing compounds should be avoided completely because of their association with renal papillary necrosis and chronic renal failure. Although other analgesic drugs have been incriminated in producing experimental renal lesions, the case against phenacetin is proven.

Major Anti-Inflammatory Agents

In the eye we are seeking drugs which not only improve the patient symptomatically but also suppress the inflammation to the extent that the normal healing process can repair the damage caused by the inflammation. Since the major symptoms in rheumatoid arthritis are due to inflammation, drug therapy should therefore include an anti-inflammatory drug.

Whether they are given for eye disease or joint disease, it should be stressed that these drugs should be given in full dosage to achieve an anti-inflammatory effect; lower dosage merely produces analgesia.

There is no place for the use of powerful addictive drugs such as the opiates.

Aspirin (acetyl salicylic acid)

Aspirin was introduced by MacLagan in 1876 for the treatment of acute rheumatism, and the year after Germain Sée announced in Paris that salicylates relieved chronic rheumatoid arthritis.

Aspirin has been advocated for the treatment of scleritis. Adolf Alt in 1903 said that the textbooks of the time 'are unanimous in giving first place in its treatment to antirheumatic remedies, especially the salicylates, and of late, with preference, aspirin. It has also been my experience that these remedies seem to have a beneficial influence in some cases, at least as far as relieving the pain and discomfort are concerned. Yet they will do the same in non-rheumatic affections, as, for instance, in syphilitic iritis. I have tried them faithfully and sometimes, perhaps, only too persistently, in episcleritis, and I have convinced myself time and again that, as far as curing the disease is concerned, they are unreliable'—with which we certainly agree!

Despite the amount of effort that has been put into the search for an ideal antirheumatic agent, aspirin is probably still the drug of first choice, although it may be replaced by the newer anti-inflammatory drugs which have fewer side-effects and are probably more suitable for patients with mild disease.

Not only has aspirin been the 'sheet anchor' of treatment for acute rheumatoid arthritis, it is also a drug with proven therapeutic qualities and is frequently employed as a yardstick whereby the effectiveness of newer antirheumatic drugs is compared. Why it is so ineffective in most patients with scleral disease of similar aetiology is uncertain.

Aspirin suppresses the two main symptoms, pain and stiffness; the latter occurs particularly in the morning and after periods of inactivity. For an adequate anti-inflammatory effect, blood levels of 25 to 30 mg/100 ml are needed and this may mean an oral dose of 3 to 6 grams per day, according to body size. One of the main objections of the patients, therefore, is the large number of tablets which they are required to take; failure to ingest the pre-scribed dose is not an infrequent cause of therapeutic failure. The therapeutic dose is near that at which toxic side-effects occur, namely nausea, anorexia, deafness and tinnitus. The plasma salicylate concentration is the best guideline to dosage. The patient is not a good judge of dose 'sufficient to be effective' as he is usually unfamiliar with and concerned about aspirin dosage of this magnitude. Tinnitus, whilst it may set the ceiling, is too rough a guide. In particular children and older adults may have other manifestations of toxicity without tinnitus. An adequate trial of several weeks at the therapeutic dosage should be tried before the drugs are rejected. Too often one sees patients who have tried a variety of drugs, when the full dose of any one would have been effective. The major complication of aspirin therapy is dyspepsia and nearly one-third of patients find full doses unacceptable because of this (Lee et al, 1974). Preparations in soluble form, in combination with antacids or enteric-coated are available, and are often effective in reducing this complication. Ocular damage is unusual but rare instances of allergic conjunctivitis or keratitis have been described.

There is no doubt that aspirin prolongs the bleeding time to a small but significant extent and this is due to an alteration in the platelet function. Symptomless bleeding from the gut is common, but the amount of blood lost is usually less than 5 ml a day and severe bleeding is rare. It has been found that about 70 to 80 per cent of patients will lose 2 to 10 ml of blood per day, ten per cent will lose less than 2 ml of blood per day and ten per cent will lose much more, are liable to develop iron deficiency anaemia, and are particularly susceptible to gastric irritants. Unfortunately, there is no way of identifying this group. The bleeding seems to be due to local factors, as it does not occur following experimental injections of intravenous aspirin. Aspirin is lipophilic in the acid gastric contents and is adsorbed onto the mucosal cell wall. Acetyl salicylate causes acetylation of proteins, including membrane proteins, with con-sequent damage. Dyspepsia and gastrointestinal haemorrhage are not closely related and serious bleeding can occur without any dyspeptic symptoms. Taking the aspirin with meals will reduce the incidence and severity of dyspepsia but does not reduce occult bleeding (Scott et al, 1961; Wood et al, 1962). Taking it with antacids causes a reduction in both dyspepsia and blood loss. There is a variety of different formulations on the market designed to try to minimise these side-effects: acetylsalicylic acid (Aspirin), enteric-coated aspirin, soluble aspirin, glycinated aspirin (Paynocil), aloxiprin (Palaprin Forte), microencapsulated aspirin (Levius), paracetamol-coated aspirin (Safoprin), and paracetamol ester (Benorylate).

Aspirin also has the disadvantage of occasionally causing allergic reactions, including asthma and urticaria, and any patient who has previously suffered such a reaction should avoid the drug.

Aspirin BP contains 300 mg and is seldom used as it causes gastric mucosal injury. Soluble aspirin is better tolerated, as are enteric-coated preparations. Aspirin has been combined with other substances, for example aluminium oxide (aloxiprin) and glycine (Paynocil), and both have the advantage of containing

500 mg and 600 mg of aspirin respectively which reduces the number of tablets required. The paracetamol ester of aspirin (Benorylate) has been found to cause minimal gastrointestinal bleeding. It is given as a suspension, and can be added to drink such as tea or coffee. Because of its long half-life, it only has to be given twice a day. There is some evidence that unhydrolysed benorylate has additional anti-inflammatory properties of its own.

Indomethacin

Both the non-steroidal anti-inflammatory drugs indomethacin (Indocid) and oxyphenbutazone (Tanderil) have been shown to be effective in suppressing the inflammation in both recurrent episcleritis and in the majority of patients with scleritis (Watson et al, 1966). Trials with other anti-inflammatory agents, aspirin and aspirin derivatives, flufenamic acid (Arlef) and ibuprofen (Brufen) have been found to be ineffective: the reason for this is unclear.

There is little to choose between the non-steroidal anti-inflammatory analgesics in terms of pain relief; nor is it likely that using combinations of these drugs, such as aspirin and indomethacin, will provide more relief than using them singly. Because of the increasing evidence of pharmacokinetic interaction between these drugs, pain should, whenever possible, be controlled with single drugs rather than combinations. A recent study showed that about one-third of patients with rheumatoid arthritis treated in hospital received two or more non-steroidal anti-inflammatory drugs at the same time (Lee et al, 1974).

Indomethacin is an indoleacetic acid derivative and has achieved widespread popularity as an effective anti-inflammatory agent, being considered as equal in efficacy to aspirin. It is a potent inhibitor of prostaglandin synthetase in certain experimental systems.

The drug is particularly useful in reducing morning stiffness at a dosage of 50 to 100 mg at night. A 100 mg suppository is available. An initial dose of 25 mg b.d. with food can be gradually increased up to 150 mg b.d. Higher doses have been used but the subsequent increase in side-effects is not worth the mild gain in therapeutic efficacy; side-effects occur in ten to 20 per cent of patients. The two common problems are gastric irritation and ulceration (even with a suppository) or cerebral symptoms which include headaches, muzziness and dizziness and seem to be dose-related.

There are several recorded, but not necessarily significant ocular complications: decreased visual acuity, corneal opacities, constricted visual fields, pallor of the optic discs and 'night blindness'. Improvement generally occurs on discontinuing treatment (Burns, 1968). However, Carr and Siegel (1973) were unable to confirm these observations. Occasional blood dyscrasias and skin rashes can occur.

Phenylbutazone

Phenylbutazone (Butazolidin) and its metabolite oxyphenbutazone (Tanderil) are powerful anti-inflammatory drugs with similar therapeutic and toxic properties. Part of their action is attributed to lysosomal membrane stabilisation. They are widely used for short-term treatment of many musculoskeletal

showing anti-inflammatory activity in experimental models of inflammation has been isolated from human plasma, it still remains to be demonstrated that there is an abnormal low concentration of the free form of this substance in active rheumatoid arthritis.

When antirheumatic drugs bind to serum proteins, then by competitive interaction protein-bound substances will be released from their binding sites. L-Tryptophan is an amino acid which is displaced by clinically effective anti-rheumatic drugs, and it has been shown that other drugs which also bind strongly to plasma proteins but have no anti-inflammatory activity, fail to displace L-tryptophan from plasma proteins. Aylward and Maddock (1973) have shown that an abnormally high proportion of L-tryptophan is bound to circulating proteins and that there is a correspondingly decreased level of the free form in patients with active rheumatoid disease. They have also shown that although this amino acid is displaced by anti-inflammatory drugs, there is a reduced displacement in patients with rheumatoid arthritis when compared to controls. L-Tryptophan should only be regarded as a convenient 'marker' for other anti-inflammatory peptides, since it has not been shown to have anti-inflammatory properties of its own. However, these studies support the hypothesis than an endogenous anti-inflammatory molecule exists in the circulation in both the free and bound form and would also support the hypothesis that there are greater binding affinities of plasma proteins in rheumatoid disease. Conditions associated with remission of arthritis, namely jaundice and pregnancy (Hench, 1949), have also been shown to have a higher proportion of the free form in the serum. Certainly anti-inflammatory drugs given in therapeutic dosages are virtually completely protein-bound, for example 90 per cent of salicylate is bound to plasma proteins, and it seems that the protein-bound rather than the free forms of these drugs are concerned with the anti-inflammatory action.

McConkey, Crockson and Crockson (1972) have demonstrated that measurements of the serum acute-phase proteins provide an accurate and objective method of assessing disease activity in rheumatoid arthritis. They also provide a method of assessing response to treatment, as improvement is accompanied by a decline in acute protein levels. C-reactive protein and fibrinogen, both acute-phase proteins, are found to be lower after treatment with gold salts or penicillamine whereas levels are not influenced by treatment with aspirin or indomethacin. It seems therefore that the former drugs have a more profound effect on reducing inflammatory activity than salicylates. They also inhibit the action of connective tissue activating particle (CTAP) present in high concentration in synovial lining cells in rheumatoid arthritis (Castor, 1972).

Non-steroidal anti-inflammatory agents are uncoupling agents for mitochondrial oxidative phosphorylation (Whitehouse, 1965). Oxidative phosphorylation (Lardy and Ferguson, 1969) is the biochemical mechanism whereby the final breakdown products of food, such as succinate or α-ketoglutarate, are transformed into reserve energy by the formation of ATP. In the first inflammatory phase energy is largely needed for the secretion of various mediators, for the migration of numerous phagocytic cells and for phagocytosis itself. In the presence of anti-inflammatory agents, the lack of inflammation would thus be explained by the lack of energy supply. It seems certain, however, that this uncoupling effect of these drugs cannot be a prime factor in their action for concentrations required in vitro are often higher than those present in the patient's plasma.

The stabilising effect of drugs on various biological membranes, especially lysosomal membranes, has also been suggested as the main cause of their clinical anti-inflammatory and analgesic effects (Weissmann, 1968) but this effect can usually only be shown in vitro at concentrations slightly higher than those found during therapy in man.

The most recent and generally accepted theory for the mode of action of these drugs is based on their inhibiting effect on prostaglandin synthesis. Vane (1971) has shown that indomethacin and aspirin inhibit prostaglandin synthesis in lung homogenates and the ability to observe this inhibiting effect with concentrates similar to those detected in the plasma of patients treated with these drugs is one of the main arguments for the clinical relevance of this mechanism (Ferreira and Vane, 1973). However, products with no real anti-inflammatory property are good inhibitors of prostaglandin synthesis and prostaglandins are sometimes also anti-inflammatory agents by themselves.

Corticosteroids

Corticosteroids may produce a rapid and dramatic relief in eye and joint inflammation and have been used for over 20 years. However, initial enthusiasm soon passed into disillusionment when their toxic side-effects were appreciated. They are strongly anti-inflammatory and they also stabilise lysosomal enzymes. Steroids strongly inhibit the manifestations of cell-mediated immunity in man and are used as such in transplantation surgery. It is not known how much of the anti-inflammatory effect is due to suppression of the specific allergic response and how much to suppression of nonspecific mechanisms, but whatever the underlying mechanism, they suppress inflammation predictably and dramatically in both eye and joint. Continued high dosage is precluded by toxic effects, and results of low dosage are sometimes disappointing. Although steroids give a marked and rapid relief to many patients, progress of the underlying joint disease is not arrested by steroids even though it is in many patients with scleral disease. The ultimate results are often little or no better than anti-inflammatory drugs (MRC Joint Committee, 1960).

The relatively high doses necessary to achieve suppression, and the long-term therapy that is required produce such serious side-effects that this form of therapy should only be used for selected patients and rarely should a maintenance dose of more than 10 mg prednisone be prescribed per day.

Corticosteroids were responsible in a Glasgow study for five per cent of hospital admissions and 12 per cent of deaths in patients with rheumatoid arthritis (Brooks et al, 1975). Complications include: infection, dyspepsia and peptic ulceration, perforation of the stomach and intestines, gastrointestinal haemorrhage, adrenal suppression, osteoporosis, psychoses, nitrogen depletion, diabetes mellitus, myopathy, sodium retention with oedema and hypertension, potassium depletion, avascular bone necrosis, and cataract and glaucoma. Steroids are specifically contraindicated in active tuberculosis and in other infections or when there is a history of psychosis. They should be avoided if possible in patients with previous peptic ulceration or gastrointestinal bleeding, diabetes mellitus and osteoporosis.

Side-effects which are common but not usually of serious consequence, include: gain in weight, fat distribution of cushingoid type, acne and hirsutes, amenorrhoea, striae, and increased bruising tendency.

Prednisolone has the advantage of familiarity and is manufactured in 1 mg as well as 5 mg tablets, allowing for small dose reductions. If gastric side-effects occur, then 2.5 mg enteric-coated tablets can be used.

Glaucoma is the most feared ophthalmological complication of steroids, but this rarely occurs with systemic therapy. Cataracts are probably the most common side-effect. Exudative macular lesions have been described after cortico-trophin therapy and a nonspecific conjunctivitis has been reported following sudden withdrawal of steroids. There is a suggestion that steroids may intensify vasculitis where already present and induce it in those who do not already have it, particularly if the doses are intermittent and high (Bywaters, 1957; Sokoloff and Bunim, 1957). However, to withhold steroids altogether may derive many patients the benefit of the suppression of inflammation, the pre-vention of the destructive changes this causes and in many instances necessary symptomatic relief. Steroids are useful in the presence of systemic disease and are valuable in a patient severely incapacitated by acute disease when there is an urgent need for symptomatic relief. Incapacitating morning stiffness is relieved and the elderly rheumatoid may be kept independent on a small dose of prednisone. They are also of value in necrotising scleritis in the intractable iritis which commonly accompanies juvenile ANF-positive poly-arthritis or Reiter's syndrome.

In rheumatoid arthritis the indications can be summarised as:

1. Relentlessly progressive polyarthritis uncontrolled by conservative methods.
2. In the elderly patient with a rapid functional deterioration.
3. When there are special social or family demands.
4. Unacceptable morning stiffness.
5. Threatened complete dependency.

No categorical rules can be laid down and it must be remembered that most patients who commence steroid treatment remain on it more or less permanently, although attempts at weaning a patient from the drug should be made frequently. They must only be given if it is essential to produce a dramatic response, as in the sudden onset of necrotising scleritis, or if simple anti-inflammatory drugs have been given adequate trial and have failed. Patients receiving long-term treatment should be frequently reassessed to determine the necessity of continued treatment.

If a regime of steroid treatment is decided for severe scleral disease it is vital to achieve suppression of the inflammation by high dosages of up to 80 to 100 mg prednisolone per day, reducing to a maintenance dose within three weeks. More gentle regimes have failed to produce an adequate response (Watson, 1966).

In the inflammatory arteriopathies such as polyarteritis nodosa and temporal arteritis, corticosteroids are the most effective agents we have, and there is evidence that though non-steroidal anti-inflammatory agents suppress inflam-matory symptoms in these disorders, they may not be powerful enough to stop vascular complications which ultimately lead to blindness or gangrene.

Corticotrophin (ACTH)

ACTH or adrenocorticotrophic hormone and tetracosactrin (Synacthen) have the advantage of not leading to hypoplasia of the adrenal gland and this makes it easier to withdraw treatment. There is also a relative lack of gastro-intestinal symptoms and myopathic complications as compared with conventional glucocorticoid therapy. On the other hand, they have to be given by intramuscular or subcutaneous injections and can cause allergic reactions. There is a higher incidence of electrolyte disturbance, hypertension and androgenic effects. In children with systemic manifestations of arthritis, ACTH is extremely useful and, provided it is given at suitably spaced intervals for the type of preparation used, suppression of the hypothalamic–adrenal axis does not occur and growth continues (Freidman and Greenwood, 1967) as do corticosteroids given on alternate days (Soyka, 1972).

Immunosuppressive Therapy

If immunosuppressive drugs are to be used the following criteria must apply:

1. Evidence of excessive immune activity.
2. This immune activity must play a central role in the pathogenesis of the disease.
3. The hope that the immune activity can be suppressed (Currey, 1971).

These compounds were synthesised especially for their ability to interfere with the proliferation of rapidly dividing cells, either by affecting further synthesis of DNA or interfering with the transmission of the message from DNA to the RNA involved in protein synthesis. However, in connective tissue diseases there is some doubt whether the effect of these drugs is due to suppression of an immunological mechanism or is purely due to an anti-inflammatory effect. Most of the compounds so far discovered have little effect on an immune response once it has already developed. The phase of the immune response which is most sensitive to the drug is the phase of cellular proliferation which precedes the circulation of immunologically active lymphocytes or the secretion of humoral antibody. In rheumatoid arthritis a fall in rheumatoid factor and a lowering of serum immunoglobulin levels have been observed, but such changes do not in themselves establish that the drugs are acting as immunosuppressive agents.

Azathioprine seems to have a more profound anti-inflammatory effect than cyclophosphamide, whereas the latter seems more effective in suppressing a secondary or on-going immune response.

Any method of immunosuppression is potentially dangerous and Schwartz and Gowans (1971) have proposed the following guidelines for the use of these drugs in the rheumatic diseases:

1. Failure to respond to, or intolerable side-effects from conventional therapy.
2. Absence of active infection.
3. No haematological contraindication.
4. Meticulous follow-up for signs of acute or long-term toxicity.

5. Careful objective evaluation.
6. The patient must be informed of the reason for this therapy and his consent obtained.
7. The use of these drugs during the child-bearing year is contraindicated.

These formidable limitations are necessary when one remembers that, once started, treatment may be life-long and when one considers the numerous and serious side-effects of these drugs. These include alopecia, gastrointestinal symptoms with nausea, hepatitis, leucopenia, sterility and haemorrhagic cystitis. There have also been disturbing reports of lymphoma developing within the central nervous system in renal transplantation patients. This does not mean that they have no place in the treatment of scleral and rheumatoid disease. It is possible to reduce the amount of systemic steroid necessary to keep the disease under control by combining azathioprine with the systemic steroid (Mason et al, 1969). Immunosuppressives are therefore of value in patients with severe disease requiring high doses of steroids for prolonged periods, or in those patients with severe and rapidly progressive disease where all other measures have failed.

Hurd and Ziff (1974) have recently examined the laboratory parameters during treatment with cyclophosphamide. Clinical improvement correlated well with a decrease in the monocyte and small lymphocyte counts. These findings suggest that levels of these cells in the blood rather than the development of leucopenia can be used as a guide to therapy.

Cyclophosphamide

Clinical trials of cyclophosphamide, which have included a controlled study by the American Rheumatism Association (Co-operating Clinics of the American Rheumatism Association, 1972), have given guidelines for dosage regimes. Patients were randomly assigned to a 'high-dose' (up to 150 mg /day) or a 'low-dose' (up to 15 mg /day) group and treatment was continued for 32 weeks. The 'high-dose' patients showed objective improvement in disease activity, and in particular a reduction in the appearance of radiological progression of the disease. Serious side-effects were seen with one case of herpes zoster and two of haemorrhagic cystitis; gastrointestinal symptoms were common and significant loss of hair was a distressing feature. A subsequent double-blind cross-over study has confirmed the effectiveness of this 'high-dose' level. In contrast the almost completely non-toxic 'low-dose' level (0.7 to1 mg /kg daily of cyclophosphamide) has little or no beneficial effect in rheumatoid arthritis.

Azathioprine

This seems to have a more profound anti-inflammatory effect than cyclophosphamide, whereas the latter seems more effective in suppressing a secondary or ongoing immune response.

Mason et al (1969) carried out a trial of azathioprine at a dose of 2.5 mg /kg daily in patients who initially required a mean daily dose of 11 mg prednisolone.

The dose of prednisolone was periodically adjusted to the minimum required and at the end of the year it was found that the net fall in steroid requirements of patients on azathioprine was 4.3 mg per day as compared with a fall of 0.75 mg per day in patients left on their original therapy. Steroid requirements in azathioprine-treated patients remained low even 18 months after this drug had been discontinued, suggesting that it influenced the underlying disease.

A recent trial in which gold has been compared with azathioprine or cyclophosphamide has demonstrated that the drugs were equally effective after six months. Azathioprine and gold produced similar improvement, but cyclophosphamide was found to be superior to gold and seemed to prevent the progression of radiological changes when given to patients with early disease (Currey et al, 1975).

Antirheumatic Drugs

If the scleritis fails to respond to therapy with anti-inflammatory drugs, what alternatives are there? A change of occupation or neighbourhood? 'A dry soil and bracing air often works wonders, and a person who, while living on a clay soil in a river valley is continually subject to annoyance from attacks of inflammation of the sclerotic, may find himself perfectly free from trouble from this source if he can live on a sandy or gravelly soil, a few hundred feet above sea level. A period at a spa, either at home or abroad, has often excellent results; for it has the double advantage of giving the patient appropriate medical treatment and at the same time of taking him away from his business and other cares' (Maitland Ramsay, 1909). Whilst all agree a good holiday helps, it will certainly not improve severe scleral disease. What of the other drugs used in rheumatology and for the treatment of connective tissue disease?

If an adequate trial of treatment with anti-inflammatory drugs fails to reduce inflammation, then treatment with gold salts, chloroquine or penicillamine can be considered. Of the three, gold salts are particularly popular and effective although their side-effects have led to periods when their use has fallen into disfavour. All these drugs have the major disadvantage in treatment of scleral disease that there is a prolonged interval, often several weeks, before the beneficial effect becomes apparent. With the progressive and sometimes rapid changes found in patients with scleral disease, this delay can be serious. Their use is therefore confined to patients with either chronic, severe, but not destructive scleral disease or to those who have failed to respond to previous treatment, or are going to require prolonged therapy as an alternative to systemic steroids. Our experience of these drugs indicates that penicillamine, especially if used with another anti-inflammatory drug, is the most effective in the treatment of scleral disease. Gold therapy has been disappointing and chloroquine only very rarely effective.

Gold salts

Gold salts have been used in the treatment of rheumatoid arthritis for over 40 years as a result of the belief in their value in the treatment of pulmonary tuberculosis. Forestier in 1932 claimed encouraging results and similar reports soon followed. It was difficult to evaluate results as there were no controlled trials of patients, but this was rectified in 1961 when a controlled trial by the Empire Rheumatism Council demonstrated improvement in clinical and laboratory parameters after three months. Patients received 20 weekly i.m. injections of sodium aurothiomalate (Myocrisin) to a total of one gram. Gold compounds are all given parenterally because they are not absorbed orally. Improvement was maintained until the eighteenth month from the start of treatment. After discontinuation of gold, the difference between treated and control groups in this trial disappeared by the thirtieth month. There was a reduction in sedimentation rate and rheumatoid factor titre and subcutaneous nodules tended to disappear but there was no influence on radiological changes. For this reason, fortnightly maintenance injections should continue after the initial one gram and the beneficial effects are prolonged. Those who fail to respond after one gram are unlikely to respond at all, and gold should not be continued. In fact about 70 per cent of patients improve. Since gold compounds have no immediate effect on inflammation, they are used in conjunction with conventional anti-inflammatory drug therapy. The conventional dosage schedule is a 10 mg i.m. test dose followed one week later by 20 mg and, provided there are no side-effects, 50 mg is given weekly until a total dose of approximately one gram has been given. This total dose is arbitrary and is based on the original controlled trials. The beneficial effects of therapy are prolonged if fortnightly or monthly maintenance injections continue. In contrast to other reports, a recent report has shown a significantly slower progression of erosive changes (Sigler et al, 1974).

It is now difficult to decide when to stop gold therapy. Many maintain treatment for at least two years after remission.

Gold is more than a slow-acting anti-inflammatory agent. Response to gold therapy ensues only after several weeks, is subtle in onset and may simulate a natural remission from rheumatoid arthritis. It actively suppresses joint inflammation, but is least effective in the chronic stages of the disease. The fact that it takes three months to become fully effective makes it valueless in the acute treatment of scleritis which initially presents as an urgent problem. It is very occasionally of value in those patients who have not been able to tolerate other forms of therapy, especially if they also have rheumatoid arthritis. If the patient is already receiving gold therapy when he develops scleritis, this is continued; many maintain therapy for at least two years after a remission has been achieved.

If gold is being used it must be remembered that 20 to 30 per cent of patients develop toxic reactions, but in most cases these are mild; reactions include leucopenia and thrombocytopenia, proteinuria, pruritus or even exfoliative dermatitis. Skin rashes often resemble pityriasis rosea or lichenoid eruptions but can mimic virtually any dermatological condition (Penneys, Ackerman and Gottlieb, 1974). The mechanisms responsible for the dermatitis are unclear, but several observers have noted the presence of eosinophilia and, more recently, elevated serum immunoglobulin E levels have been reported (Davis et al, 1973). Eosinophilia is also noted frequently in patients without toxic effects of gold and should alert the therapist to watch especially carefully for side-effects. A second course of gold may not result in dermatitis. Proteinuria occurs in four per cent of the patients, but renal damage is rarely serious and there is complete reversal in discontinuing the drug. Biopsies show a membranous type of nephritis with immune complex deposition (Strunk and Ziff, 1970). Blepharitis and conjunctivitis may be a manifestation of gold toxicity, and corneal deposition of gold salts can occur which does not elicit an inflammatory reaction. This is not a contraindication to further gold therapy (Thiel and Langness, 1970).

A mild dermatitis clears spontaneously if no more gold is given. Agranulo-cytes and hypoplastic anaemia may necessitate blood transfusion, but the bone marrow can recover even after severe depression for many weeks. Marrow depression with agranulocytosis or thrombocytopenia occurs in up to three per cent of cases, and gold has the unenviable reputation of being responsible for more deaths per million prescriptions than any other drug (Girdwood, 1974). Hence the importance of careful control.

The most important precaution is to emphasise to patients that they must report at once on the appearance of any untoward symptoms, especially sore throat or pruritus which may precede changes in the blood. If injections are stopped immediately on the suspicion of an adverse reaction, serious trouble may be avoided. Monthly estimation of haemoglobin, white cells and platelets is desirable and the urine should be tested for protein before each injection.

Gold suppresses joint inflammation after several months of use but is least effective in the chronic stages of disease. The mechanism of action is still unknown; it does not seem to modify the immune response but has been shown to stabilise lysosomal membranes. It has also been suggested that gold may compete for the −SH radical in such a way as to alter cellular metabolism. Phagocytic activity of macrophages and neutrophils is elevated above control populations in rheumatoid arthritis and is decreased by treatment with gold compounds (Jessop, Vernon-Roberts and Harris, 1973).

Chloroquine

Antimalarial drugs have been widely prescribed in rheumatoid arthritis following their successful use in discoid lupus erythematosus. Most clinical trials have shown that they have a slight anti-inflammatory activity and a fall in rheumatoid factor titre occurs (Hamilton and Scott, 1962).

Improvement should not be expected until about the third month of treatment and this again precludes the use of chloroquine for the treatment of scleritis quite apart from the well-known occurrence of toxic manifestations which include skin rashes, gastrointestinal upsets and leucopenia. Both the therapeutic and toxic effects of the drug are dose-related. The most serious side-effect is the bull's eye macular changes which result from the progressive accumulation of the drug at the macula. It is not only irreversible but the retinopathy may progress even following withdrawal of the drug and can result in blindness. Chloroquine and hydroxychloroquine cause irreversible retinal damage in one in every 1000 to 2000 patients on long-term treatment. The corneal deposits which are more common do, however, disappear when the drug is stopped. Chloroquine is the most commonly used member of this group. It is suggested that 250 mg daily is sufficient to produce a therapeutic response and at this dose retinal toxicity is less commonly observed. Regular eye examination is required at three-monthly intervals so that the drug can be discontinued before irreversible damage occurs.

Because of the ophthalmic complications and its weak anti-inflammatory activity, the place of chloroquine in the management of rheumatoid arthritis is still controversial. It can be considered if for any reason gold or penicillamine cannot be used.

D -Penicillamine

Penicillamine (Distamine, Cuprimine) is a sulphur-containing amino acid related to cysteine. As a chelating agent it is used in the management of Wilson's disease and the treatment of lead poisoning, gold poisoning and cystinuria. More recently it has been used in the treatment of rheumatoid arthritis. Penicillamine is a sulphydryl reducing agent and is able to split the disulphide bridges holding together subunits of rheumatoid factor. Rheumatoid factors are mainly IgM class antibodies and although the role of rheumatoid factor in the pathogenesis of rheumatoid arthritis is still controversial, rheumatoid factor is found more commonly and in higher titre in rheumatoid arthritis than in other conditions. There is a recognised correlation between vasculitis and the other extra-articular features of rheumatoid arthritis and the presence of a high titre on rheumatoid factor. However, it now appears that the action of penicillamine in rheumatoid arthritis depends on actions much more complex than simple dissociation of rheumatoid factor, and it is still not certain how penicillamine acts. It is known that total skin collagen may be reduced (Harvey, Henderson and Grahame, 1974) and penicillamine has been shown to prevent the initial formation of cross-links between collagen molecules (Francis and Mowat, 1974). Penicillamine has also been shown to result in lowering of serum IgG and IgM levels and to a lesser extent of IgA (Huskisson and Berry, 1974).

In 1973 a British double-blind multicentre controlled study (Multicentre Trial Group, 1973) showed that penicillamine undoubtedly benefited patients with severe rheumatoid arthritis. In this trial 105 patients were allocated randomly to treatment with either penicillamine or identical placebo; their drug therapy was otherwise unchanged. After one year, the penicillamine-treated group showed a significant advantage in terms of pain scores, duration of morning stiffness, grip strength, articular index, functional grade and reduction in ESR.

A recent trial in which gold was compared with penicillamine found that both drugs were equally effective after six months (Huskisson et al, 1974) and both drugs produced highly significant improvement in all clinical measurements. Penicillamine has been found to be particularly useful in treating some of the non-articular manifestations of rheumatoid arthritis such as tenosynovitis, neuropathy and skin ulceration (Multicentre Trial Group, 1973). It is also claimed to be helpful in patients with vasculitis and gangrene (Jaffe, 1970).

The side-effects are similar to gold and the use of this drug requires careful monitoring. About 20 per cent of patients develop skin rashes and two types are recognised (Huskisson et al, 1974b): one appears within four months of therapy and resembles an ampicillin rash whereas that appearing after six months consists of lichenoid plaques.

As many as 30 per cent of cases develop temporary loss of taste about six weeks after starting therapy. This can be very distressing but returns in six to eight weeks whether or not penicillamine is continued.

Proteinuria, which occurs in 10 to 15 per cent of cases, is reversible but can take up to one year to disappear after discontinuing the drug. The nephrotic syndrome can occur and, despite the changes characteristic of immune complex nephritis, there have been no signs of impaired renal function. In patients who develop heavy proteinuria penicillamine should be stopped.

The Multicentre Trial Group noted a mean fall of 27 per cent in the platelet count; in all cases recovery was rapid after treatment was stopped. Neutropenia occurs less often. Penicillamine can also cause drug-induced lupus syndrome with joint pains (Oliver, Liberman and de Vries, 1972). It is therefore worth remembering that a patient complaining of joint pains may need less penicillamine and not more.

Despite this daunting list of side-effects, penicillamine is a useful drug in the management of rheumatoid arthritis. When used, careful account must be taken of the possibility of proteinuria and thrombocytopenia. It is suggested that starting at the low dose of 125 mg per day and increasing it at intervals of two to four weeks reduces the incidence of side-effects; clinical benefit is usually achieved by 750 mg daily and often 375 mg produces improvement (Day, Golding and Lee, 1974).

Penicillamine in high doses has proved useful in the treatment of rheumatoid vasculitis and there is some evidence that patients with scleritis also improve, but it should be reserved as an adjunct for other therapy or when other therapy is contraindicated. On its own the improvement in scleral disease to date has not been impressive, partly because of the long time it takes to produce its therapeutic effects. However, one or two patients have been maintained in prolonged remission or have been able to reduce the dosage of their other drugs by the addition of penicillamine to the regime.

Present experience suggests that gold and penicillamine are equally effective, but Huskisson et al (1974) found a lower withdrawal rate on penicillamine than on gold and for this reason suggested that it should be the first line of therapy. It should be reserved for patients who have failed to respond to or have progressed despite the optimal use of anti-inflammatory drugs. To obtain the best results it should be used before irreversible structural changes have developed in either eye or joint.

MEDICAL TREATMENT OF SCLERITIS AND EPISCLERITIS

Treatment of Episcleritis

A few patients who have tumours, infiltrations or granulomas of the episclera due to small foreign bodies require to have the lesion excised for treatment and diagnosis. The majority require no treatment at all because the condition is self-limiting and does not damage the eye. Some demand treatment and there are a few who need some help because of the severity and duration of the attacks. The patients fall into two groups. The first, the majority, usually have simple episcleritis and intermittent bouts of moderate or severe inflammation at one- to three-month intervals lasting seven to ten days, occurring more commonly in the spring or autumn than in the summer or winter. Only rarely can a precipitating factor be found, attacks usually related to family upsets or worries at work. A second group of patients gives no history of periodicity but rather of mild, prolonged attacks of inflammation. In this category come almost all the patients who had some intercurrent systemic disease. Surprisingly it is this second mild group, not the more florid group, who require treatment, which will often completely cure the episcleritis; at worst local inflammatory agents may be required in addition from time to time.

Occasionally, a clear history of exogenous sensitisation can be obtained and, if this is so, the patients will sometimes improve following removal from the environment which precipitated the attack. Unfortunately, this does not always work, neither does desensitisation to the allergen, because it appears that once the tissues have been sensitised they often respond thereafter to a multitude of nonspecific antigenic stimuli.

Every now and again episcleritis will go into remission and even disappear completely simply by explaining to the patient the nature and natural history of the condition and emphasising its benign nature and that it is known to flare up with undue stress. More often, the patients will not accept a simple explanation or that the lesion is self-limiting and demand some therapy to provide subjective comfort or occasionally, in the severe recurrences, to reduce the intensity of the inflammation.

The traditional therapy for episcleritis has been steroids applied locally in the form of eye drops in the conjunctival sac (Duke Elder, 1951a, 1951b) given at frequent intervals, sometimes half-hourly, whilst the inflammation was present, gradually tailing the treatment off as the patients improved. A rise in intraocular pressure will occur in up to 16 per cent of patients treated in this way and as 64 per cent of patients will develop recurrences at intervals from as short a period as three weeks or less for as much as 30 years, the chances of them developing an intractable and practically untreatable glaucoma are very high. In addition, at least 15 per cent of patients with episcleritis receiving local steroids for over one year will develop posterior cortical cataracts. In view of these long-term hazards of using local steroid therapy, double-blind control studies were undertaken to determine whether any steroid treatment was effective and, if so, whether any of the other available non-steroid anti-inflammatory agents, which did not have these disastrous side-effects, were as effective in controlling the inflammation. A double-blind control study was set up to compare the effect of betamethasone 0.1 per cent ointment, oxyphenbutazone (Tanderil) ten per cent ointment and placebo eye ointment (Watson et al, 1973). This trial showed that episcleritis is a self-limiting condition in that the inflammation improved by 50 per cent within seven days of the onset without any treatment at all, and that well over 80 per cent of these patients were free of all traces of episcleritis in 21 days. Resolution was faster when drugs were used, a 75 per cent improvement having occurred with oxyphenbutazone, a 63 per cent improvement with betamethasone and a 51 per cent improvement with placebo within the three weeks (Figure 10.1). From every point of view oxyphenbutazone would be the treatment of choice. Unfortunately, it is only available in ointment form and although the effective

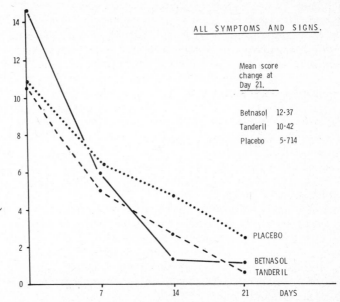

ALL SYMPTOMS AND SIGNS.

Mean score change at Day 21.

Betnasol   12·37
Tanderil   10·42
Placebo   5·714

PLACEBO

BETNASOL

TANDERIL

7   14   21   DAYS

Figure 10.1. A double-blind control trial in episcleritis between Betnasol, oxyphenbutazone and placebo ointments. The patients on the active drugs improved only slightly faster than those on placebo.

dose is increased by this method of application, many patients are handicapped for an hour or so after the ointment has been applied, because the grease on the cornea blurs the vision. Some patients also develop redness of the conjunctiva and lids, possibly as a reaction to the ointment base, which means that therapy has to be curtailed. From this trial it appeared that the sooner treatment was started the quicker it was brought under control, so we have asked a few patients to use the drops or ointment just as soon as the symptoms appear and in many cases the attacks have been aborted. It seems, therefore, that in most patients with episcleritis, treatment is unnecessary, but if given, it should be oxyphenbutazone (Tanderil) ten per cent ointment at the very beginning of an attack, steroids only being used if the condition fails to respond, if the patient is intolerant of the ointment, or if side-effects appear.

In the few patients who have recurrent attacks of episcleritis which are not adequately controlled by local therapy or whose attacks are so severe, or recurrences so frequent as to cause considerable distress, then systemic therapy may be indicated. In 1965 a double-blind control trial was carried out in patients who had recurrent episcleritis to compare the effects of oxyphenbuta-zone (Tanderil) and systemic prednisolone (Watson et al, 1966). These two drugs were equally effective in relieving the episcleritis. The rate of resolution was similar to that found later with the trial of local drops. Fifty per cent had very much improved by seven days and 70 per cent by 21 days, but the improvement was maintained after the oxyphenbutazone was withdrawn at the end of the three-week period, whereas those receiving prednisolone tended to deteriorate after the treatment was withdrawn, particularly between days 28 and 24 and was thought to be due to a rebound phenomenon (Figure 10.2). Oxyphenbutazone has a half life of three days and the persistence of the drug in the circulation in reducing quantities may be important in preventing recur-rences. When the patients were reviewed a year later, it was found that each

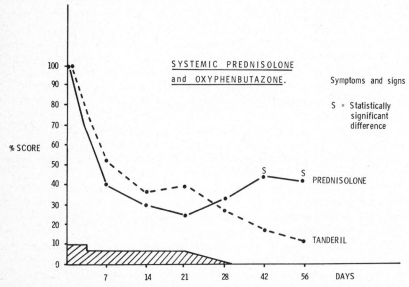

Figure 10.2.　A double-blind trial of oxyphenbutazone and prednisolone. Both drugs are effective in suppressing the signs and symptoms but the effect was prolonged with oxyphenbutazone whereas the symptoms recurred after the withdrawal of the prednisolone.

group had had the same number of recurrences, but that those who had received oxyphenbutazone had remained free of trouble for an average of five months. The doses used in the trial were prednisolone 30 mg per day for the first two days and 20 mg daily for three weeks and 600 mg of oxyphenbutazone for two days and 400 mg thereafter. We have recently completed a double-blind trial designed in the same way between oxyphenbutazone (Tanderil) 400 mg daily and indomethacin (Indocid) 75 mg daily in patients with recurrent episcleritis. This shows that both are equally effective in the suppression of episcleral inflammation in the majority of patients, but that some patients have a better response to one drug than the other when they are crossed over.

Because both these drugs have been shown to be effective, it is probably never necessary to resort to the use of systemic steroid preparations in the treatment of episcleritis and we would recommend a course of 21 days of either oxyphenbutazone starting at 600 mg per day for seven days and then reducing to 400 mg per day or indomethacin 100 mg daily for seven days and 75 mg daily thereafter. Both can be used in the first attack or in recurrences and although both drugs have side-effects which must be looked for, these are not ocular and not as severe as those induced by long-term steroid therapy.

Treatment of Scleritis in Patients in whom no Systemic Disease is Discovered

Whilst with episcleritis the question is whether one should treat or not, the situation is quite different with scleral disease, which must be treated symptomatically to relieve the very severe pain and discomfort and to suppress potentially destructive inflammation. Local steroid therapy and local oxyphenbutazone therapy are ineffective in suppressing the inflammation but they increase the patient's comfort considerably. This is unexpected because the concentration which can be achieved in the eye by local application is much higher than that which can be produced by systemic therapy. Treatment only suppresses the inflammation sufficiently to allow normal repair of tissues to occur and must be continued while the disease follows its natural course which is usually between six months to six years but occasionally lasts a lifetime.

In the less severe anterior diffuse, nodular and posterior scleritis, the anti-inflammatory drugs are tried first. Our preference is for oxyphenbutazone (Tanderil) 600 mg in divided doses, reducing to 400 mg in divided doses as soon as the pain is relieved and the inflammation begins to subside. It is a characteristic of all patients with scleritis that the pain is relieved as soon as the inflammatory reaction is suppressed even though the external appearance appears the same. The presence or absence of pain may even be used to titrate the dosage of the drug in some patients.

If there is no response or a very weak response to oxyphenbutazone, then indomethacin (Indocid) 100 mg daily is used, reducing to 75 mg daily in divided doses as soon as the condition is under control. Many patients will respond to indomethacin who will not respond to Tanderil and vice versa; it is therefore worth trying both.

Although not usually recommended, systemic anti-inflammatory drugs may be used together with local steroid drops or ointment of prednisolone 0.5 per cent or betamethasone 0.1 per cent, or local oxyphenbutazone ointment ten per cent. This gives subjective relief and comfort to some patients. Once the disease has been suppressed, certain patients can stop the tablets and can then keep the inflammation under control by using drops infrequently, occasionally as little as 0.1 per cent prednisolone drops once or twice a week.

If local steroid therapy is continued the side-effects of glaucoma and cataract need to be looked for continuously and the treatment stopped should any of these changes occur. If the scleritis is either very severe, obviously necrotising, or if any avascular areas appear in the sclera or episclera, and it does not respond to oxyphenbutazone or indomethacin treatment within a week or two (Figures 10.3 to 10.7) then systemic steroids must be given in heavy suppressive doses. The sclera is an avascular structure and therefore high concentrations

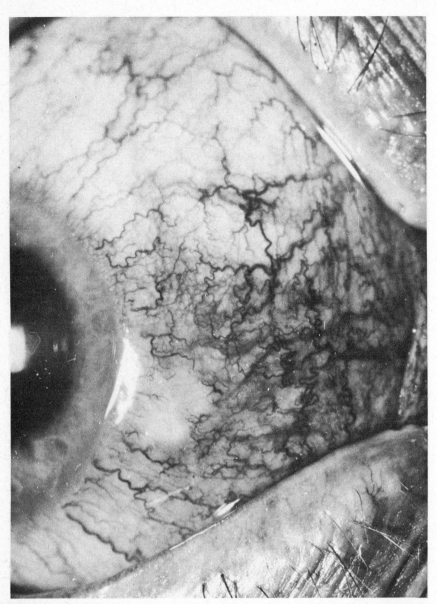

Figure 10.3. Day 1. This 35-year-old female patient gave a week's history of a painful red eye and pain in the face. She has an obvious anterior scleritis but an avascular patch has appeared adjacent to the limbus indicating an early necrotising disease. She was given 600 mg oxyphenbutazone daily.

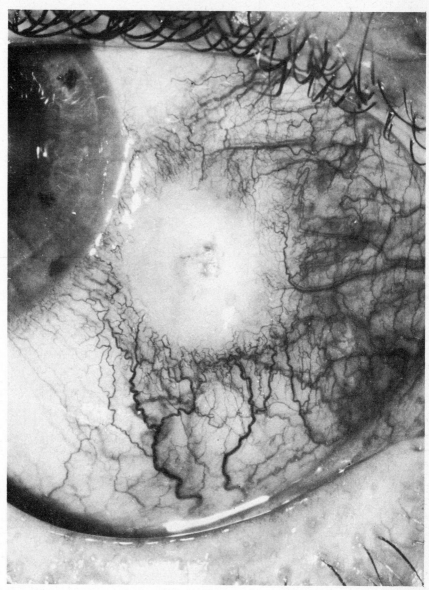

Figure 10.4. The appearance on day 7. A large area of the sclera is necrosic and the avascular patch is much increased. The pain was very severe so she was admitted to hospital and was given 60 mg of prednisolone. The oxyphenbutazone was discontinued.

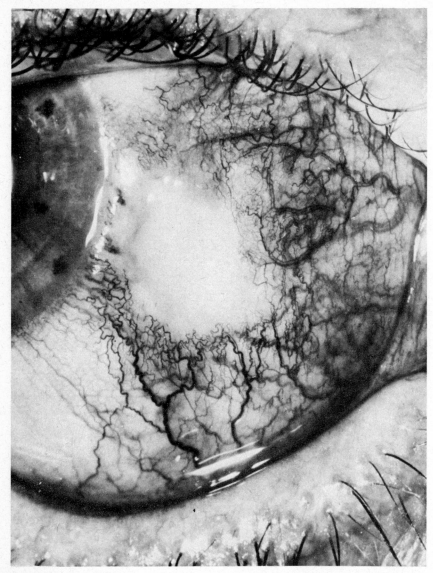

Figure 10.5. Day 9. The external appearance appeared almost unchanged but all the pain had disappeared.

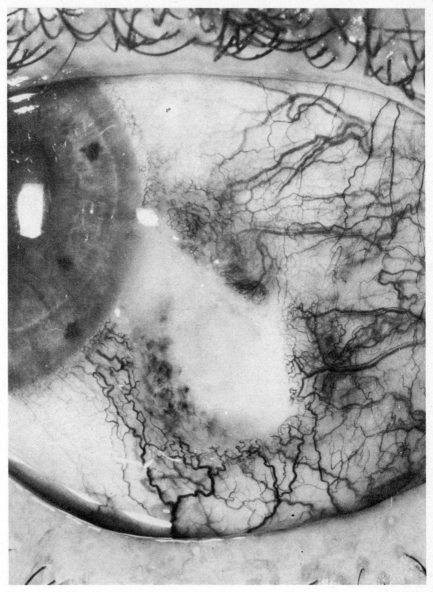

Figure 10.6. Day 14. The eye was still comfortable and the prednisolone had been reduced to 30 mg per day. New vessels can be seen entering the necrotic area from all sides.

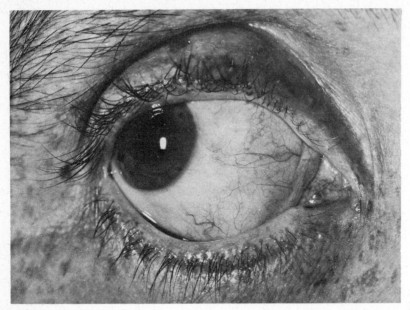

Figure 10.7. One month later. All treatment has stopped and the eye is apparently normal apart from some distortion of the vascular pattern.

are required to produce a therapeutic effect. It has been noticed many times that one of the first signs of necrotising scleral disease is an avascular patch in the sclera which, if it extends, will eventually slough leaving a dehiscence within the sclera itself. However benign the rest of the inflammatory signs, if such an area is seen it should be taken with the greatest seriousness because this does indicate a necrotising scleral disease and requires systemic therapy for its control. In order to determine what the effective suppressive dose should be in these circumstances, some patients were given 20 mg prednisolone and the dose was increased by 20 mg every third day until a response was obtained. Using this approach, most of our patients responded at 60 mg but some required 80 mg and a few even 120 mg before suppression occurred. Since then, we have started all our patients on 60 mg prednisolone and only rarely have we needed to increase this dose. The response is dramatic; within a few hours and certainly within 48 hours the pain disappears and the physical signs start to improve within a further 48 hours. As soon as there is a clinical response, the dose is reduced by 20 mg per day to a maintenance dose of 20 mg daily in divided doses. The dose is reduced further with great caution. Another anti-inflammatory drug is often added at this stage and the patient then weaned off the steroid in 2.5 mg steps. If a rebound of the inflammation does occur, it is necessary to restart the course at the same high dose that is known to suppress the inflammation. The policy, which will not always be achieved, should be to take patients off steroids as soon as possible, recognising the fact that this may possibly induce a systemic vasculitis, but, because of the chronicity of scleritis and because of the fear of side-effects, long-term steroid therapy is not justified if it can be avoided.

There are a few patients with anterior and posterior scleritis who fail to respond adequately to prednisolone but respond to Sintisone (prednisolone 21-steatoryl-glycolate). This was confirmed in a small trial which was conducted to discover the effect of this drug in scleritis (Hayreh and Watson, 1970). One tablet of Sintisone contains 6.65 mg of prednisolone 21-steatoryl-glycolate and is equivalent to 3.5 mg of prednisolone. It is therefore convenient to think of treatment in terms of tablets.

Treatment is usually started with eight tablets (12 or 16 occasionally being necessary) and reduced to two a day as soon as possible. Table 10.1 shows how quickly complete resolution of the scleritis was achieved on this regime in the 21 patients in the trial.

Table 10.1.   *Complete resolution of scleritis with Sintisone*

Time of onset	No. of cases
2 days	1
4 days	7
5 days	3
6 days	1
1 week	6
2 weeks	1
4 weeks	2
Total	21

Two patients were removed from this trial because they developed an acute steroid psychosis with suicidal tendencies at the end of the first week of treatment which disappeared as soon as the drug was discontinued. One of them had no tendency to psychotic symptoms on prolonged treatment with prednisolone given both before and after treatment with Sintisone. Another patient showed no response to Sintisone but was completely controlled on prednisolone. In the same way that oxyphenbutazone and indomethacin are complementary in the treatment of the milder forms of scleritis, prednisolone and Sintisone are complementary in the more severe forms.

In the patients with very severe necrotising scleritis which is only controlled with very high dosages of steroids or is never controlled either with prednisolone or Sintisone, it is reasonable to add immunosuppressive therapy to the steroid therapy. Azathioprine is the drug of choice and is started at 100 mg daily increasing the dose to 150 mg or 200 mg over the next two weeks. Hurd, Snyder and Ziff (1970) and Brubaker, Font and Shepherd (1971) have reported regression of lesions in both anterior and posterior scleritis using cyclophosphamide and prednisolone. To suppress the inflammatory reaction Hurd, Snyder and Ziff found it necessary to use 60 mg prednisolone and 100 mg cyclophosphamide reducing eventually to 7.5 mg and 75 mg daily respectively. The improvement in clinical condition was correlated with a fall in IgG and IgM levels to normal. Whatever immunosuppressive agent is used, constant monitoring of the platelet and white counts is necessary and any reduction in these necessitates the withdrawal of the drug. In necrotising disease we have seen the disease progress even though the patients are symptom-free and the disease itself seems to be in a quiescent stage. Very careful observation is therefore required in these patients as any sign of further destruction should be an indication for further treatment.

It might be thought that to give steroids subconjunctivally was the most effective method of delivering it in high concentration to the eye in scleral disease. The reverse is the truth. It is uncertain whether it was because of the high concentration of the steroid or whether it was the result of the base in which it was suspended which caused the extreme thinning at the site of subconjunctival injection in two patients (Figure 10.8). Whatever the cause, it was sufficiently alarming for us to recommend that this method of steroid delivery should not be used in the treatment of scleritis unless the circumstances are very exceptional. One of the objects in reviewing the cases which had come to histology with a primary diagnosis of scleritis (Fraunfelder and Watson, 1976) was to determine whether subconjunctival injections predisposed to scleral perforation. Tooker (1931) and Swan and Butler (1950) related the focus of necrogranulomatous scleritis to the 'trauma' of subconjunctival injections of atropine and Sevel and Abramson (1972) also say that in one case in the series it was the opinion of the ophthalmic surgeon that the necrogranulomatous scleritis corresponded to the location of the subconjunctival injection of cortisone.

In our series of 30 patients six did not receive any steroids at all and none perforated. Eleven of the 19 received steroids and did perforate; of these, two out of the five who had subconjunctival steroids perforated at the site of the subconjunctival injection. The data are insufficient to differentiate which form of therapy was more often associated with scleral perforation.

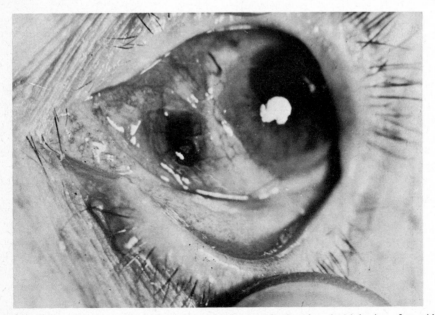

Figure 10.8. Scleral necrosis which occurred at the site of subconjunctival injection of steroid in a patient with necrotising scleritis.

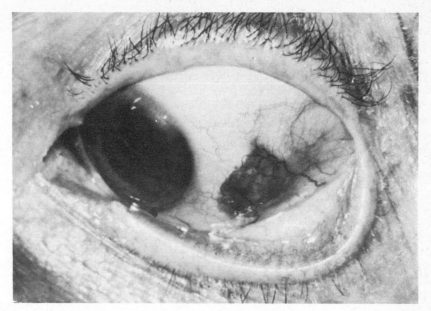

Figure 10.9.   Extreme thinning at the site of a biopsy of a scleral nodule.

Although the evidence is circumstantial, Sevel found the incidence of corneal perforation to be the same in those cases in which the eyes had been enucleated before the general introduction of steroids as afterwards. Whilst the case is unproven, we have avoided giving subconjunctival steroid injections at all, but we have, from time to time, given intraorbital steroid injections to patients unable to take steroids systemically. The effects are transient and the injections have to be repeated frequently, often at weekly intervals to be effective. As most patients will not tolerate this type of regime it is not satisfactory for routine use.

Patients who are unable to tolerate systemic steroids or the anti-inflammatory agents, or who, for any reason, are unable to continue them, can be given penicillamine or rarely gold therapy. It must be remembered that not only do these drugs have side-effects, but also it may be three months before the beneficial effects become apparent, so that some other form of anti-inflammatory or immunosuppressive therapy must be given in addition.

Anticoagulants and inhibitors of fibrinolysin

There is histological evidence of a vasculitis occurring within the vessels which transgress the sclera and in the new vessels near a scleral granuloma. Intra-vascular coagulation can be seen to have occurred in some of those vessels. On the assumption that thrombus formation which led to ischaemia was the cause of necrosis of the scleral tissue, Aronson and Elliott (1974) have advocated the use of local heparin therapy if corticosteroid therapy fails. Heparin is known to block new clot formation and interrupt the fibrinogen–fibrin pathway. They suggest using subconjunctival heparin 450 to 750 units as much as once a week for at least a year or until improvement occurs. They feel that they have had success from this method of treatment, but we have no personal experience of it.

Epsilon-aminocaproic acid also inhibits fibrinolysin and theoretically should help to prevent intravascular clotting. In those few patients in whom we have used this drug there has not been a convincing improvement.

Avascularity of the episcleral tissue precedes the necrosis of the sclera in some patients but Sevel (1966) failed to induce necrosis by total occlusion of the anterior ciliary circulation in rabbits. The role of the perivasculitis and intravascular clotting in necrotising scleral disease is still unclear but may be very significant. Methods of treatment designed to prevent the vascular occlusion may be helpful as an adjunct to other therapy in the resistant patient.

Sodium versenate (EDTA)

On the grounds that collagenase is released when scleral destruction occurs, Jameson Evans and Eustace (1973) used the collagenase inhibitor sodium versenate (EDTA) in a patient who had necrotising scleritis, Crohn's disease and arthritis. The patient had previously had heparin injections without improvement and a scleral graft had been placed over the necrotic patch of sclera.

Postoperatively EDTA 0.5 per cent solution was given four times a day. Following the graft and EDTA the response was dramatic; the conjunctival congestion disappeared and the defects filled in. After three weeks the patient was given systemic steroid and maintained on these thereafter.

This is an isolated report and whilst collagenase is certainly activated and released in necrotising scleral disease, inhibiting the action of this enzyme alone has not in our experience had any effect on preventing the extension of the destructive process. This is not saying that it should not be tried in the patient who is not responding to other therapy. The success in Jameson Evans' patient may be because a large area of necrotic tissue or perhaps a source of antigen had also been removed, in the same way that a corneal gutter in a patient of ours filled in once a large area of necrotic corneoscleral tissue was removed from the opposite side of the cornea.

X-ray therapy

From time to time small doses of x-rays have been used on the assumption that in some way they alter the immune response. Doses of 100 to 300 R cause transient changes in the proteoglycans of connective tissue and given in the region of the trabecular meshwork can induce a fall in intraocular pressure which lasts about one week (Mitchell and Cairns, 1970, personal communication). It may be that temporary alteration of the proteoglycan molecules in the inflamed sclera may prevent further destruction or assist in repair.

Contardo (1952) used, with success, doses of 100 to 300 R on 12 patients with scleritis who had failed to respond to other therapy. Nonnenmacher

(1952) also quoted a patient with scleroperikeratitis and lacrimal gland swelling which resolved with similar doses of x-rays. We have not used this method of therapy and feel unable to do more than report its use.

SURGICAL TREATMENT OF SCLERAL DISEASE

Although the literature contains many reports of surgical therapy in scleral disease, the treatment of scleritis is primarily medical and not surgical, because if the condition is seen early and treated vigorously, scleral necrosis can be largely prevented. Surgery is, however, sometimes necessary either for diagnosis, threatened perforation or strengthening an expanding eyeball, repair of peripheral corneal guttering or descemetocele, conjunctival excision to aid in the healing of corneal gutter and occasionally for patching the sclera, strengthening a staphyloma, removing a cataract or performing a trabeculectomy in order to reduce the intraocular pressure. None of these procedures should be undertaken unless really necessary because, not only is the surgery technically difficult, but also if the surgery is in any way complicated, the eye may rapidly become phthisical.

Scleral biopsy

The advantages and disadvantages of scleral biopsy have been discussed in Chapter 5. Because many scleral nodules contain nothing but the fluid necrotic products of scleral destruction, little is gained by surgical attack on them and, because this material can no longer be used as a framework for repair, a permanent scleral defect or even scleral rupture may result (Figure 10.9).

Nevertheless, to establish a diagnosis in the very puzzling patient it is sometimes necessary to resort to biopsy (Friedman and Henkind, 1974). If this is done, it is very important that a precise surgical technique is used because handling the conjunctiva in the same quadrant as the lesion to be biopsied alters the cellular content of the histological specimen.

Anaesthesia for episcleral lesions. Lesions confined to the episclera can be removed under local anaesthesia. One drop of 1/1000 adrenaline is first instilled into the conjunctival sac. Amethocaine one per cent drops are then used at one-minute intervals for at least five minutes over the site of the lesion. One drop of 1/1000 adrenaline is also instilled before surgery is started and repeated if the conjunctiva becomes congested during the procedure. Adrenaline is used because vascular constriction inhibits cellular migration induced by the surgery.

Anaesthesia for scleral lesions. Not only will local anaesthesia be insufficient to anaesthetise a scleral lesion, but further reparative surgery may become necessary. It is therefore necessary either to give a retrobulbar injection of 2 ml amethocaine two per cent, or to give a general anaesthetic. The only eye drops instilled should be 1/1000 adrenaline.

Operation. The lids are held open with a speculum which is put in place as gently as possible so that no congestion of the conjunctiva is induced and there is no pressure on the globe.

It is *most important* that no instruments or sutures are placed within 90° of the lesion to be biopsied. Fixation can be achieved either by sutures or by forceps at the limbus in two positions on the opposite side of the globe from the lesions. We prefer to use two sutures because the forceps can get in the way of subsequent procedures. If the lesion is at 3.0 o'clock the sutures are inserted through the deep episcleral tissue at the limbus at 11 and 7 o'clock. The eye is thus held firm and can be rotated to obtain the most satisfactory position for the biopsy.

Again, no forceps are used in the region of the tissue to be biopsied before the specimen is removed. To obtain the very best histological material a very sharp blade is used as in Figure 10.10. The conjunctiva is incised remote from the site

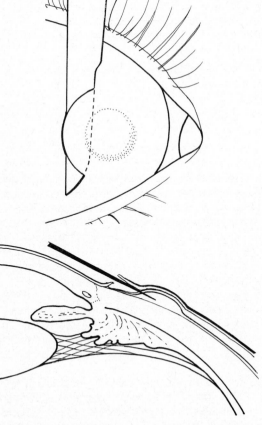

Figure 10.10.   Technique of biopsy of scleral nodule. No sutures or forceps are placed anywhere near the lesion as this alters the cellular content of the specimen. The tissue is removed by a sawing action with the blade of the knife.

of the lesion with a long stroke of shaft of the blade up to and then through the nodule itself. Once an adequate piece of scleral tissue has been removed the blade is then rotated to cut vertically through the remaining conjunctiva. Because of the mobility of the conjunctiva, this may roll on the knife during the final part of the procedure. If this happens then the knife with the attached specimen is held forwards and the base snipped off with scissors. The whole specimen, still attached to the knife blade, is placed in fixative, the nature of which will depend on the type of investigation to be undertaken and the preference of the histologist. The specimen floats off the blade and is not handled further.

This method of biopsy inevitably leaves a large bare area of conjunctiva and episclera. The episclera is important in the healing of scleral wounds and the defect needs to be covered by a flap of conjunctiva and episclera drawn from an adjacent area of the globe. The area selected is undermined with spring scissors over twice the area to be covered. If necessary, the conjunctiva at the limbus can be incised to give adequate mobility to the flap. Hooks are inserted in the edge of the flap which is brought to the opposite edge without tension and the incision closed with vertical mattress sutures of 8.0 virgin silk which if possible are made to engage the normal deep episclera. Antibiotic drops are instilled and an eye pad placed on the eye.

Postoperative care. Local antibiotics are given for three to seven days, supplemented by local steroids after the fourth day if the inflammatory response is intense.

Scleral Patching

Spontaneous scleral rupture is rare; terrible looking scleral defects which look as if they should rupture are relatively common. Staphylomas, i.e. bulging forward of the uveal tissue through a thin or absent sclera, are very unusual unless the intraocular pressure is raised above 35 mm Hg, and will largely regress if the pressure is restored to normal. Although covering an active area of necrotising scleritis with a patch can sometimes dramatically relieve otherwise intractable pain, this should only be carried out as a last resort; nor should it be imagined that simply covering an area of necrosis with a patch will in any way alter the underlying disease process. Although certainly some eyes do settle down after the patch has been applied, the majority of patches become invaded by the granuloma (Sevel and Abramson, 1972) and are eventually eroded from the edges. The indications, therefore, for patching the sclera are very limited, but it is nevertheless the correct procedure in a few patients.

Many materials have been used for scleral patches, e.g. mucous membrane (van der Hoeve, 1934), fascia lata (Armstrong and McGovern, 1955), aorta (Merz, 1964) and auricular cartilage (Nicolas, 1972). Sclera, if available, is excellent for the purpose. It can readily be fashioned from donor eyes and, because it has no active cellular components, it does not necessarily have to be fresh for the graft to be accepted. The graft is only supplying a collagen framework and will continue to give support even if none of the donor cells remains.

The site and extent of the lesion determine the exact surgical approach and, because no two patients are alike, the surgery is very interesting and exacting. There are several broad principles which must be followed if surgery is to be successful and they depend on doing everything possible to keep the globe intact, or if spontaneous rupture has occurred to restore the normal intraocular pressure as soon as possible.

Indications for scleral patching are as follows:

1. Spontaneous or traumatic scleral rupture in a patient with necrotising scleral disease or following chemical injury or burns.
2. Progressive circumferential necrotising scleritis which is unresponsive to all forms of medical therapy. Progressive true thinning of the sclera in a localised affected area of necrotising scleritis is not necessarily an indication for surgery, because once a sequestrum has formed, the inflammation may well subside. A staphyloma will not form nor leakage of intraocular fluid occur through this defect unless it is very large or the intraocular pressure becomes raised.
3. Intractable pain from areas of necrotising scleritis or chemical burns.

Anaesthesia. General anaesthesia should be given if at all possible. Scleral rupture can occur simply from the pressure of the fluid from a retro-ocular injection, which may be relatively ineffective if there is any significant posterior scleritis or orbital inflammation. Inflamed scleral tissue is extremely sensitive and if compressed in the unanaesthetised or poorly anaesthetised eye, will give rise to severe boring pain in eye and head. This effect is noticed even if the conjunctiva has been removed.

Operation. The lids are held open by a speculum, lid clamps or sutures.

Fixation. Because of the danger of perforating the eye by manipulation, no superior rectus or other traction sutures should be inserted unless it is impossible to see the site of grafting without them.

Conjunctival and episcleral reflection. Because it is important to have vascular tissue in apposition with the graft, as large a conjunctival flap as possible must be fashioned. This can be the most difficult part of the procedure because of the extreme attenuation of this structure in these patients. Dissection is best achieved with the use of the operating microscope at $\times$ 10 magnification. If the necrotising process involves or is adjacent to the limbus, the dissection is started here, the tissue being removed by a razor fragment from its underlying attachment. Only large bleeding points are stopped at this stage. The conjunctival dissection is carried over the affected area and then as far as practicable over normal sclera using Westcott's spring scissors and non-toothed forceps or cellulose swabs for fixation. The dissection is also carried out for at least 20° on either side of the affected tissue. If the necrotic area is away from the limbus then either two flaps, one limbus-based and one fornix-based, or a large limbus based flap which starts 12 mm back from the limbus are made to include the conjunctiva over the necrotic area.

Size 5/0 or 6/0 sutures are placed in the edge of the conjunctival flap which is retracted away if it overlaps the area to be grafted.

Selection of the area for grafting. The graft should cover the necrotic tissue and an area of at least 3 mm on all sides of it. This adjacent scleral tissue is not necessarily normal but is of such consistency as will hold any suture placed in it.

The perimeter of the selected area is marked with dots of methylene or Bonney's blue or gentian violet. A piece of oiled silk is placed over the area and the dots will be seen on its underside. A template is then fashioned in the oiled silk of the exact size and shape required.

Preparation of the donor tissue. A whole eye, or preserved scleral tissue can be used as the donor. The whole eye should be placed in a suitable holding device such as a Tudor Thomas stand and the conjunctiva removed. The template is then placed over a similar area to that which is to be grafted and the area to be removed marked with dye. This ensures that the curvature of the donor is similar to that of the host. A full thickness scleral graft is now fashioned by incising through the sclera around the marked area. The posterior margin of the graft is lifted first and the dissection is carried forward, teasing off the underlying choroid and ciliary body with a spatula. The anterior margin is removed last. The excised piece is left in place on the donor eye under wet gauze until required.

Preparation of the host. The approach at this stage depends on the individual circumstances. If the edges of the host tissue are firm and normal it is reasonable to prepare a lamellar bed especially adjacent to the limbus, or to shelve the posterior edge towards the wound (Figure 10.11), but as is usually the case, the tissue is soft and difficult to work so it is better to make no effort to shape the graft posteriorly but only to make sharp edges for suturing close to the limbus and at the lateral extensions. Whatever is done, as little normal host tissue as possible is excised.

We have always been very loath to remove the necrotic tissue from the deep layers of the damaged sclera as this has been known to lead to perforation, and have confined debridement to those pieces of tissue obviously dead.

Placing the graft. Once a satisfactory bed has been made then the graft is taken from the donor and made to lie snugly in it. This may require the thinning of the underside posteriorly to form a wedge (Figure 10.11). This is particularly important if the eye is perforated or if it is soft.

10/0 Perlon or Ethilon or 8/0 virgin silk sutures are placed first in the edge close to the limbus, the number used being determined by how satisfactory the fit of the graft. These sutures must be deep and have a long bite into host tissue otherwise they will tend to cut out. Two or three sutures are placed in the outer edges of the graft, but it is usually unnecessary to suture the posterior edge because this will be held in place by the conjunctiva. Perlon or Ethilon sutures are preferred as they do not react in the tissues and are less likely to cause erosion or to cut out.

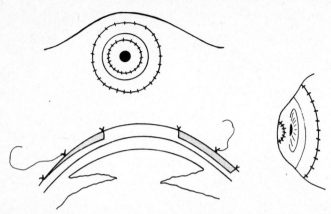

Figure 10.11. Technique of scleral patching. In this instance a 360° corneoscleral lamellar patch has been applied but the same technique is used for any patch. Depending on whether the tissue is thin or normal a lamellar bed is fashioned (right side of cross-section diagram) or the donor tissue is shaped to a wedge shape. It is not always necessary to suture the posterior edge of the donor as this is covered by conjunctiva sutured at the new limbus.

The conjunctival flap is now replaced and sutured at the limbus or, if two flaps have been used, on the limbal side of the graft, with 8/0 virgin silk. Antibiotic drops are placed on the conjunctival sac and an eye pad placed on the eye.

Postoperative care. The eye is left undisturbed for at least 48 hours. Antibiotic drops are used postoperatively twice daily after the first 24 hours. Any systemic therapy which had been given preoperatively is continued. Local steroids, atropine or other cycloplegics are given if there is any evidence of uveitis. Conjunctival suture removal is usually unnecessary and only undertaken if the sutures cause irritation. The deep sutures are left undisturbed unless they cut out or erode through the overlying conjunctiva. Over the succeeding months, vessels derived from the conjunctiva pass into and occasionally through the scleral graft which eventually takes on an almost normal appearance (Figure 10.12).

Conjunctival Excision

After taking pieces of limbal conjunctiva to study the proteolytic enzymes of patients with limbal ulceration, Stuart Brown (1975) discovered that some of the ulcers healed without requiring any other medication. He describes some ulcers which appear to be the same as those we have seen in patients with scleritis and connective tissue disease. Certainly one of his patients had rheumatoid arthritis and the ulceration in another followed herpes zoster. It is possible that excision of the conjunctiva could remove the site of immune complex deposition which might, adjacent to the ulcer, have either caused or at least have been responsible for the perpetuation of the ulceration. We have now performed conjunctival excision in three patients with limbal ulceration, two with periarteritis nodosa

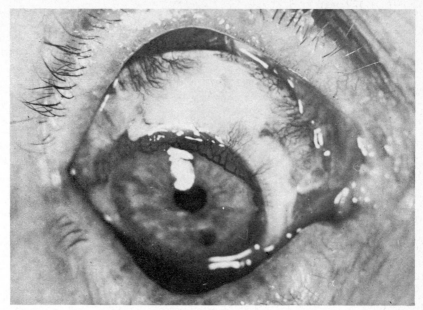

Figure 10.12.   The appearance of a scleral patch graft three months after the operation. The vessels derived from conjunctiva are invading the graft.

and one from an unknown cause. So far we have not produced any improvement by performing this procedure. It is, however, relatively atraumatic, it gives valuable histological evidence of the cell types present, and it is a useful procedure before proceeding to corneoscleral grafting.

Operation. Local amethocaine one per cent drops are instilled into the conjunctival sac at one-minute intervals for five minutes or until the conjunctiva is fully anaesthetised. Just before the operation is started, one drop of adrenaline 1/1000 is instilled.

Using the operating microscope the conjunctiva and underlying episclera, which is usually swollen, are dissected for a distance of 3 to 4 mm from the limbus in the region of the ulcer and 2 or 3 mm above or below the ulcer.

A razor fragment is used and the limbal conjunctival insertion gently raised from the underlying corneoscleral margin and dissected back away from the limbus until it is entirely free. The affected conjunctiva is excised with scissors and sent for histological section. The area is not covered by a flap but is allowed to epithelialise over the next few days.

Antibiotic drops are instilled and an eye pad placed over the eye. The antibiotics are used for about two weeks in addition to any other therapy which may be felt necessary.

Corneoscleral and Corneal Grafting

Spontaneous corneal and limbal perforations, although unusual, are more common than spontaneous scleral perforations and corneal grafting is more often undertaken. In all instances, these grafts are of the overlay type and although perforations may occur during the course of the surgical procedure, every attempt should be made to insert only lamellar material.

Indications for corneoscleral and corneal grafting are similar to those for scleral patching:

1. Spontaneous or traumatic corneal rupture.
2. Impending rupture following the rapid development of a descemetocele.
3. Rapidly progressing circumferential guttering which is unresponsive to medical therapy.
4. Intractable pain.
5. For restoration of vision following sclerosing keratitis in active disease with central corneal distortion, and after overlay transplantation.

Limbal guttering in association with connective tissue disease is usually amenable to medical therapy and surgery should never be attempted until medicines have been found to fail. The differential diagnosis of the various types of limbal gutters is still poorly worked out, and there are certain types, e.g. Mooren's ulcer and the peripheral gutters associated with some types of systemic allergic vasculitis, in which the gutter will recur at the limbus of the donor tissue. The patient may then be even worse off than before the operation.

Limbal Corneoscleral Grafting

This seems to be a much more satisfactory procedure than simple conjunctival excision although it is probably best reserved for those patients in whom conjunctival excision and medical treatment have failed. It may be necessary to continue systemic therapy throughout the postoperative period and for years thereafter. With modern suturing techniques we have had no difficulty with healing even with prolonged and high dosage steroid therapy.

Operation. General anaesthesia and surgery under microscopic control are obligatory to obtain the best results. Intravenous mannitol 1.5 g/kg body weight is given at the start of the anaesthesia to soften the eye for surgery.

Preliminary preparation of the host. Again, as with scleral grafting, the chance of rupturing the globe by even slight distortion means no traction sutures are inserted. If a conjunctival excision has not already been performed, the conjunctiva is removed from the limbus with a razor-blade knife and dissected about 3 mm beyond the area to be grafted and then undermined to prepare a conjunctival flap. Any heaped-up conjunctiva is removed at this stage. Traction sutures of 5/0 silk are placed in the edge to retract it from the operative field. The area to be grafted is determined by the need to suture into firm cornea and sclera and must therefore include at least 2 mm of firm relatively normal tissue. Once the area is decided it is then marked with methylene or Bonney's blue dye (Figure 10.13). A corneal trephine, usually 9 or 10 mm is selected of the appropriate diameter to enter normal thickness corneal tissue adjacent to the ulcer (Figure 10.14). A mark is made with this trephine on the cornea and the distance measured from this mark to the blue marks at the posterior edge of the graft.

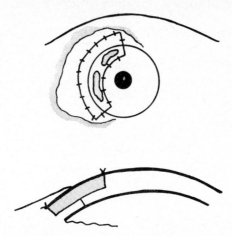

Figure 10.13.   Limbal corneoscleral graft. The conjunctiva is dissected 3 mm from the edge of the proposed graft, the area of which is marked with a sharp pen or knife dipped in methylene blue. This enables the size of the graft to be measured so that an exactly similar patch can be cut from the donor eye.

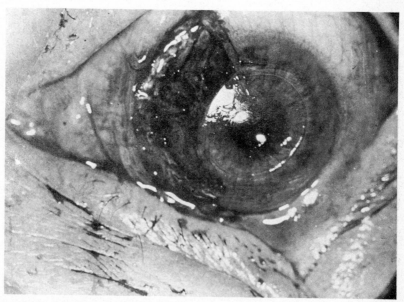

Figure 10.14.   Limbal corneoscleral graft. Here a trephine has been used to cut the inner corneal margin. The distance to the scleral edge is then measured with calipers. The very soft cornea can be seen in the region of the ulcers marked on Figure 10.13. A gutter, which can just be seen at 3 o'clock, healed spontaneously within a week of operation even though it was not touched.

Preparation of the donor. The donor eye is placed in a Tudor Thomas or similar stand. The conjunctiva is removed. The same corneoscleral trephine used to mark the host is now used on the donor, trephining at least two-thirds thickness of the cornea. As the width of the graft is known the posterior extent and the lateral margins of the graft are measured and marked with blue dots. A freehand incision is then made through two-thirds thickness of the sclera over the line of the dots.

A Paufique starter knife is used to start a lamella Y dissection of the cornea at two-thirds depth or deeper if the ulcer on the host is very deep or a descemetocele has formed. A lamellar dissection of the cornea is then undertaken with a hockey-stick lamellar dissecting knife and this dissection is continued at the same depth into the sclera to its posterior edge.

Rather than a corneoscleral donor graft, an entirely corneal graft can be fashioned if the cornea to be covered is small enough. These grafts have the advantage that they are much easier to cut. The technique of measuring is the same but the posterior margin of the graft is placed at the limbus and the position of the trephine cut measured from the limbus. When in place the white sclera shows through the cornea and the cosmetic appearance is excellent (Figures 10.15 and 10.16).

Once a satisfactory graft has been prepared it is left in the donor eye until required.

Preparation of the host. If at all practicable a bed is cut for the graft with a sharp edge for ease of suturing. This manoeuvre is always difficult when

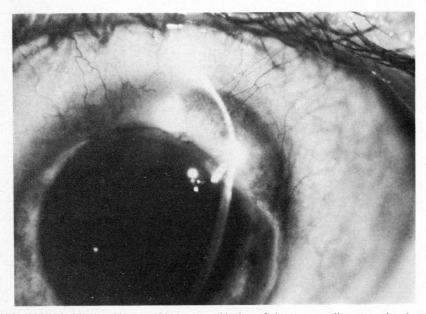

Figure 10.15. 32-year-old man with extreme thinning of the cornea adjacent to the site of intense scleritis which had been present for 16 years before the globe started to expand.

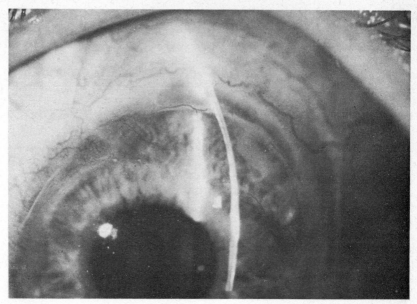

Figure 10.16.   The same patient as Figure 10.15. 12 months after a lamellar graft of corneal tissue had been placed over the thin area and 5 mm into adjacent sclera. The normal thickness of the cornea has been restored and the astigmatic error halved. The underlying sclera can be seen through clear cornea. The cosmetic appearance is so good that it is difficult to see the edges and extent of the graft.

the cornea is involved in the necrotising process as it is always extremely soft and of mushy consistency.

The mark of the trephine is deepened, either with the trephine itself or with a razor blade knife to the same level as the depths of the ulcer. If the ulcer is very deep then no more than two-thirds depth of cornea should be removed. A very careful lamellar dissection is then made through the cornea to the limbus. In soft tissue such as this the hockey stick knife works badly and it may be necessary to use the razor knife to cut the strands. Dissection is assisted considerably by working in a completely dry field. The slit beam on the microscope can be invaluable in detecting and avoiding areas of extremely thin cornea. Dissection of the sclera is continued from the limbus and does not need to be very deep as long as there is a good sharp posterior scleral margin.

If a perforation occurs at any stage during the dissection it is ignored provided no iris prolapses through the perforation. If iris comes through the rupture rather than just plugging it a small iridotomy will allow it to fall back into the anterior chamber. Iris plugging a rupture is helpful because it prevents the eye becoming soft and will usually fall away spontaneously later.

Perforation makes further dissection difficult because the eye is soft; also the deep cornea in necrotising scleral disease tends to split and the rupture can become very large. It is therefore most important to prevent this complication if at all possible. Theoretically it would be helpful to have a preplaced paracentesis puncture in order to put air in the anterior chamber if rupture occurred; unfortunately, it more often is the case that attempting to do a paracentesis ruptures the ulcer.

Once a satisfactory base has been fashioned, the donor tissue is placed in the base and sutured to it by deep 10/0 Perlon sutures which are tied with four throws and cut on the knot. The knot is then rotated in the suture track to lie deep and buried in the cornea. It is important to take a good bite of normal corneal tissue otherwise the sutures will tend to cut out. It is, however, important that these sutures do not cut the optic axis and so interfere with vision. The conjunctival flap is then brought to the limbus and sutured to it with 8/0 virgin silk sutures.

This type of overlay graft can be enlarged to cover the whole of the eye anterior to the insertion of the recti muscles. If this is undertaken (Figure 10.11) then there is the chance of anterior segment necrosis because the anterior ciliary arteries are compromised. This is rarely severe and can be treated with Rheomacrodex and steroids.

Penetrating Corneal Grafts

Simple penetrating corneal grafting is sometimes necessary for the replacement of cornea which has opacified as a result of sclerokeratitis, or has become irregularly distorted from corneoscleral disease, or has been covered by an overlay transplant at an earlier date.

The techniques involved are the same as for any other penetrating corneal graft for the restoration of vision, but because of the nature of the inflammation which has given rise to the corneal disease, there are a few special considerations. Very fresh material is essential because the endothelium is often very unhealthy in patients suffering from scleral disease. Because of the iritis which may have accompanied the original attack, the iris has a great tendency to become adherent to the cornea, thus the smallest graft compatible with a good visual result should be used, i.e. not more than 7 mm.

The host cornea is often irregularly thin, sometimes vascularised, but always softer than normal. Because of this, we think it essential to use interrupted 10/0 Perlon or Ethilon sutures rather than, or as well as, a continuous suture. Each suture must be at least 1 mm into donor tissue and taken right to the limbus or even into the sclera of the host. The knots should either be buried or tied over the sclera.

Postoperatively local steroids will usually suppress any recrudescence of inflammation caused by the surgery as well as the rejection phenomena inevitable in a heavily vascularised cornea.

Overlay Full Thickness Corneal Grafting

If there is a central descemetocele it is often better to cover the whole of the cornea up to the limbus or just inside it with a large full thickness corneal overlay and then perform a penetrating corneal graft when the scleritis is under control. The chance of perforating the globe by even the most minor trauma under these circumstances is so high that it is essential to have two eyes available before the operation starts, because it may be necessary to alter the type of operation half way through and convert an overlay procedure to a formal full thickness graft of a different size. Full thickness grafts done during the active stage of the disease have, in our experience, all become opaque, but if the host endothelium can be retained, remarkably good visual results can eventually be obtained. Full thickness material is used as it is much easier to work with and better optically than very deep lamellar material.

Operation. General anaesthesia and intravenous Mannitol (1 g/kg body weight) are given, and the operation performed with the aid of the operating microscope. No fixation sutures are used.

Central descemetoceles. If only the central cornea is involved then the graft should extend 2 mm from the limbus. This area is marked with a trephine, the depth of the cut being determined by the assessment of the strength of the cornea to be dissected away. Very carefully and gradually a peripheral bed is made in corneal tissue as deep as is safe and this dissection contained in this plane to within 2 mm of the descemetocele or the adjacent very thin stroma. It is sometimes prudent not to do a lamellar dissection but simply to remove the epithelium with alcohol and place the patch directly on the corneal surface. In any case no attempt is made to make the deep lamellae optically clear; too much attention to this sort of detail can easily lead to perforation of an area of adjacent thin cornea.

A full thickness corneal disc is cut from a donor eye of the same size as the host and the button sutured with about 20 interrupted 10/0 sutures to the host, each suture being taken up to the limbus or beyond and the knot tied over sclera. The manipulation of the eye when suturing may cause the cornea to rupture but provided the descemetocele is covered and the periphery watertight this will not matter. If the rupture extends beyond the line of the graft margin then a new graft will have to be fashioned.

Peripheral and central descemetoceles. If it is going to be impossible to suture the graft at the limbus, then a graft needs to be prepared which has a full thickness cornea and a partial thickness sclera.

The same preparation for operation is given as for other full thickness overlay grafts. No fixation sutures are used.

The conjunctiva together with all the underlying episclera through 360° is dissected from the limbus and is split by radial incisions at 12, 9, 6 and 3 o'clock into four flaps which are retracted. A superficial lamellar scleral dissection may be necessary to keep the deep episcleral tissue with these flaps. The epithelium is removed from the cornea where possible with cellulose swabs, but no attempt is made to do a lamellar dissection unless it is to remove dead tissue. The sclera already cleared of all episcleral tissue is cut to produce a small sharp edge for suturing about 3 or 4 mm from the limbus.

A donor eye is held in a clamp. The conjunctiva is removed and an incision throughout 360° made halfway through the sclera the same distance from the limbus as has been marked in the host. A wedge shaped incision aimed to penetrate the sclera at this limbus is made forwards from this cut with the razor knife and corneal scissors.

The resulting graft of a lamellar scleral graft and full thickness cornea is placed over the whole of the anterior segment and sutured to normal sclera with either Perlon 10/0 or silk 8/0. The conjunctiva and episclera are replaced at the new limbus.

The results of these grafts are most unpredictable. One we have done has been extremely successful. The severe pain from which the patient had been suffering disappeared from the time of the graft. The inflammation gradually regressed and he saw reasonably well (6/60) through his central double cornea, there being a water cleft between new cornea which was of normal thickness and old thin cornea. Another did reasonably well. Her own cornea ruptured centrally spontaneously six weeks after surgery and although the donor cornea is thickened and scarred she can count fingers and has a pain-free eye. Central penetrating corneal grafting is planned later. The other two have done less well. Shortly after surgery both corneas became very swollen. One eye became very soft, presumably because it perforated and he refused further surgery. The other has had an anterior segment replacement.

Anterior Segment Replacement

Total anterior segment replacement was attempted in one patient who ruptured his globe spontaneously in two places after full thickness corneoscleral replacement. He had an almost opaque cornea with limbal guttering and circumferential anterior necrotising disease, the sclera at and beyond the equator being apparently normal. Technically the operation was successful and he retains a normal size comfortable eye with normal intraocular pressure. As is universal experience with anterior segment grafts, the cornea rejected after six months and is now oedematous with slight limbal guttering. The sclera is still congested behind the tissue of the graft but the junction sutures are still holding. He still requires oxyphenbutazone to control the scleritis. If the rejection problem can be overcome, anterior segment replacement might be a good procedure for the very severe case where nothing else is practical, but is used at present as a last resort.

The operation aims to remove all the necrotic tissue anterior to the insertion of the rectus muscles, the iris up to its roots and the lens, but preferably leaving the vitreous intact and to replace this with cornea and sclera.

Operation. The operation requires full anaesthesia and intravenous mannitol (1 to 1.5 g/kg body weight) in an attempt to shrink the vitreous.

Preliminary preparation of the host. Two scleral Fleiringer rings are sutured to the globe behind and at the level of the insertion of the rectus muscles. The conjunctiva and underlying episcleral tissue is reflected from the limbus up to the level of the rings by incising it at 12, 3, 6 and 9 o'clock. The level of penetration of the sclera must not be behind the insertion of the iris and the site of this can be accurately determined by transilluminating the eye from the front. This level is marked on the sclera and any sclera which has to be dissected behind this removed by lamellar dissection. If this is done then a template of oiled silk must be made for the donor eye (page 416) otherwise the size of the donor can be determined by measurement.

Preparation of the donor. A donor eye is fixed in a Tudor Thomas clamp and the conjunctiva removed. The size and shape of the graft is marked out on the sclera with dye and the sclera is then incised through its full thickness with a razor knife through 360°. The underlying ciliary body and iris is removed by dissection with an iris spatula and the whole anterior segment lifted forwards. This is surprisingly easy to do. 8/0 virgin silk sutures are now placed in the edge at 12, 3, 6 and 9 o'clock. The graft is left on the eye till required.

Preparation of the host and grafting. The scleral incision is commenced between the muscles and extended around the globe. Bleeding points are coagulated by electrocautery or diathermy as they are encountered. This process is continued until the whole circumference has been cut. The underlying scleral spur is dissected free over the upper half until a 180° flap is formed. α-Chymotrypsin is now injected beneath the iris. If the iris bulges into the wound at this stage, a small iridotomy is performed and it immediately settles back. The lens is removed with the cryo probe. The scleral spur dissection is carried through the remaining 180° and the corneoscleral tissue removed. The iris is incised with Vannas scissors leaving only a small frill at the edges. Bleeding occurs at this stage from iris vessels but usually stops spontaneously. The donor graft is placed over the defect when all bleeding points have been stopped and is sutured in place with multiple interrupted 8/0 virgin silk sutures after tying and placing those already preplaced in the graft. The conjunctiva is then sutured at the new limbus.

In our case and those we have heard about, the vitreous has remained intact. Should it break a generous anterior vitrectomy should be undertaken. This will probably not affect the final result.

Postoperative care. We know of no anterior segment graft which has survived over 18 months without becoming opaque. This is because of the homograft reaction, suppression of which is a major problem still unsolved. Glaucoma does not occur even though the whole trabecular meshwork has been removed. Local steroids are normally given together with local antibiotics in the immediate postoperative period and a combination of azathioprine and steroids given from the fourth postoperative day onwards in an attempt to suppress the homograft reaction. The patient is kept at rest in bed for seven days because any bleeding which occurs during this time tends to be from choroidal vessels and leads to expulsive haemorrhage.

Imbrication of the Sclera

This operation is for staphylomas which have expanded the anterior segment of the globe to such an extent that the eye is distorted. Such staphylomas may be so large that the lids cannot close over them. The procedure is only possible if there is normal cornea and sclera adjacent to the defect, the intraocular pressure is uncontrollably high and the eye can see.

Two techniques are commonly used. Both depend on the use of sutures to close the defect. In patients with ciliary staphylomas Stallard (1965) used a technique in which he excised the sclera intervening between the arms of the sutures. Murube del Castillo (1966) folds the sclera inwards to treat equatorial and intercalary staphylomas.

Stallard's operation for ciliary staphylomas. A conjunctival hood is fashioned at the limbus over the area of the staphyloma and on either side of it so that it can be drawn over the operation site at the end of the procedure. 6/0 silk sutures are passed transversely through normally thick sclera and cornea adjacent to staphyloma (Figure 10.17). One suture is used for every 4 mm of staphyloma. A stay knot is placed in the end of each suture at its corneal end and then this is drawn up to the cornea. The loops of the mattress sutures are laid away from the staphyloma. The centre of the staphyloma is then lifted up with blocked iris forceps and a 5 mm incision made on either side of the base of the staphyloma through its entire thickness. This is excised together with the adherent iris from one end, the sutures being closed as the operation progresses. The remaining iris is reposited from the wound which can be closed with further sutures if necessary. The conjunctival hood is brought down over the wound.

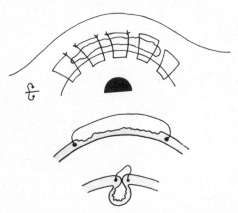

Figure 10.17. Scleral imbrication or excision for the treatment of staphylomas. The sutures are laid in the same place for both procedures. 6.0 silk is used and one suture placed for each 4 mm of staphyloma. In ciliary staphylomas the tissue between the sutures is excised. In inter-calary and equatorial staphylomas the sclera is indented after aspiration of vitreous.

Equatorial staphylomas. Because these are of extreme thinness and are often attached to ciliary body and choroid, excision of scleral tissue is unwise. The eye is prepared and a similar set of sutures is placed on either side of the defect as in Stallard's procedure. Space to close the sutures is provided by aspiration of vitreous which is performed through a separate incision (Figure

10.17). As vitreous is removed, with either a large bore aspiration needle or a vitreous suction cutter, the sutures are drawn up and the sclera indented with a large flat spatula (Figure 10.17). There should be no tension on the sutures at the end of the operation.

Cataract Extraction

It is extraordinary but nevertheless a fact that surgically produced limbal wounds heal normally in spite of active scleritis in the region provided the actual piece of sclera cut is not already replaced by granuloma. As a result of this, cataract extraction is perfectly feasible even in patients with severe necrotising scleritis. It is advisable to choose an area of sclera away from the site of active scleral destruction and this may mean removing the cataract from below or from the side. The operation is otherwise not modified but because of the tenuous nature of the sclera and the tendency to form granulomata we prefer to use multiple 10/0 Perlon sutures to close the wound. This is particularly important if the corneoscleral wound is not covered by the upper lid. Whether α-chymotrypsin is used is a matter for consideration.

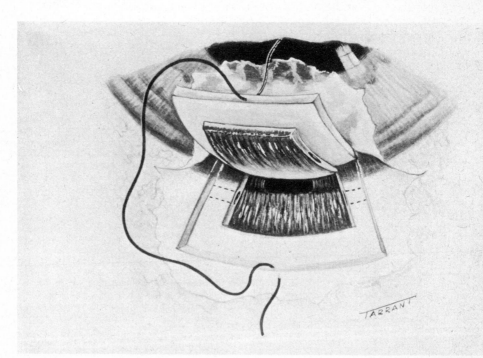

Figure 10.18. Trabeculectomy. A superficial flap of between 4 and 5 mm² sclera about two-thirds thickness is lifted forwards to the limbus. A suture is placed in this flap which is held forwards over the cornea by an assistant. A deep flap is then fashioned incising just behind the scleral spur and cutting forwards to the limbus to include the trabecular meshwork. This flap is excised, an iridectomy performed and the superficial flap replaced and sutured with three 8/0 virgin silk sutures.

It has been shown that α-chymotrypsin can produce anaphylactic reactions (Watson, 1963) and we have seen scleritis start at the site of the corneoscleral wound used for cataract extractions. The enzyme had been used in all these patients. Theoretically it would seem α-chymotrypsin should be avoided, but it makes the extraction so much easier and prevents further complications that we prefer to take the slight risk involved.

Glaucoma Surgery

Glaucoma, as a complication of scleritis, is usually treatable medically by treating the scleritis with or without the aid of specific glaucoma medication. Every now and again, however, surgical relief of the glaucoma becomes necessary.

Where the glaucoma is of the chronic open angle type and the sclera of normal thickness, any of the standard glaucoma procedures can be used. Many of the patients, however, have very thin sclera and uveal tissue prolapses into and through the wound if the sclera is penetrated in one plane, as in the trephine or Scheie operation. Since the introduction of trabeculectomy (Cairns, 1968) this problem has been very much reduced. In this operation a superficial flap of sclera is raised. A piece of tissue which contains the trabecular meshwork and in some the scleral spur is excised and the superficial flap replaced and sutured (Figures 10.18 and 10.19). If the sclera is truly

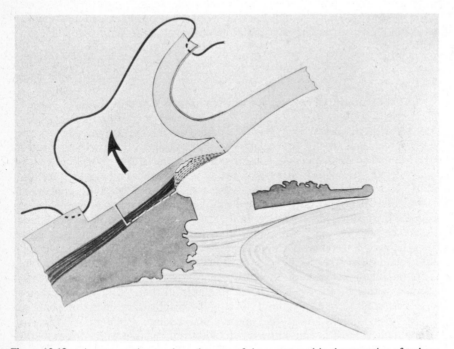

Figure 10.19. A cross-section to show the area of tissue removed in the operation of trabeculectomy.

thin and not just transparent, the superficial flap may be very thin indeed but replacing it in its original position under its conjunctival cover prevents uveal protrusion and allows subconjunctival drainage of fluid and a reduction of intraocular pressure. Provided a relatively normal area of sclera is chosen the wounds heal normally and the operation can be repeated at different sites in the same eye. In certain patients in whom the glaucoma is due to circumferential scleral oedema, the operation is modified by not suturing the posterior flap (Figure 10.20). Angle closure glaucoma can be precipitated by oedema of the anterior segment in patients at risk of developing closed angle glaucoma and by forward movement of the lens iris diaphragm by a posterior scleritis (Figure 10.21). Medical treatment with steroids together with pilocarpine drops, Diamox (acetazolamide) and osmotic agents will usually reduce the intraocular pressure and allow the angle to open again. Occasionally however a peripheral iridectomy is necessary to relieve persistent angle closure. The operation has been entirely uncomplicated when the incision has been made through an area of active scleritis and in very inflamed eyes. Mannitol has been given preoperatively in all our cases and the pupil constricted with miotics prior to surgery.

Patients with secondary angle closure glaucoma due to dense peripheral anterior synechiae (a rare occurrence), and in whom trabeculectomy has failed, should be treated by Krasnov's (1971) iridocyclo retraction operation. In this procedure two tongues of sclera 3 mm apart, 8 mm long and 3 mm wide are cut from the superficial sclera and folded into the anterior chamber through an incision just anterior to or just behind the scleral spur (Figure 10.22) with a view to holding the angle open between the two tongues. In most patients in whom the operation is successful, drainage of aqueous also occurs from the base.

Treatment of Scleritis for which a Specific Cause is Known

The treatment of the specific bacterial infections of the sclera, whether they be granulomatous or non-granulomatous and pyogenic, differ in no way from the treatment of these infections elsewhere. Once the organism has been identified, systemic treatment is given with the appropriate bacteriostatic or bacteriocidal preparation. This may need to be supplemented by local applications of antibiotics or even by subconjunctival injections, adding steroids or atropine if there is intraocular inflammation. In the few patients in whom the inflammation of the sclera is an allergic response to original infection, then it is necessary to treat these patients with anti-inflammatory drugs in addition to the specific anti-bacterial therapy. Treatment of the underlying systemic manifestations is not modified because of the presence of scleral disease. Treatment with systemic penicillin for syphilis is an example of this. Although there may be a dramatic response without local eye treatment, it may be necessary to give local steroid drops to suppress the ocular inflammatory response. Also, although scleritis caused by tuberculosis will respond to the usual therapy with streptomycin and para-aminosalicylic acid (PAS, isonicotinic acid hydrazide (INAH), antituberculous drugs and local steroids may need to be

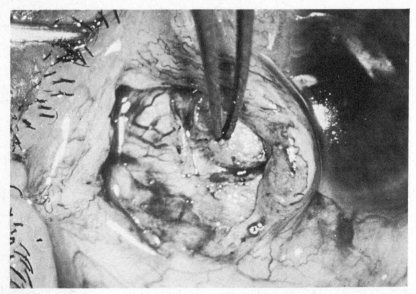

Figure 10.20. Trabeculectomy in scleritis. The superficial flap is just being dissected. The sclera is greatly thickened in the affected area but the trabeculectomy functioned satisfactorily. No sutures were placed in the superficial flap in this patient.

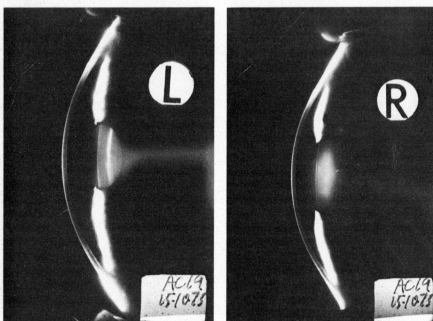

Figure 10.21, A and B. A slit-lamp photograph of the normal anterior chamber depth of the left eye contrasted with the very shallow anterior chamber of the right eye in a patient who presented with an acute angle closure attack in the right eye. The angle closure was found to be due to a anterior shift in the lens iris diaphragm caused by a posterior scleritis.

Courtesy of Nicholas Brown, London.

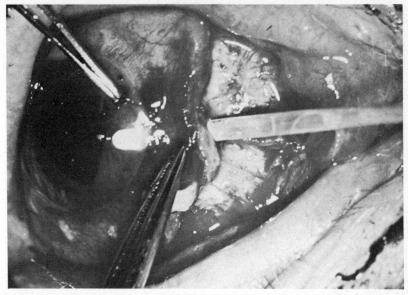

Figure 10.22. Iridocyclo retraction (Krasnov) for secondary closed angle glaucoma. Two separate pillars 8 mm long by 2 mm wide and 2 mm from each other are fashioned from the superficial sclera. One of the pillars can be seen below the lower forceps. The pillars are inserted into the anterior chamber with Pierce Hoskin curved forceps through the incision just in front of the scleral spur; this incision is made just wider than the flaps. The pillars must be visible through clear cornea. The upper one can be seen lying on the iris repositor. Although drainage may occur subconjunctivally, holding the angle open between the two pillars relieves the angle closure in about half the patients.

given as well. Improvement in tuberculous scleritis starts after two to four weeks and the patient recovers in two months but may regress if the systemic therapy is stopped too soon (Chrzanowska Srzednicka, 1954; Kesavacher, 1954). In this case the drugs may need to be changed using Rifampicin systemically and subconjunctival streptomycin which is well tolerated by this route.

Connective tissue disease

Rheumatoid arthritis

> *'Nothing hinders a cure so much as frequent change of medicine; no wound will heal when one salve is tried after another,' Moral Epistles to Lucilius* (Seneca, ?4 BC−65 AD).

Numerically, socially and economically rheumatoid arthritis is by far the most important of the connective tissue diseases; the cause of these diseases remains unknown and treatment is thus symptomatic. Scleral disease appears to be more common in rheumatoid arthritis than in the other connective tissue diseases but this only reflects the relative frequency of the various types.

Rheumatoid arthritis is often badly treated; patients are either kept on anti-inflammatory drugs for long periods in the face of obvious deterioration, or corticosteroids are given early with considerable immediate effect but at a great cost later on. It is essential to set guidelines, but these should be constantly reviewed. The general principle governing one's use of available drugs is to use the least number of drugs in the lowest effective dosage, in order to suppress the inflammatory response. The drug regime must be tailored to the needs of the individual patient because the indications for a particular drug will vary throughout the course of the disease, which can be both variable and unpredictable for the individual patient.

Rheumatoid arthritis is not a disease the patient can suffer alone; a comprehensive programme of management is required, but also considerable understanding by patients of their own part in it. Sufferers from any chronic disease must know something of their disability, how to control it, and how to live with and adapt to it.

Eye disease is uncommon in rheumatoid arthritis, its incidence varying between 0.15 and 0.83 per cent, and there is a very much stronger association between scleritis and rheumatoid arthritis in those patients who had severe erosive seropositive arthritis, extensive vasculitis and a high mortality. If therefore a patient with rheumatoid arthritis develops eye disease this should be taken seriously and the treatment regimes reassessed to take account of this extra-articular manifestation of the disease, and also to be sure that the disease has not changed in character to a more severe form.

The majority of the inflammatory joint diseases, painful and disabling as they may be, are relatively non-lethal and are compatible with a well-maintained functional level for many years. For instance, Duthie et al (1964) studied over 300 patients with rheumatoid arthritis for over nine years. Sixty-two patients on admission were confined to bed or a chair; after treatment only one patient remained in this category. After nine years 60 per cent were socially and economically independent, and only 15 per cent were confined to bed or chair. These patients received conventional treatment which included rest, splinting, aspirin and physiotherapy. Claims for other types of therapy must be measured against such results and side-effects of drugs must be taken into consideration.

It is a disease characterised by spontaneous remissions and relapses and may be lifelong, and this is important when one considers the use of potentially harmful drugs in management; nevertheless, they must not be withheld if a potentially destructive disease, like necrotising scleritis, supervenes. The progressive destructive inflammatory process in rheumatoid arthritis causes not only crippling, but systemic illness and changes outside the joints that may prove fatal. In its early stages before crippling has occurred, it can be a reversible disease.

It is important too to remember that drug treatment plays but a part in the total management of these arthritic patients (Table 10.2).

It should be stressed that management must also include advice about rest and exercises, splintage, the provision of various appliances designed to reduce dependence upon others, and advice about employment. There is an understandable tendency to keep increasing drug therapy to alleviate the patient's symptoms. This is both dangerous and often unnecessary. Increasingly, surgical

Table 10.2.   *Management of rheumatoid arthritis*

Medication: anti-inflammatory, simple
analgesics, correction of
anaemia, antidepressants

Rest: local, general, mental
Graduated exercise
Explanation and reassurance
Other physical treatment

techniques are playing an important part in the management of patients with arthritis at all stages of the disease. The objectives of treatment are to reduce inflammation and pain, maintain function and prevent deformity. No therapeutic agent or programme is 'curative' and therefore 'suppression' of disease activity is the goal. Rest is a valuable form of treatment and about 50 per cent of patients with severe active arthritis benefit from admission to hospital. There is a reduction both in local inflammation, in systemic disease and general well-being.

Therapeutic objectives. We cannot effectively suppress the inflammatory disease; we can produce symptomatic ease, better function, less stiffness and considerable pain relief but we cannot cure the disease. Hence adequate patient education from the outset, stressing the importance of controlling the disease will often help immensely in moderating the patient's expectations.

The aims of treatment are to reduce inflammation, maintain function and prevent deformities. The need to tailor the dose of any drug to suit each patient cannot be over-emphasised. In this regard aspirin has the advantage over the other drugs in that plasma salicylate levels can be readily measured. Because sometimes only partial suppression of the disease is possible, the development of joint deformity may occur, and early local treatment is required. It should be remembered that adequate suppression of the chronic inflammation will allow the secondary manifestations such as anaemia to revert to normal.

Certain clinical features indicate a worse prognosis and require more aggressive therapy. These include an insidious onset, sustained disease activity (more than one year), high titres of rheumatoid factor, and extra-articular features. The early appearance of bone erosions in radiographs is clear evidence of swiftly progressive disease.

Aspirin, gold and chloroquine have no part to play in the treatment of the scleral complications and, as with the treatment of scleritis for which no cause is found, the anti-inflammatory drugs oxyphenbutazone and indomethacin should be tried first, accepting the fact that some patients will have side-effects. Local steroids may give subjective comfort.

Corticosteroid drugs are the only preparations that will predictably suppress rheumatoid activity, but should not be used unless absolutely necessary. They are, however, valuable in a patient severely incapacitated by acute disease when there is an urgent need for symptomatic relief. Incapacitating morning stiffness is also relieved and the elderly rheumatoid may be kept independent on a small dose of prednisone. Necrotising scleral disease may be one indication for its use because it is often associated with the onset of rheumatoid vasculitis.

Rheumatoid arthritis can be complicated by vasculitis which can produce various clinical syndromes, such as peripheral neuropathy (Lyne and Pitkeathley, 1968). Vasculitis can undoubtedly occur in the absence of steroid therapy but most patients are found to be taking corticosteroids and it has been suggested that they may have a potentiating effect (Bywaters, 1957; Sokoloff and Bunim, 1957). Certainly fluctuating dosages of corticosteroids have been shown to precipitate immune complexes and complexes of rheumatoid factor have been demonstrated on vessel walls in vasculitis. There has been much work recently carried out on the effect of steroids on hypothalamic–pituitary–adrenal function during and following treatment. The results show that there is suppression of activity in a substantial proportion of patients, that the variation is wide, but that suppression is generally proportional to the dosage and duration in therapy.

Although corticosteroids are undoubtedly the most powerful agents in the control of inflammation in arthritis and scleritis, there is little evidence that they affect the ultimate course of generalised disease. Eyesight can, however, be preserved by their use. For the suppression of necrotising scleritis they must be given in high dosage initially—80 mg daily until the pain or inflammation comes under control. The dose is then reduced by 20 mg daily to as low a maintenance level as possible, adding other anti-inflammatory agents, local steroids or even immunosuppressives to achieve this desired effect.

Cortisol metabolism. There is in vitro evidence that rheumatoid synovial tissue cells are hyporesponsive to the regulatory actions of glucocorticoids (Castor, 1971). Murphy and West (1969) have shown that rheumatoid tissue tends to convert unusual amounts of cortisol to cortisone, possibly leading to a decrease in the effective concentration of the active agent in the inflamed tissue. Cortisol acts on normal synovial cells to reduce the rate of hyaluronic acid synthesis by approximately 50 per cent, and the rate of collagen formation by approximately 80 per cent (Castor, 1971). The effect of cortisol on energy metabolism of synovial tissue is conflicting, and this may be due to the varying responsiveness of different cell types as well as interactions between them. For instance, high concentrations of hydrocortisone (250 pg/ml) inhibit glycolysis and oxygen uptake of rheumatoid tissue in vitro (Page Thomas and Dingle, 1958) and intra-articular glucocorticoids reduce lactate production, blood flow and hyaluronate formation by rheumatoid joint tissue in vitro (Goetzl et al, 1971). On the other hand, $1.0 \mu g$/ml of hydrocortisone added to monolayer cultures of normal or rheumatoid synovial lining cells both depresses hyaluronate synthesis and stimulates glucose consumption and lactate formation.

This probably accounts for the need for such high doses of corticosteroids to control eye and joint involvement. High concentrations intra-orbitally are possible, but the results are only transitory as the steroid is washed away fairly quickly, and the strictures against subconjunctival injections apply.

Intra-articular therapy. Corticosteroids can be given as an intra-articular injection usually following the aspiration of fluid; 12.5 to 50 mg hydrocortisone acetate is commonly used depending on the size of the joint.

The role of immunosuppressive drugs. Jayson and Jones (1971) found that some of their patients with scleritis who remained resistant to treatment with corticosteroids did respond to treatment with immunosuppressive therapy alone or in combination with steroids (pages 392, 408). There have been several controlled studies, which have demonstrated clinical improvement, but generally the use of these agents has proved disappointing. The potential side-effects are numerous, serious and contraindicate the wide acceptance of these drugs, which should be reserved for patients with severe and progressive disease in whom other forms of treatment have been unsuccessful.

Treatment of seronegative arthritis

These patients have generally much more in the way of intraocular signs than those with seropositive arthritis and, as a consequence, respond much better to local steroids. It is often worth starting these patients on local prednisolone 0.5 per cent eye drops half-hourly when they present with eye signs, whether they are intraocular or scleral, and a gratifying and dramatic response will be obtained in the majority. A mydriatic should also be used to prevent the iris adhering to the lens. Atropine eye drops one per cent twice or three times a day are used by tradition, but cyclopentalate 0.5 per cent or mydriacyl 0.5 per cent three or four times a day will probably achieve the same object and allow the pupil to remain mobile. In very severe anterior uveitis in which there is a fibrous exudate in the anterior chamber, 0.5 ml subconjunctival soluble hydrocortisone one per cent together with mydricaine No. 2 is the best initial treatment. Systemic therapy with the anti-inflammatory agents helps in those who respond poorly to local steroid therapy but systemic steroid therapy is rarely if ever necessary to control the scleral disease in any of this group other than Behçet's syndrome and occasionally Reiter's syndrome. The combination of steroid and azathioprine has been recommended if the eye disease becomes difficult to control.

The general management of this group of diseases depends on careful assessment of the patient. Spinal involvement requires active and specific physical management to maintain mobility and prevent deformity. The polyarthropathy of the synovial joints is managed in a similar manner as rheumatoid arthritis and the treatment of the associated features is unaffected by the occurrence or presence of the arthritis.

Unlike rheumatoid arthritis, the end result of which is destruction, increased deformity and unnatural mobility with occasional fibrosis but only rarely bony ankylosis, the inflammation of ankylosing spondylitis leads to fusion and ankylosis, particularly if the patient is rested overmuch.

The aim is to ease pain and stiffness, to keep deformity to a minimum and to maintain spinal mobility as much as possible. Rest is positively harmful and lumbar supports should not be prescribed. The patient should be taught a series of spinal and breathing exercises and it is incumbent on the doctor to make sure that the patient understands that they must be done daily for the rest of his life. Indomethacin and phenylbutazone are usually effective anti-inflammatory drugs and corticosteroids are rarely required. Gold salts are also used in treating non-rheumatoid inflammatory joint disease such as psoriatic arthritis.

Deep x-ray treatment applied locally to the spine in conservative skin dose of 1000 R or less is helpful, but because of the risk of leukaemia it is now reserved for patients not responding to other measures. Applied locally to, for instance, heels or iliac crests in skin doses of 200 to 400 R this treatment is still often helpful in relieving tenderness in these areas.

The Arthritis and Rheumatism Council supply excellent booklets to assist the patient's understanding of the condition.

Treatment of systemic lupus erythematosus

The high incidence of emotional and neuropsychiatric problems together with the unpredictability of the disease call for particularly sympathetic care of patients with SLE. There is no evidence that treatment during periods of remission alters the long-term prognosis, and it is usual policy not to treat patients in remission with normal serum complement levels.

Chloroquine salts should still be considered before corticosteroids in patients where the skin and joint manifestations predominate, although many of the joint symptoms respond to salicylates alone.

The management of active SLE mainly consists of monitoring prednisone dosage to the lowest level sufficient to control symptoms and signs. Some features, such as pericarditis or haemolytic anaemia, respond regularly to corticosteroids. Others, particularly central nervous system manifestations are difficult to manage. Lowered serum complement levels have serious implications and in a patient previously known to have had normal complement level it is justifiable to assume that this finding represents renal involvement and to treat it accordingly. The evidence for the clinical value of immunosuppressive drugs in this condition is slim, and most controlled studies relate to renal lupus. It appears that the combination of prednisone with an immunosuppressive drug is superior to the use of either drug alone because when azathioprine, heparin and prednisone singly and in combination were recently compared in a three-way trial, in 50 patients with proliferative lupus nephritis, prednisone alone was far less effective in influencing mortality, renal function and serum complement levels than a combination of either azathioprine or heparin and prednisone (Cade et al, 1973). Similar claims have also been made for cyclophosphamide.

Sztejnbock et al (1971) compared patients given azathioprine 2.5 mg/kg/day plus prednisone for one to four years with those on prednisone alone. The former patients improved and none died, none had serious infections and their creatinine clearance improved. Of the control patients six out of 19 died, six had serious infections and renal function deteriorated.

For over a decade cyclophosphamide and azathioprine (and to a lesser extent chlorambucil) have been widely used in the management of SLE, particularly in those patients with severe renal disease. Use of these drugs seemed logical in a disease characterised by such widespread immunological over-activity, and the dramatic improvement in prognosis achieved by similar therapy in another vasculitic disease (Wegener's granulomatosis; Reza et al, 1975) suggested that it might have potential benefit in SLE. Unfortunately, the widespread clinical experience now accumulated with the drug in SLE has not been matched by a parallel number of clinical trials.

Recently the results of two larger trials have been published (Decker et al, 1975; Hahn, Kantor and Osterland, 1975) in which the benefits produced were marginal. Hahn could not demonstrate a steroid sparing effect with azathioprine and Decker added cyclophosphamide or azathioprine to low dose corticosteroid therapy in 38 patients with diffuse lupus glomerulonephritis and the cytotoxic drugs added only marginally to the control of the disease, although no SLE-related disease occurred amongst the 12 patients treated with cyclophosphamide.

The severity of the scleral disease seen in SLE lies mid-way between that seen in seropositive arthritis, in which it is sometimes severe, and that seen in seronegative arthritis when it is rarely so. Unfortunately, the scleritis of SLE rarely responds to local therapy. If it is controlled by any form of medication the eyes do not seem to become affected, and in one or two patients the flare-up of the scleritis is the first sign of a recrudescence of the disease. It is very unusual for it to be necessary to treat the scleritis as a separate entity; it is the general condition which requires treatment.

Treatment of gout

Treatment has three main aims:
1. Reduction of acute synovitis
2. Prevention of further crystal formation
3. Identification of associated disease.

Reduction of acute synovitis. The treatment of acute gout is aimed at relieving the severe pain as rapidly as possible. The earlier treatment is started in the course of the acute attack, the easier it is to abort. It is important, therefore, that patients at home are given a supply of tablets and instructions so that they can begin treatment as soon as the attack starts. In addition to early treatment, the other essentials for rapid and effective control are a high initial dose and 24 hour cover for two to four days; apparent resistance to treatment is often due to too little being given too late.

The traditional remedy is colchicine 0.5 mg given two-hourly for a maximum of 24 hours, until the pain subsides or diarrhoea or vomiting occurs. These side-effects often occur at about the same time as clinical improvement and therefore this treatment has been superseded by phenylbutazone or indomethacin.

With indomethacin night cover with a 100 mg suppository is effective and by day 150 mg with food by mouth in divided doses is sufficient; seldom is it necessary to give more than this. Phenylbutazone or oxyphenbutazone are also highly effective; 600 to 800 mg in divided doses should be given by mouth on day 1, with subsequent reductions by 100 to 200 mg daily over four to five days. Boardman and Hart (1965) found indomethacin rather quicker in action than phenylbutazone and therefore marginally preferable, both drugs proving superior to colchicine. On short-term treatment, toxic changes in the blood are extremely unlikely on these drugs. Although much is known about the inflammatory reaction in gout, little is known about why some agents work so much better than others.

Control of acute episodes may occasionally prove difficult and bed rest and ACTH therapy will be required. Treatment of the acute attack of pyrophosphate arthropathy is similar to that for acute gout, although drugs are less effective; joint aspiration together with the injection of corticosteroid gives relief.

Prevention of crystal formation. Most physicians now commence uricosuric or allopurinol treatment after the second episode of gout, or if there is marked overproduction of uric acid. Once started the therapy will be life-long. All patients must be instructed in the necessity for continued therapy and a high fluid intake. Treatment is aimed at keeping the serum uric acid below the solubility level (7.0 mg/100 ml).

Uricosuric drugs (probenicid and sulphinpyrazone) act by blocking the renal tubular transport of uric acid which allows the filtered load to be excreted. Side-effects are rare, but include nephrotic syndrome and skin rashes. Their main disadvantage is that the amount of uric acid excreted through the kidneys is increased, with the theoretical possibility that uric deposition there may also be increased.

The effect of aspirin on uric acid excretion is also important. In low doses below 4 g per day, it causes retention of uric acid. In doses above this level, it enhances uric acid excretion. As few patients take aspirin in doses greater than 4 g daily, it is usual to advise patients with gout not to take aspirin, particularly if they take uricosuric drugs as aspirin antagonises the effect of probenecid and sulphinpyrazone.

Allopurinol, a xanthine oxidase inhibitor, reduces the oxidation of hypoxanthine to xanthine and of xanthine to uric acid. The more soluble xanthine is excreted. Indications for this drug include extensive tophaceous gout, renal impairment, antimitotic drug therapy and intolerance or failure of response to uricosuric therapy. Side-effects are few and include dyspepsia and skin rash. Allopurinol may also be used prophylactically in situations where a sudden increase in serum uric acid is anticipated, as in the treatment of leukaemia with cytotoxic agents.

When long-term treatment is introduced, the patient must be warned that an acute attack of gout may take place during the early weeks of therapy. In order to reduce the chance of such an acute attack taking place, it is usual to add a small dose of colchicine (0.5 mg twice daily) for the first three to six months of long-term therapy. Acute attacks occurring at any time while on long-term treatment are treated as before but with elimination of the long-term regime.

Dietary management is not so important with the advent of effective drugs, but the obese patient should be encouraged to lose weight. However, a strict diet should be avoided because it causes urate retention if ketoacidosis occurs. Nevertheless patients should be advised to moderate alcoholic intake and to refrain from high purine foods.

Unfortunately there is no effective means of preventing further attacks of pyrophosphate arthropathy, although colchicine may sometimes prove helpful. Management is that of osteoarthrosis with analgesics and physiotherapy.

Drug interactions. In any programme of long-continued therapy, drug interactions may occur. Phenylbutazone, for instance, displaces warfarin from protein binding sites and may precipitate bleeding episodes. As mercaptopurine and azathioprine are inactivated by xanthine oxidase, its inhibition by allopurinol will increase plasma levels of these drugs. Probenecid may cause an increase of levels of free and conjugated sulphonamide in the blood and precipitate over-dosage effects.

Identification of associated disease. It is important to ensure that there is no associated disease such as myeloproliferative disorders or chronic haemolytic state. It is also wise to be aware of this type of arthritis in patients with these diseases.

Asymptomatic hyperuricaemia merits treatment if the serum uric acid is consistently above 9.0 mg/100 ml (Hall et al, 1967). Gouty arthritis is very likely to occur in these patients. They are also exposed to the risk of developing chronic hyperuricaemic nephropathy.

Treatment of the scleral and episcleral changes. Identification and treatment of the gout will often completely suppress the episcleral inflammation which is sometimes due to deposition of crystals in the episcleral tissue. Treatment with uricosuric drugs of some patients who are hyperuraemic without any other manifestations of clinical gout will also suppress some attacks of episcleritis. Unfortunately, this does not cure all the patients, some of whom develop episcleritis regardless of whether their clinical gout is under control or not. These patients, however, usually do well with local steroid drops or at worst with systemic oxyphenbutazone.

Scleritis which occurs in gout is rare but usually responds to treatment with systemic anti-inflammatory drugs. If these fail to produce a response, one must suspect the even rarer gouty tophus which produces an indolent inflammation of the sclera and is difficult to treat and may need excision. Systemic steroids are not indicated as they do not produce any greater improvement than the systemic anti-inflammatory drugs.

Treatment of chronic juvenile polyarthritis

The treatment of the eye changes of chronic juvenile polyarthritis depends on its type. There are no eye changes in the classic seronegative disease described by Still, but they occur in all the other types. The acute iritis found in seronegative patients with chronic juvenile polyarthritis is exactly the same as that found in adult ankylosing spondylitis and, as in that condition, responds very rapidly to local steroid therapy.

The scleritis in seropositive juvenile rheumatoid arthritis is of the diffuse anterior variety and responds rapidly to local steroid therapy. Only once have we had to use systemic oxyphenbutazone and then only for two weeks. Uveitis does not occur in this type.

True scleritis does occasionally accompany the chronic iridocyclitis in juvenile ANF-positive arthritis and has even been the presenting feature in a child who developed arthritis five years later. Its treatment is as unsatisfactory as that of chronic iritis. As the scleritis does not seem to contribute to the visual deterioration which is due to intraocular inflammation, no specific therapy is necessary to control it. Local steroids may precipitate steroid glaucoma and both local and systemic steroids can induce cataract formation which is difficult to distinguish from cataract induced by the uveitis. As a consequence, systemic and local steroids must be used with great circumspection, and only for the iritis.

The general care of the patient does not differ with the various types and is aimed at achieving a state in which the child lives at home under adequate supervision, and is left with minimal residual joint deformity. A successful outcome depends on two main factors: first, support from the child's family who must be told of the good ultimate general prognosis and understand the aims of treatment, and second, liaison between general practitioner, hospital, social and educational services. Drugs are used to suppress inflammation, but they form only part of the treatment. Daily exercises are important and must be taught to the parents. Bed rest is only indicated in children with severe systemic features since it can result in muscle wasting and joint ankylosis. Weight-bearing is only restricted if there is severe pain or a flexion deformity which requires correction by serial splinting. Hip and knee flexion is discouraged by daily periods of lying prone. Night splints are used during the acute phase to rest the joints in a good position.

Aspirin in anti-inflammatory dosage is the drug of choice and usually controls the fever. This means approximately 90 mg/kg body weight per day in divided doses which produces a blood salicylate level of 25 mg/100 ml. Young children rarely complain of tinnitus or deafness, so it is important to monitor the blood level and to look for over-breathing, drowsiness and vomiting. If necessary, ibuprofen or indomethacin can be added. Indomethacin will reduce stiffness as well as fever in older children but is not well tolerated by the under-fives. If the disease continues to progress, gold or penicillamine should be tried before resorting to steroids.

The indications for the use of corticosteroids are few. They do not influence the ultimate prognosis nor prevent complications and can cause alarming iatrogenic effects which cannot be justified in a disease with such a good prognosis. They are indicated in severe systemic disease, chronic iridocyclitis not responding to local steroids and in progressive disease resistant to other drugs. ACTH is useful for short periods in acute systemic disease. If prednisone is used, alternate day dosage is preferred because this does allow for some skeletal growth and does not suppress growth spurts, sexual maturation or reaction to stress.

Eye surgery is restricted to the removal of cataracts, control of glaucoma, and occasionally removing calcium deposits from the corneas of children with ANF-positive arthritis. The visual results are generally only fair. Orthopaedic surgery is restricted to synovectomy in children old enough to cooperate with postoperative physiotherapy, at least seven to eight years old. Correction of joint deformities or joint replacement is done in adolescence or adult life after growth has ceased. The ultimate prognosis is favourable. In one series followed for 15 years, 80 per cent were able to lead useful independent lives, although one-third still required anti-inflammatory drugs to control pain. Ten per cent died from infection or chronic renal disease secondary to amyloidosis (Ansell and Bywaters, 1969).

SUMMARY OF TREATMENT OF SCLERITIS AND EPISCLERITIS

Medical Treatment

Treatment should be given to infections and other conditions for which there is a specific therapy before any anti-inflammatory agents are administered. If no cause is found or the condition is associated with a connective tissue disease, then anti-inflammatory agents should be administered, as well as treating the underlying condition.

Episcleritis

Simple. This condition is self-limiting and requires no treatment.

Nodular. This is also self-limiting but is more indolent and may require local steroid drops or anti-inflammatory agents for its control.

In rare instances where episcleritis is unresponsive then systemic oxyphenbutazone or indomethacin should be given.

Scleritis

Systemic therapy is necessary. Local treatment is ineffective.

Diffuse anterior and nodular scleritis

Systemic oxyphenbutazone or indomethacin will control most attacks. Stronger anti-inflammatory agents are rarely necessary.

Necrotising scleritis, posterior scleritis

Some will respond to oxyphenbutazone or indomethacin but most need systemic steroids for its control. These must be given in high initial doses and many require a continuous maintenance dose to suppress the inflammation. Either prednisolone or sintisone can be used, some patients responding to one and some to the other.

Subconjunctival steroids are contraindicated in the treatment of scleritis.

Treatment of patients resistant to or unable to tolerate systemic steroids

Treatment may be tried with other anti-inflammatory agents, e.g. aspirin, Arlef, Brufen, etc., the antirheumatic drugs, e.g. penicillamine, gold and chloroquine, or the immunosuppressives, azathioprine, cyclophosphamide, either alone or in combinations in which there is no known harmful drug interaction. Anticoagulation, sodium versonate and x-ray therapy may also have a place in the resistant patient.

Surgical Treatment

Biopsy should *only* be performed if it is essential to establish an obscure diagnosis. Surgery is also reserved for those patients who are resistant to medical treatment, have perforated the globe, or whose disease is so extensive when first seen that too much tissue has been lost to be replaced by the normal reparative processes. The surgery which varies in severity from conjunctival excision to full anterior segment replacement is always difficult and full of unrecognised hazards because of the softness of the inflamed tissues and its limited powers of healing.

Cataract extractions and glaucoma operations (particularly trabeculectomy) can be performed unmodified, provided the tissue operated upon is uninflamed.

REFERENCES

Alt, A. (1903) Episcleritis and scleritis. *American Journal of Ophthalmology*, **20**, 101–111.

Ansell, B. M. & Bywaters, E. G. (1969) Prognosis in Still's disease. *Bulletin of the Rheumatic Diseases*, **9**, 139.

Armstrong, K. & McGovern, V. J. (1955) Scleromalacia perforans with repair grafting. *Transactions of the Ophthalmological Society of Australia*, **15**, 110–121.

Aronson, S. B. & Elliott, J. H. (1974) Scleritis. In *Ocular Inflammatory Disease* (Ed.) Golden, B. 43 pp. Springfield, Illinois: Charles C. Thomas.

Aylward, M. & Maddock, J. (1973) Total and free plasma tryptophan concentration in rheumatoid disease. *Journal of Pharmacy and Pharmacology*, **25**, 570–572.

Boardman, P. L. & Hart, F. D. (1965) Indomethacin in the treatment of acute gout. *Practitioner*, **194**, 560–565.

Brooks, P. M., Stephens, W. H., Stephens, M. E. et al (1975) How safe are anti-rheumatic drugs? A study of possible iatrogenic deaths in patients with rheumatoid arthritis. *Health Bulletin*, **33B**, 108–111.

Brown, S. I. (1975) Mooren's ulcer. *British Journal of Ophthalmology*, **59**, 675–682.

Brubaker, R., Font, R. L. & Shepherd, E. M. (1971) Granulomatous sclero-uveitis; regression of ocular lesions with cyclophosphamide and prednisone. *Archives of Ophthalmology*, **86**, 517–524.

Burns, C. A. (1968) Indomethacin, reduced retinal sensitivity and corneal deposits. *American Journal of Ophthalmology*, **66**, 825–835.

Bywaters, E. G. L. (1957) Peripheral vascular obstruction in rheumatoid arthritis and its relationship to other vascular lesions. *Annals of the Rheumatic Diseases*, **16**, 84–103.

Cade, R., Spooner, G., Schlein, E. et al (1973) Comparison of azathioprine, prednisone and heparin alone or combined in treating lupus nephritis. *Nephron*, **10**, 37–56.

Cairns, J. E. (1968) Trabeculectomy: preliminary report of a new method. *American Journal of Ophthalmology*, **66**, 673–679.

Carr, R. E. & Siegel, I. M. (1973) Retinal function in patients treated with indomethacin. *American Journal of Ophthalmology*, **75**, 302–326.

Castor, C. W. (1971) Abnormalities of connective tissue cells cultured from patients with rheumatoid arthritis. II. Defective regulation of hyaluronate and collagen formation. *Journal of Laboratory and Clinical Medicine*, **77**, 65–75.

Castor, C. W. (1972) Connective tissue activation. IV: Regulatory effects of anti-rheumatic drugs. *Arthritis and Rheumatism*, **15**, 504–514.

Chrzanowska-Srzednicka, K. (1954) Results of isonicotinic acid hydrazide therapy in scleritis. *Klinika Oczna*, **24**, 191–193.

Contardo, R. (1952) X-ray treatment in ophthalmology. *IVth Congreso Pan-Americano Oftal-mologica*, **2**, 735–840.

Co-operating Clinics of the American Rheumatism Association (1972) A controlled trial of high and low doses of cyclophosphamide in 82 patients with rheumatoid arthritis. *Arthritis and Rheumatism*, **15**, 434.

Currey, H. L. F. (1971) Immunosuppressive drugs in rheumatoid arthritis. In *Modern Trends in Rheumatology* (Ed.) Hill, A. G. S. 2nd edition, pp. 174–194. London: Butterworth.

Currey, H. L. F., Harris, J., Mason, R. M. et al (1975) Comparison of azathioprine and cyclophosphamide and gold in the treatment of rheumatoid arthritis. *British Medical Journal*, **iii**, 763–766.

Cuthbert, M. F. (1974) Adverse reactions to non-steroid anti-rheumatic drugs. *Current Medical Research and Opinion*, **2**, 600–609.

Davis, P., Ezeoke, A., Munro, J. et al (1973) Immunological studies on the mechanism of gold hypersensitivity reactions. *British Medical Journal*, **iii**, 676–678.

Day, A. T., Golding, J. R. & Lee, P. M. (1974) Penicillamine in rheumatoid disease: a long term study. *British Medical Journal*, **i**, 180–183.

Decker, J. L., Klippel, J. H., Plotz, P. H. et al (1975) Cyclophosphamide or azathioprine in lupus glomerulonephritis. *Annals of Internal Medicine*, **83**, 606–615.

Duke Elder, S. (1951a) The clinical value of cortisone and ACTH in ocular disease. A preliminary report. *British Journal of Ophthalmology*, **35**, 637–671.

Duke Elder, S. (1951b) Series of cases treated locally by cortisone. Report to the M. R. C. on ophthalmological applications of cortisone and ACTH. *British Journal of Ophthalmology*, **35**, 672–694.

Duthie, J. J. R., Brown, P. E., Truelove, L. H. et al (1964) Course and prognosis in rheumatoid arthritis: a further report. *Annals of the Rheumatic Diseases*, **23**, 193–204.

Empire Rheumatism Council Research Sub-Committee (1961) Gold therapy in rheumatoid arthritis: final report of a multi-centre controlled trial. *Annals of the Rheumatic Diseases*, **20**, 315–333.

Ferreira, S. H. & Vane, J. R. (1973) Inhibition of prostaglandin biosynthesis: an explanation of the therapeutic effects of non-steroid anti-inflammatory agents. In *Prostaglandines, 1973*, pp. 345–357. Paris: INSERM.

Fowler, P. D. (1967) Marrow toxicity of the pyrazoles. *Annals of the Rheumatic Diseases*, **26**, 344–345.

Fowler, P. D. (1972) *Adverse Drug Reactions, their Prediction, Detection and Assessment* (Ed.) Richards, D. J. & Randal, R. K. London: Churchill.

Francis, M. J. O. & Mowat, A. G. (1974) Effects of D-penicillamine on skin collagen in man. *Postgraduate Medical Journal*, **50**, supplement 2, 30–33.

Fraunfelder, F. T. & Watson, P. G. (1976) Evaluation of eyes enucleated for scleritis. *British Journal of Ophthalmology*, **60**, 227–230.

Freidman, M. & Greenwood, F. C. (1967) The effect of prolonged ACTH or corticosteroid therapy in children on growth and on pituitary–adrenal and pituitary function. *Proceedings of the Royal Society of Medicine*, **60**, 910–911.

Friedman, A. H. & Henkind, P. (1974) Unusual causes of episcleritis. *Transactions of the American Academy of Ophthalmology and Otolaryngology*, **78**, 890–895.

Girdwood, R. H. (1974) Death after taking medicaments. *British Medical Journal*, **i**, 501–505.

Goetzl, E. J., Falchuk, K. H., Zieger, L. S. et al (1971) A physiological approach to the assessment of disease activity in rheumatoid arthritis. *Journal of Clinical Investigation*, **50**, 1167–1180.

Hahn, B. H., Kantor, O. S. & Osterland, C. K. (1975) Azathioprine plus prednisone compared with prednisone alone in the treatment of systemic lupus erythematosus. *Annals of Internal Medicine*, **83**, 597–605.

Hall, A. P., Berry, P., Dawber, T. R. et al (1967) Epidemiology of gout and hyperuricemia. *American Journal of Medicine*, **42**, 27–30.

Hamilton, E. B. & Scott, J. T. (1962) Hydroxychloroquine sulfate 'plaguenil' in treatment of rheumatoid arthritis. *Arthritis and Rheumatism*, **5**, 502–512.

Harvey, W., Henderson, D. R. F. & Graham, R. (1974) Observations on in vivo skin elasticity and skin thickness of patients with rheumatoid arthritis treated with D-penicillamine and gold salts. *Postgraduate Medical Journal*, **50**, supplement 2, 33–36.

Hayreh, S. S. & Watson, P. G. (1970) Prednisolone-21-stearoglycolate in scleritis. *British Journal of Ophthalmology*, **54**, 394–398.

Hench, P. S. (1949) Potential reversibility of rheumatoid arthritis. *Annals of the Rheumatic Diseases*, **8**, 90.

Hurd, E. R. & Ziff, H. (1974) Parameters of improvement in patients with rheumatoid arthritis treated with cyclophosphamide. *Arthritis and Rheumatism*, **17**, 72–78.

Hurd, E. R., Snyder, W. B. & Ziff, M. (1970) Choroidal nodules and retinal detachments in rheumatoid arthritis. *American Journal of Medicine*, **48**, 273–278.

Huskisson, E. C. & Berry, H. (1974) Some immunological changes in rheumatoid arthritis among patients receiving penicillamine and gold. *Postgraduate Medical Journal*, **50**, supplement 2, 59–61.

Huskisson, E. C., Balme, H. W., Berry, H. et al (1974) A comparison of D-penicillamine and gold in rheumatoid arthritis. *Proceedings of International Symposium on Penicillamine*. In press.

Huskisson, E. C., Gibson, T. J., Balme, H. W. et al (1974) A trial comparing D-penicillamine and gold in rheumatoid arthritis. *Annals of the Rheumatic Diseases*, **33**, 532–535.

Jaffe, I. A. (1970) The treatment of rheumatoid arthritis and necrotising vasculitis with penicillamine. *Arthritis and Rheumatism*, **13**, 435–443.

Jameson Evans, P. & Eustace, P. (1973) Scleromalacia perforans associated with Crohn's disease. *British Journal of Ophthalmology*, **57**, 330–335.

Jayson, M. I. V. & Jones, D. E. P. (1971) Scleritis and rheumatoid arthritis. *Annals of the Rheumatic Diseases*, **30**, 343–347.

Jessop, J. D., Vernon Roberts, B. & Harris, J. (1973) Effects of gold salts and prednisolone on inflammatory cells. *Annals of the Rheumatic Diseases*, **32**, 294–300.

Kesavachar, K. R. (1954) Use of isonicotinic acid hydrazide in ocular tuberculosis. *Journal of the All-India Ophthalmological Society*, **1**, 113–118.

Krasnov, M. M. (1971) Iridocycloretraction in narrow angle glaucoma. *British Journal of Ophthalmology*, **55**, 389–395.

Lardy, H. A. & Ferguson, S. M. (1969) Oxidative phosphorylation in mitochondria. *Annual Review of Biochemistry*, **38**, 991–1034.

Lee, P., Ahola, S. J., Grennan, D. et al (1974) Observations on drug prescribing in rheumatoid arthritis. *British Medical Journal*, **i**, 424–426.

Lyne, A. J. & Pitkeathley, D. A. (1968) Episcleritis and scleritis: association with connective tissue disease. *Archives of Ophthalmology*, **80**, 171–176.

MacLagan, T. J. (1876) Treatment of acute rheumatism by salicin and salicylic acid. *Lancet*, **i**, 342.

Mason, M., Currey, H. L. F., Barnes, C. G. et al (1969) Azathioprine in rheumatoid arthritis. *British Medical Journal*, **i**, 420–422.

McArthur, J. N., Dawkins, P. D., Smith, M. J. H. et al (1971) Mode of action of anti-rheumatic drugs. *British Medical Journal*, **ii**, 677–679.

McConkey, B., Crockson, R. A. & Crockson, A. P. (1972) The assessment of rheumatoid arthritis. Study based on measurements of the serum acute phase reactants. *Quarterly Journal of Medicine*, **41**, 115–125.

Medical Research Council & Nuffield Foundation Joint Committee (1960) A comparison of prednisolone with aspirin or other analgesics in the treatment of rheumatoid arthritis. *Annals of the Rheumatic Diseases*, **19**, 331–337.

Merz, E. H. (1964) Scleral reinforcement with aortic tissue. *American Journal of Ophthalmology*, **57**, 766–770.

Multicentre Trial Group (1973) Controlled trial of D-penicillamine in severe rheumatoid arthritis. *Lancet*, **ii**, 275–280.

Murphy, D. & West, H. F. (1969) Catabolism and interconversion of cortisol and cortisone in human synovial tissue in vitro. *Annals of the Rheumatic Diseases*, **28**, 637–643.

Murube del Castillo, J. (1966) Operation in a case of equatorial scleral staphyloma. *Archives de la Sociedad Oftalmologica Hispano-Americana*, **26**, 860–862.

Nicolas, J. G. (1972) Cure of a necrotic nodular scleritis by auricular cartilaginous graft. *Bulletin des Sociétés d'Ophtalmologie de France*, **72**, 981–982.

Nonnenmacher, H. (1952) The treatment of progressive sclero-perikeratitis. *Klinische Monatsblätter für Augenheilkunde*, **121**, 707–712.

Oliver, I., Liberman, V. A. & DeVries, A. (1972) Lupus like syndrome induced by penicillamine in cystinuria. *Journal of the American Medical Association*, **220**, 588.

Page Thomas, D. P. & Dingle, J. T. (1958) Studies on human synovial membrane in vitro. The metabolism of normal and rheumatoid synovia and the effect of hydrocortisone. *Biochemical Journal*, **68**, 231–238.

Penneys, N. S., Ackerman, A. B. & Gottlieb, N. L. (1974) Gold dermatitis. *Archives of Dermatology*, **109**, 372–376.

Ramsay, A. M. (1909) *Diasthesis and Ocular Disease*. London: Balliere Tindall & Cox.

Reza, M. J., Dornkeld, L., Goldberg, S. et al (1975) Wegener's granulomatosis. Long term follow up of patients treated with cyclophosphamide. *Arthritis and Rheumatism*, **18**, 501–506.

Rooney, P. J., Lee, P., Brooks, P. et al (1973) Reflections on possible mechanisms of action of anti-inflammatory drugs. *Current Medical Research and Opinion*, **1**, 501–516.

Schwartz, R. S. & Gowans, J. D. C. (1971) Guidelines for the use of cytotoxic drugs in rheumatic diseases. *Arthritis and Rheumatism*, **14**, 134.

Scott, J. T., Porter, I. H., Lewis, S. M. et al (1961) Studies on gastrointestinal bleeding caused by corticosteroids, salicylates and other analgesics. *Quarterly Journal of Medicine*, **30**, 167–188.

Sée, G. (1877) *Bulletin de l'Academie de Médécine de Paris*, **26**, 689.

Sevel, D. (1966) *Necrogranulomatous Scleritis. A Clinical, Pathological and Experimental Study*. Thesis, University of London.

Sevel, D. & Abramson, A. (1972) Necrogranulomatous scleritis treated by an onlay scleral graft. *British Journal of Ophthalmology*, **56**, 791–799.

Sigler, J. W., Bluhm, G. B., Duncan, H. et al (1974) Gold salts in the treatment of rheumatoid arthritis. *Annals of Internal Medicine*, **80**, 21–26.

Smiley, W. K. (1974) The eye in juvenile rheumatoid arthritis. *Transactions of the Ophthalmological Societies of the United Kingdom*, **94**, 817–829.

Smith, M. J. H. & Dawkins, P. D. (1971) Salicylates and enzymes. *Journal of Pharmacy and Pharmacology*, **23**, 729.

Sokoloff, L. & Bunim, J. J. (1957) Vascular lesions in rheumatoid arthritis. *Journal of Chronic Disease*, **5**, 668–687.

Soyka, L. F. (1972) Alternate day corticosteroid therapy. *Advances in Pediatrics*, **19**, 39–52.

Stallard, H. B. (1965) *Eye Surgery*. pp. 469–471. Bristol: Wright.

Strunk, S. W. & Ziff, M. (1970) Ultrastructure studies of the passage of gold thiomalate across the renal glomerular capillary wall. *Arthritis and Rheumatism*, **13**, 39–52.

Swan, K. C. & Butler, J. B. (1950) Brawny type of scleritis following sub-conjunctival injections. *Transactions of the Pacific Coast Oto-Ophthalmological Society*, **31**, 111–116.

Sztejnbock, M., Stewart, A., Diamond, H. et al (1971) Azathioprine in the treatment of systemic lupus erythematosus. A controlled study. *Arthritis and Rheumatism*, **14**, 639–645.

Thiel, H. J. & Langness, U. (1970) Augensymptome bei parenteraler Goldtherapie der chronischen Polyarthritis. *Medizinische Klinik*, **65**, 1366–1368.

Tooker, C. W. (1931) Annular scleritis: report of a case. *American Journal of Ophthalmology*, **14**, 911–914.

van der Hoeve, J. (1934) Scleromalacia perforans. *Archives of Ophthalmology*, **11**, 111–118.

Vane, J. R. (1971) Inhibition of prostaglandin synthesis as a mechanism of action for aspirin-like drugs. *Nature New Biology*, **231**, 232–235.

Watson, P. G. (1963) Anaphylactic reaction caused by intra-muscular injection of lyophilized alpha-chymotrypsin. *British Journal of Ophthalmology*, **48**, 35–38.

Watson, P. G. (1966) Management of scleral disease. *Transactions of the Ophthalmological Societies of the United Kingdom*, **86**, 151–167.

Watson, P. G. (1969) Trabeculectomy. *Transactions of the Ophthalmological Societies of the United Kingdom*, **89**, 523–526.

Watson, P. G., Lobascher, D. J., Sabiston, D. W. et al (1966) Double-blind trial of the treatment of episcleritis–scleritis with oxyphenbutazone or prednisolone. *British Journal of Ophthalmology*, **50**, 463–481.

Watson, P. G., McKay, D. A., Clemett, R. S. et al (1973) Treatment of episcleritis. A double-blind trial comparing betamethasone 0.1%, oxyphenbutazone 10% and placebo eye ointments. *British Journal of Ophthalmology*, **57**, 866–870.

Weissman, G. (1968) Effect on lysosome of drugs useful in connective tissue disease. In *The Interactions of Drugs and Sub-cellular Components in Animal Cells* (Ed.) Campbell, P. W. pp. 203–207. Boston: Little Brown.

Whitehouse, M. W. (1965) Some biochemical and pharmacological properties of anti-inflammatory drugs. *Progress in Drug Research*, **81**, 321–429.

Wood, P. H. N., Harvey Smith, E. A. & Dixon, A. St. J. (1962) Salicylates and gastrointestinal bleeding: acetylsalicylic acid and aspirin derivatives. *British Medical Journal*, **i**, 669–675.

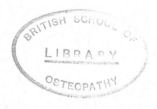

Index